Contents

LIST OF FIGURES, v

PREFACE, vii

1
WHAT IT MEANS TO HAVE A SPEECH DISORDER, 1

2
THE DISORDERS OF SPEECH, 27

3
THE DEVELOPMENT OF SPEECH, 53

4
DELAYED SPEECH AND LANGUAGE, 82

5
VOICE DISORDERS, 130

6

Disorders of Articulation, 171

7

Stuttering, 248

8

The Organic Disorders of Speech, 341

9

Hearing Problems, 392

10

Speech Pathology as a Profession, 422

Glossary, 433

The Phonetic Alphabet, 443

Index, 445

List of Figures

1. *Human Waste and Wasted Humans,* 8
2. *Even Birds Can Talk,* 10
3. *Copy of a Crayon Drawing of Himself by a Cleft-Palate Child,* 19
4. *The Field of Speech Pathology,* 31
5. *Articulation Disorders,* 34
6. *Disorders of Time,* 40
7. *Voice Disorders,* 44
8. *Symbolization Disorders: Aphasia, Language,* 48
9. *Percentage of Different Types of Cases Referred to WMU Speech Clinic in a Ten-Year Period,* 50
10. *Testing the Child's Comprehension of Pluralization,* 75
11. *Causes of Delayed Speech and Language,* 88
12. *Diagram of Interaction between Clinician and Child,* 109
13. *The Motokinesthetic Method,* 114
14. *Pictures for Receptive Distinction between "This is Mother's cat" and "This is a mother cat.",* 118
15. *Artificial Larynx; How the Electrolarynx Is Used,* 133
16. *Vocal Nodules,* 156
17. *Tongue-tie: Laller,* 179
18. *Mouth of a Child Who Suffered a Severe Lye-Burn,* 182
19. *Types of Sibilant Errors,* 188
20. *The Most Common Types of Consonantal Errors,* 196
21. *Design for Articulation Therapy,* 207
22. *Ear Training,* 212
23. *Nonsense Syllables,* 223

24. *The Sooba Family,* 227

25. *Checking Progress,* 233

26. *An Old Stutterer,* 249

27. *Origin and Development of Stuttering,* 277

28. *MIDVAS,* 308

29. *A Thank You Note Written by an Aphasic to His Therapist, Miss Josephine Simonson,* 344

30. *Representations of the Most Common Clefts of the Lip and Palate,* 358

31. *Clefts of the Lip and Palate,* 361

32. *Pharyngeal Flap,* 363

33. *A Prosthesis,* 364

34. *A Panendoscopic Examination,* 368

35. *Reflex-Inhibiting Patterns for Cerebral Palsy,* 384

36. *Structure of the Ear,* 393

37. *Audiogram Showing Conductive Hearing Loss,* 396

38. *Sensori-neural Hearing Loss,* 396

39. *Air and Bone Conduction Thresholds for a Typical Mixed Hearing Loss,* 396

40. *Bilateral Otosclerosis Resulting in a Conductive Loss in the Left Ear and a Mixed Loss in the Right Ear,* 404

41. *Drug-Induced, Bilateral Sensori-neural Hearing Loss,* 407

42. *Noise-Induced Hearing Loss,* 410

43. *Bilateral Sensori-neural Hearing Loss Diagnosed as Presbycusis,* 412

Preface

This book is an invitation. Those of us who have labored long in the field of speech pathology and know its challenges and fascinations invite others who are younger to join us in our continuing exploration of ways to serve those who have been deprived of that most fundamental of all human rights—the ability to speak out without fear of displaying abnormality. We have revised the text extensively, adding much new material on cerebral palsy, hearing problems, language development, and applications of learning theory. We have prepared guides for exploring the literature through the questions on the references at the end of each chapter. We think it is a better book than its four predecessors, and we hope that this new generation of students will find it intriguing.

C. Van Riper

1

What It Means To Have
a Speech Disorder

If there is any real hope for mankind in these troubled times it is to be found in the swelling tide of belief that somehow we must change this planet from a polluted sphere into one where man can fulfill his destiny with some grace. We are sickened from the ugliness in which we live and die. We are appalled by the way we have raped the good earth and anointed its wounds with human waste. We protest the human cruelty and exploitation we see all about us. We are angry with those who preceded us for handing down to us this heritage, and we are utterly determined to reverse this evil course, for we see very clearly where it will end.

This is a book about people troubled by the way they speak, about children and adults who stutter, or who cannot utter a sound because they have lost their vocal folds, or who possess some other speech disorder. At first glance, it might seem as though its contents could have no bearing on this generation's compelling need to make the world a fit place for man to fulfill his infinite potential for something other than evil. But there are many kinds of pollution, and some of the worst are those that reflect man's inhumanity to man. Perhaps all other evils flow from this befouled spring. If so, the study of speech pathology should help us discern what must be done.

It is important to realize that speech is the unique feature that distinguishes man from animal. Had he not talked, man would still be in Eden or the cave. In the dark mirror of speech pathology we will find reflected his fears, his frustrations, his shame, and the way he is treated by others; but the profession of speech therapy also provides the hope that somehow, someday, we can solve our problems. The author has been privileged to spend his life seeking to reduce, prevent, and heal that special kind of human misery found in defective speech, and it has given him a sense of meaningfulness he hungers to share. He is under no illusions about the extent of his own personal contribution. By any measure it is infinitesimal, but at least it has been directed toward eliminating some of the human pollution that surrounded the people who have felt his impact. Each of us must do what we can so that our children's children will find a better world and better individuals to inhabit it.

Sometimes it seems that there are so many human ills and evils that anyone who dedicates his life to their diminishing is dooming himself to a life of futility and frustration. We have not found it so. Though our individual efforts may seem at times to have no more effect than those of an ant carrying a grain of sand away from the seashore, we have before us the example of atomic fission in which one active particle triggers those about it, and these then fire others until incredible forces are released. Each human being has within his lifetime a host of opportunities to trigger forces for good or evil which lie latent in his fellows. We believe that it is therefore possible for any one of us to start chain reactions which may finally result in the kind of world and the kind of men we hope for.

Speech Deviancy. All societies develop value systems and a corresponding set of controls to insure that their members respect them. These value systems vary widely from culture to culture, and so do the controls that implement them. While all human societies place a premium upon effective communication as a primary bond holding them together, certain societies seem to prize it more than others. In our own, a highly competitive, upwardly mobile one, verbal skill is greatly rewarded. We swim in a vast ocean of words all of our lives. Effective speech in such a society is of the utmost importance if one is to gain and maintain membership or to get the status and material possessions which are constantly held up to us as goals to be desired.

It is very hard for normal speakers to comprehend how difficult it is to live in a culture such as ours without possessing the ability to speak in an acceptable fashion. Perhaps a few glimpses into the lives of the speech-handicapped may help. Here are some excerpts from autobiographies:

> After they found out I had cancer the doctors took out my voice box, and suddenly I was in a new, terribly strange world. I'd open my mouth to talk and nothing came out, just a rush of air out of the hole in my neck. I was mute. I could move my mouth and tongue but only silence came. And I got terribly afraid and depressed and wanted to die. How was I ever to work again? How was I to have friends? I was a stranger even to my wife and to myself. I tried to pray for strength and my mouth moved but no words came.

My friends tell me I'm attractive, but at twenty-four years of age I can count all the dates I've had on the fingers of one hand. Boys don't want to go out with girls who talk through their nose like I do. The doctors fixed my cleft lip so you can't hardly see the scar, but my voice is nasal and they say they can't help me with that. In grade school the kids called me "Honker" or "Nosey" and mocked the way I talked. People don't do that now that I'm grown up, but they look at me funny and shy away. Or they are extra kind to me and that's worse. I don't want pity. I just want to live like everybody else. I wonder how many nights I've cried myself to sleep over these miserable years.

Maybe the best way I can tell you how my stuttering covers my life is by writing some of what happened today. I was OK until I had breakfast, because I didn't talk. Then I went down to the corner drugstore because I had overslept, or rather just lay there in bed, dreading the day. I wanted coffee and rolls, but I ordered milk and oatmeal because I knew I'd stutter hard on those other words and I didn't want the old lady who waited on me to feel sorry for me. I hate oatmeal, and I had a little block on it anyway, dammit. Then I walked back to school and once went over to the other side of the street so I wouldn't have to say hello or to talk to a girl in my class who knows me. I remembered the times I've stopped someone in their tracks waiting for me to get the hello out. In my first class the instructor called on me out of the blue, and although I knew the answer, I played dumb and shook my head no, and then felt like a dog. A cur, a mongrel! After class I hurried away up to the library, got a book, and pretended to study hard when anyone I knew passed by. I also had to tie my shoestring which then broke and broke again when I fixed it. I thought of going downtown to get a new pair of shoestrings, but I didn't know where I could just point to them without saying anything. Maybe at Kresge's, but maybe not. So I finally tied enough knots to hold, though it looked lousy. Felt ashamed that I didn't even have the guts to ask for shoestrings. Put it off like I always do. I'm broke and wrote a letter to my Dad asking for money. Wanted to put a special delivery stamp on it, but remembered the last time I tried to buy one at the post office, and the sp-spsp-sp-sp-sp just kept going forever, and the clerk got impatient and the people in line behind me too, and well, I couldn't face it, so I got a regular stamp out of the machine and mailed it. Got thirty cents left to eat on and hope Dad isn't as slow as he often is in answering. Maybe I can borrow from my roomie—but God, that'll mean a mess of stuttering too. Hate to ask favors. I'll be making faces and jump around. I've got over about fifteen ways of saying it to him but can't find one combination that has any chance of being said without stuttering. . . .

This glimpse into the inner world of a stutterer as he reacts to his speech deviancy may seem to present an exaggerated and distorted picture. Unfortunately, it is not distorted. We have heard literally thousands of similar tales in one form or another. These people have been hurt deeply and repeatedly because they did not and could not conform to the speech standards of our society. The tragedy lies in the fact that they *could not*. They were not responsible for their defective speech, but those who hurt them acted as though they were, as though they had a choice. This assumption is the core of the problem not only of the person with a speech disorder but also of the poor, the insane, and most of the other kinds of deviancy.

Once, on Fiji in the South Pacific, we found a whole family of stutterers. As our guide and translator phrased it: "Mama kaka; papa kaka; and kaka, kaka, kaka, kaka." All six persons in that family showed marked repetitions and prolongations in their speech; but they were happy people, not at all troubled by their stuttering. It was just the way they talked. No hurry, no frustration, no stigma, indeed very little awareness. We could not help but contrast their attitudes and the simplicity of their stuttering with those which would have been shown by a similar family in our own land, where the pace of living is so much faster, where defective communication is rejected, where stutterers get penalized all their lives. To possess a marked speech disorder in our society is almost as handicapping as to be a physical cripple in a nomadic tribe that exists by hunting. Lemert, the sociologist, found a similar contrast in the way stutterers were treated among Polynesians as compared to the Japanese.[1] He writes, "In common with the Hawaiians and Samoans, Manganians neither laugh at nor ridicule the stutterers. The individuals who stutter are not socially rejected and are under no handicap as to marriage or occupation. No attempt is made by the Manganians to treat or correct stuttering since it is accepted as an inborn characteristic." Lemert showed that the Japanese, on the other hand, reacted to stuttering much as we do.

All societies demand a certain amount of conformity of their members. Only in anarchy could all members theoretically "do their own thing." The patterning of this conformity varies, of course, from culture to culture, and the demands change within any specific one from time to time. One needs only observe the variance in fashion or dress to understand that this is true. The hemlines go up and the hemlines come down. Beards disappear only to reappear after a generation or two. Moral values ebb and flow, a Reformation yielding to a Restoration. When the tyranny of conformity becomes too onerous, there are always a few mavericks to lead a revolt. They usually take a beating, but their impact sets off a counter-

[1] E. M. Lemert, "Stuttering and Social Structure in Two Pacific Societies," *Journal of Speech and Hearing Disorders*, XXVII (1962), 3–10.

reaction that spreads throughout the society until a new set of rules and demands predominates. Some societies are more rigid than others and change slowly, but ours seems to oscillate rather easily. The current youth movement may be viewed as the culmination of a fairly long trend against the excessive controls for conformity which dominated the value systems of preceding generations. Certainly our society is now in flux, and many of the old values are being strongly challenged. If this is disturbing, it is also exciting in its promise that we may yet create a world in which men can live not only in harmony with an unpolluted environment but with themselves.

If so, the major change must come in the way we interact with others. We must come to have concern for those less fortunate than ourselves. In our emerging affluent society in which machines do most of the work and leisure time becomes increasingly available, our energies must find creative outlets. If we merely use that leisure and affluence to indulge our appetites, we shall become decadent and corrupt, thereby inviting our inevitable extinction. If, on the other hand, we seek to alleviate human misery wherever and in whatever form it exists, we shall flower beyond all vision. It is with these thoughts in mind that we present the problems of those handicapped by disordered speech, for, in a small way, in speech therapy we find a minor model of things to come, a template of the future.

The speech therapist dedicates himself to the reduction of a special kind of misfortune. There are other human ills, of course: poverty, hunger, disease, war, intolerance, injustice. When the whole pool of human misery is surveyed, it might seem that those who are handicapped in communication must represent little more than an adjacent and insignificant puddle. How can we have the nerve to present the field of speech pathology as the shape of things to come, as a possible promise of a better future? All we can answer is that those who have concerned themselves with the untangling of tongues do seem to feel this way. They are concerned about the unfortunate; they devote their lives to the relief of human distress. But there is something more—and it is difficult to put into words. When we deal with speech, we deal with the essence of man. Only human beings have mastered speech. It is what sets us apart from all other species. Because we can speak, we can think symbolically; and it is this which has enabled man to conquer the world and space and every other creature. Dimly we believe or at least hope that someday it may enable us to master ourselves.

We who have spoken so much so easily and for so long find it hard to comprehend the miraculous nature of speech—this peculiarly human tool. It seems as natural and as easy as breathing. But those of us who try to help those who have been deprived of normal communication soon come to know how utterly vital and necessary speech is to human existence. Not only do we use it in thinking and in the sending and receiving of messages, we also build our very sense of self out of word-stuff. We need speech to command and restrain ourselves. Our words are our means for controlling others. Verbally we express our loves and hates. It is the safety valve of our emotions, the medicine of psychotherapy. Only those who come to know the problems of those who have been denied the magical power of the spoken word can realize the tremendous scope of this marvelous instrument that man has invented. Indeed, there are times when it seems that man has just begun to exploit the latent powers inherent in his speech. Someday he may learn to employ all those powers, but now he is like an ape using a flute to scratch himself. We who deal with the speech-handicapped do not take speech for granted. We are constantly aware of the extent of their deprivation. Our task is no small one; it is to help these persons gain the tools they need to fulfill their potential; it is to help them to join or rejoin the human race.

The Handicap of Defective Speech

The pollution of human misery comes from many wells, but its composition is the same. Abnormal speech is no asset to anyone. It invites penalty from any society which prizes the ability to communicate effectively. Normal speech is the membership card that signified that its owner belongs to the human race. Those who do not possess it are penalized and rejected. Even the abnormal speaker himself often feels this rejection is justified.

Moreover, the inability to communicate, to get the rewards our society offers to those who can talk effectively, results in great frustration. To be unable to say the word when he desires to do so, as in the case of the stutterer; to say "think" when he means "sink," as in lisping; not to be able to produce a voice at all, as in the aphonic; to try to say something meaningful only to find that gibberish emerges, as in the aphasic—all these are profoundly frustrating. Anxiety, guilt, and hostility are the natural reactions to penalty and frustration. You too have known these three miseries transiently when you have been punished or met frustration, but many individuals with defective speech spend their lives immersed in these emotions.

Penalties

Let us present some illustrative penalties culled from the autobiographies of stutterers, remembering that similar tales could be told by individuals with other varieties of defective speech:

Most clerks look away when I get stuck and begin to force. It always infuriates me that they don't even have the decency to look at me. Once I even went to the manager of a store about it, and he looked away too.

My father wouldn't ever listen to me when I stuttered. He always walked off. I finally got so I'd say everything to him by having mother give him the message.

People do not usually laugh at my other kinds of stuttering, but when I begin to go up in pitch, they always smile or laugh right out loud. I was phoning a girl today and hung up when I heard her snickering.

My mother always hurried to say the word for me whenever company was in the house. I often asked her not to, but she couldn't help herself. It used to shame me so, I'd go up in my room and cry; and I never went visiting with them. Sometimes I'd eat in the kitchen when we had strangers come for dinner.

The other boys in the school used to call me "stuttercat" and imitate me whenever I came to school. At first I always managed to be tardy and stay after school to avoid them, but my folks got after me, and then I began to fight with them. I got to be a pretty good fighter, but the bigger boys always licked me, and the teacher punished me when I hit the girls. I still hate girls.

After I came to high school from the country, everybody laughed at me whenever I tried to recite. After that, I pretended to be dumb and always said "I don't know" when the teacher called on me. That's why I quit school.

Every time I'd ask for a job, a funny look would come over their faces, and some of them would say no right away away even before I finished what I was going to say. Some of the others, and one of them was a stutterer too, just waited till I finally got it out and then they'd shake their heads. One storekeeper was so sympathetic I could hardly get out of there fast enough.

The worst time I ever had was when a hotel clerk saw me jumping around and called a doctor. He thought I was having a fit.

These are but a few of the many penalties and rejections which any speech defective or any other individual with an unpleasant difference is likely to experience. Imitative behavior, curiosity, nicknaming, humorous response, embarrassed withdrawal, brutal attack, impatience, quick rejection or exclusion, overprotection, pity, misinterpretation, and condescension are some of the other common penalties.

The amount and kind of penalty inflicted on a speech defective are dependent on four factors: (1) the vividness or peculiarity of the speech difference; (2) the speech defective's attitude toward his own difference:

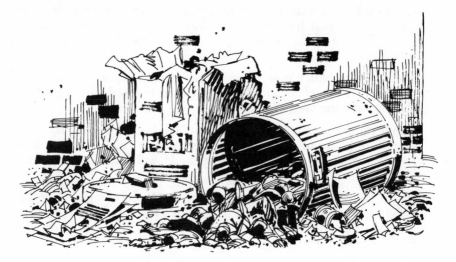

FIGURE 1: *Human Waste and Wasted Humans*

(3) the sensitivities, maladjustments, or preconceived attitudes of the people who penalize him; and (4) the presence of other personality assets.

First of all, in general, the more frequent or bizarre the speech peculiarity, the more frequently and strongly it is penalized. Thus a child with only one sound substitution or one that occurs only intermittently will be penalized less than one with almost unintelligible speech, and a mild stutterer will be penalized less than a severe one. Second, the speech defective's own attitude toward his defect often determines what the attitude of the auditor will be. If the speech defective considers it a shameful abnormality, his listeners can hardly be expected to contradict him. Empathic response is a powerful agent in the creation of attitudes. Third, the worst penalties will come from those individuals who are sensitive about some difference of their own. Since many speech defectives have parents or siblings with similar speech differences, they are often penalized very early in life by those persons.

> You ask why I slap Jerry every time he stutters? I do it for his own good. If my mother had slapped me every time I did it I could have broken myself of this habit. It's horrible going through life stuttering every time you open your mouth, and my boy isn't going to have to do it even if I have to knock his head off.

Moreover, many individuals have such preconceived notions or attitudes concerning the causes or the unpleasantness of speech handicaps that they react in a more or less stereotyped fashion to such differences, no matter how well adjusted the speech defective himself may be. Finally, as we have pointed out, the speech defective may possess other abilities or personal assets which so overshadow his speech difference that he is penalized very little.

Even though some children with a speech disorder are fortunate enough to be brought up in a family and an environment where they meet little punishment for their difference, eventually they will meet the rejection that society reserves for the person who has an unacceptable difference. Indeed, some of these protected children are more vulnerable than those whose lives have been full of penalty. Let us give a few examples from our own practice:

> A second-grade boy had been receiving speech therapy for over a year and had made excellent progress in mastering many of his defective sounds. In the third grade he met a teacher who was old and uncontrolled, who had had to return to teaching after her husband had died, and who hated the whole business. She used the boy as a scapegoat for her own frustrations. Under the guise of helping him, she ridiculed his errors and held him up to scorn before his fellows. Shortly after the fall term began, this boy's speech began to get worse, and within a few months it had lapsed to its former unintelligible jargon.

> We had been working for three years with Ted, an eight-year-old youngster. His cleft palate had been repaired surgically; but the muscles were very weak, and there was scar tissue which made it a bit difficult to close off the rear opening to the nasal passages with speed. He had improved greatly, however, and only a few bits of nasal snorting or excessive nasality remained when he talked carefully. Then one day his associates on the playground, led by the inevitable bully, began to call him "Mortimer Snerd" and "Nosey–Nosey." Within one week his speech disintegrated into a honking, unintelligible jargon, and he refused to come to the clinic for any more therapy.

Covert Penalties. Not all of the penalties bestowed upon the person who talks queerly are so obvious. Perhaps the worst ones are those that are hidden, the covert kind. One of our stutterers said this:

> In my whole life, never did my parents ever say a single thing about my stuttering, no matter how hard or badly I stuttered. Sometimes they might blink an eye or become transfixed or look away or change the conversation, but we never talked about it. It was a black shadow that always followed me, but no one looked at it. It was unmentionable, unspeakable. Mustn't talk about such dirty things. Sometimes

I wanted to shout, "I'm having trouble. Can't you see? I'm stuttering. Help me! Help me!" But I couldn't break that wall of silence.

Most of the more obvious penalties are felt by children. After a speech-handicapped person becomes an adult, few people mock him, laugh at him, or show disgust. Instead, he now finds that they shun him. Their distant politeness may hurt worse than the epithets he knew when he was young. One of our cases, a girl with a paralyzed tongue and very slurred speech who was desperately in need of work so she could eat and have a place to sleep, contacted forty-nine different prospective employers before she found one who would give her a chance to exist. "Not one of them ever said anything about my speech," she told us. "Some were extra kind, some were impatient, some were rude, but all of them had some other reason besides my speech for saying no. I could tell right away by seeing how they changed the moment I began to talk. Like I was unclean or something."

Why do such things happen? Why do we punish the person who is different? Why must he punish himself? Surely Americans are some of the kindest people who have ever lived on this earth. We show our concern for the unfortunate every day. No nation has ever known so many agencies, campaigns, foundations, and private charities. One drive for funds follows another. Muscular Dystrophy, the Red Cross, the United Fund, the Heart Association, Seeing Eye dogs, the coin bottle in the drugstore, the pleading on radio and television. Surely all of these activities seem to show that we help rather than punish our handicapped.

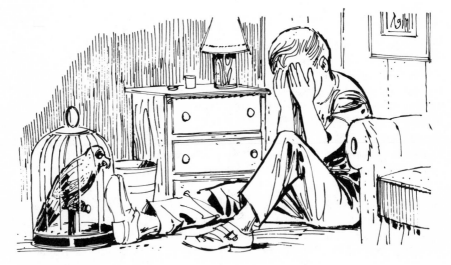

FIGURE 2: *"Even Birds Can Talk!"*

Cultural anthropologists have regarded this altruism with more than academic interest. They point out that our culture is one that features the setting up of a constant series of material goals and possessions which are highly advertised. Prestige and status seem often to be based upon winning these possessions and positions in a highly competitive struggle. We fight for security and approval, but in the process we trample underfoot the security of others. Some psychologists have felt that our need to help the handicapped is a product of the guilt feelings we possess from this trampling. Others attribute our concern for the underprivileged to fear lest someday we too will be the losers in the battle for life. They claim that we tend to say to ourselves, "There, but for the grace of God, go I," when we meet someone who has failed to find a place for himself in the world for reasons beyond his control. These organized charities do much good, but they cannot fulfill the needs of the handicapped for personal acceptance. Until we understand those needs and find ourselves able to care for each other on a person-to-person basis, the pollution of human misery will continue to exist.

Aggressive or Protest Behavior as a Reaction to Penalty.   Penalty and rejection by his associates may lead an individual to react aggressively by attack, protest, or some form of rebellion. He may employ the mechanism of projection and blame his parents, teachers, or playmates for his objectionable difference. He may display toward the weaknesses of others in the group the same intolerant attitude which they have manifested toward his own. In this way he not only temporarily minimizes the importance of his own handicap, but also enjoys the revenge of recognizing weaknesses in others. He may attempt to shift the blame for rejection. He will say, "They didn't keep me out because I stutter—they just didn't think I had as nice clothes as the rest of them wore." In this way he will exaggerate the unfairness of the group evaluation and ignore the actual cause. Another attack reaction may be to focus all attention upon himself. He can refuse to cooperate with the group in any way, can belittle its importance openly, and can refuse to consider it in his scheme of existence. Finally, he may react by a direct outward attack. A child, or an adult with an easily provoked temper, may indulge in actual physical conflict with members of the group that has not accepted him.

THE CASE OF THE GRANDMOTHER'S NOSE

Ivan, whom we straightway named "The Terrible," was a very agile little boy of six with completely unintelligible speech. He was a holy terror. Other mothers would sweep their children back into the house when Ivan came tricycling up the sidewalk. No baby-sitter ever sat twice at his house. His mother worked days, probably in self-defense; and the boy was cared for by his grandfather and grandmother, who lived upstairs. Only the grandfather could control Ivan, and when he left the house to go to the store the grandmother would flee to her bedroom and lock the door because Ivan would occasionally swarm up her and bite her, preferably on the nose. She was hard-of-hearing and found Ivan's garbled jargon quite impossible to comprehend. Ivan demanded that people understand him. If they did, he was well behaved and cooperative. But when they didn't, he went berserk; he scratched, bit, and attacked the object of his hatred. It took two years before Ivan was tamed and talking, and our speech clinic still bears certain scars as an enduring memorial to Ivan. So do this therapist's hands.

A rejected individual may spread pointed criticism of the group in a resentful manner. In any of these methods, the object of the rejection does not retreat from reality—he reacts antagonistically and attacks those who made his reality unpleasant.

Among the speech defectives few show outward signs of these reactions except attitudes of sullenness or noncooperation; in others, the protest is unmistakable. Unfortunately, these protest reactions do not solve the problem. They merely increase its unpleasantness.

The more the speech defective attacks the group, the more it penalizes him. Often such reactions interfere with treatment, for many of these speech defectives resent any proffered aid. They attack the speech correctionist and sabotage his assignments. The inevitable result of these attack reactions is to push the speech defective even further from normal speech and adequate adjustment.

FRUSTRATION

Frustration is always experienced when human potential is blocked from fulfillment. It is the ache of the giant in chains. All lives are full of frustrations. We cannot live together without inhibiting some of our impulses and desires. Circumstances always place barriers in the paths we desire to take. But for some persons, the cup of frustration is filled to the brim and more is added every day. Frustration breeds anger and aggression, and these corrupt everything they touch. Those who cannot talk normally are constantly thwarted. Consider, then, how a person must feel if he cannot talk intelligibly. Others have difficulty in understanding the messages of the stutterer, the jargon-talking child, or the person who has lost his voice forever due to cancer. Others listen, but they do not, they cannot, understand. The aphasic tries to ask for a cigarette and says, "Come me a bummadee. A bummadee! A bummadee!" This is frustration.

Or even when the listener can understand the words, he finds himself distracted by the odd contortions of the spastic's or stutterer's face, the twitching of the cleft-palate case's nostrils; and he forgets what has been said and asks that it be repeated. This is frustration too. Communication is the lifeblood of a society. When it cannot flow, the pressure builds up explosively. The worst of all legal punishments short of death is solitary confinement where no one can talk to the prisoner, nor can he talk to anyone else. There are such prisoners walking about among us, sentenced by their speech and hearing disorders to lives of deprivation and frustration.

One young stutterer diagnosed his own problem for us. His speech was full of irregular and forced repetitions. He hesitated. He seldom was able to utter even a short sentence without having wide gaps in it. One day, after he had just beaten up our plastic-clown punching bag he confided in us. "Y-y-y-you know . . . y-y-you know whuh-whuh-what's wrrrrrong with me? I-I-I-I-I'm the lllllittlest . . . child." He was. He was the runt of the litter, the weakest, smallest, most unattractive of the eight children in that family. The others were an aggressive bunch, yelling, fighting, arguing, talking. His mouth never had an ear to hear it. When his sentences were finished, it was some brother's or sister's mouth that finished them. He was constantly interrupted or ignored. He had learned a broken English, a hesitant speech.

The good things of life must be asked for, must be earned by the mouth as well as by the hands. The fun of companionship, the satisfaction of earning a good living, the winning of a mate, the pride of self-respect and appreciation, these things come hard to the person who cannot talk. Often he must settle for less than his potential might provide, were it not for his tangled tongue. Speech is the "Open Sesame," the magical power. When it is distorted, there is small magic in it—and much frustration.

We need safety valves for emotion. When we can express the angry evils within us, they subside; when we can verbalize our grief, it decreases. A fear coded into words and shared by a companion seems less distressing. A guilt confessed brings absolution. But what of the poor devils who find speaking hard, who find it difficult even to ask for bread? This wonderful function of speech is denied them. The evil acids cannot be emptied; they remain within, eating their container. For many of us it comes hard to verbalize our unpleasant emotions, even though we know that in their expression we find relief. How much more frustrating it must be for those who feel that they have only the choice of being still—or being abnormal.

Perhaps most frustrating of all is the inability to use speech as the expression of self. One of the hardest words for the average stutterer to say is his own name. Most of us talk about ourselves most of the time. We talk so people will notice us, so we can feel important. This egocentric speech is highly important in the development of the personality. Until the abnormal child begins to use it, he has little concept of selfhood, according to Piaget, the famous French psychologist. If you will listen to the people about you or to yourself, you will discover how large a portion of your talking consists of this cock-a-doodle-dooing. When we speak this way we reassure ourselves that all is well, that we are not alone, that we exist and belong. The person with a severe speech defect finds no such reassurance when he speaks. He exposes himself as little as he can. In this self-denial, too, lies much frustration.

One very severe frustration is the deprivation from social interaction which persons with speech disorders experience. It is not hard to understand why this occurs. Speech is the vital prerequisite for human interaction. It is the bond that unites us together. When it is impaired, that bonding is disrupted. Long ago the author spent a week once in a school for the deaf where all the students used sign language and did very little lipreading. He felt isolated, rejected, excluded from that miniature society; and it was with relief that he reentered a speaking world. Those who cannot talk feel much the same way. They are rejected from membership. They find it hard to belong. The worse they talk the more isolated they become. Here again we find in speech pathology a miniature model of a basic evil that pollutes mankind, the same rejecting exclusion that plagues the crippled, the poor, the insane, the old, and the minority groups.

ANXIETY

It should not be difficult to understand why people who meet rejection, pity, or mockery would experience anxiety. When one is punished for a certain behavior, and the behavior occurs again, fear and anxiety raise their ugly heads. If penalty is the parent of fear, then we might speak of anxiety as the grandchild of penalty, for the two are not synonymous. The stutterer may fear the classmate who bedevils him, or he may fear to answer the telephone since fear is the expectation of approaching evils which are known and defined. But anxiety is the dread of the unknown, of defeats and helplessness to come. In its milder form, we speak of "worrying." There is a vague nagging anticipation that something dangerous is approaching. To observe a person in an acute anxiety attack is profoundly disturbing. Often he can find no reason for his anxiety, but it is there just the same. At times it fades, only to have its red flare return when least expected. Few of us can hope to escape it completely in our lifetimes, but there are those for whom anxiety is a way of life. It is not good to see a little child bearing such a burden.

One of the evil features of anxiety is that it is contagious. When parents of a handicapped child begin to worry about his speech, the child is almost bound to reflect and share their feelings. "Will he ever be able to go to school, to learn to read, to earn a living, to get married? Who will hurt him? Will he ever learn to talk like the fellows?" Such thoughts may never leave the parents' lips, but somehow they are transmitted to the child, perhaps by tiny gestures or facial expressions or even the holding of the breath. Once the seeds of anxiety are planted, they sprout and grow with incredible speed.

Another of the evils of anxiety is that it usually is destructive. It does not aid learning or speech therapy. It distracts; it negates. It undermines the self-esteem. The person seeks to contain it, to explain it. Sometimes he invents a symptom or magnifies one already there. When speech becomes contaminated with anxiety, the way of the speech therapist is hard. One of the first things a student speech therapist must learn is to create a permissive atmosphere in which speaking is not painful, over which no threat hangs darkly. The speech therapy room of the public school must be a gay, pleasant place, so much so that some little children hang on to their defective speech sounds so they will not have to leave. All of us need such a harbor once in a while; *these* children need a haven often, one where for once they can feel free from penalty and frustration, where defective speech is viewed as a problem instead of a curse. In the presence of an accepting, understanding therapist, they can touch the untouchable, speak the unspeakable. There they can learn. Anxiety does not help in learning or relearning.

Reactions to Anxiety.   Anxiety is invisible, but it has many faces. By this we mean that it shows itself in different ways.

Edward had undergone many operations for his cleft palate, but the scars on his face and the speech that came from his mouth bore testimony of his difference. Throughout his elementary and secondary school years, he had appeared a carefree, laughing, mischievous child. He was the happy clown, the gay spirit, and by this behavior, he had managed to gain much acceptance. When other people laughed at him, he laughed with them. His grades were poor, although he was bright. Then suddenly, in the final semester of his senior year in high school, he underwent a marked personality change. He laughed no longer; he became apathetic, quiet, and morose. Formerly very much the extrovert, he now withdrew from contacts with others. He daydreamed. He walked alone. Our intensive study of this boy revealed that he had always lived with anxiety, that his gay behavior was adaptive but spurious. Underneath he had always ached. The compensatory pose of gaiety had brought him rewards, but it had not allayed the anxiety. When faced with the necessity for leaving school and earning a living, the anxiety flared up too strongly to be hidden, and the change of personality took place. Not until we were able to provide some hope through the fitting of a prosthesis (a false palate) and some information about the possibility of plastic surgery, did the anxiety decrease sufficiently to enable us to improve his speech.

One of the common methods used to ease anxiety is the search for other pleasures. By gratifying other urges we seem to be able temporarily to diminish anxiety's nagging. Some of the people with whom we have worked are compulsive eaters of sweets; they grow fat and gross. And then they worry about their weight. Others relieve their anxiety by sexual indulgences. There are others who find a precarious and temporary peace by regressing to infantile modes of behavior, trying to return to the period of their lives when they did not need to worry about speaking. We also find a few sufferers who attach themselves to a stronger person like leeches, hoping for the security of dependency. Yes, there are many ways of reducing anxiety; but unless the spring from which it flows is stopped, it always returns. That is why people with defective speech need speech therapists.

When the anxiety clusters about speaking, one way of reducing it is to stop talking. Some persons with speech defects merely become taciturn; some lose their voices; others contract what is called *voluntary mutism* and do not make an attempt to communicate except through gestures. We knew a night watchman once who claimed that he averaged only two or three spoken sentences every twenty-four hours. "It's easier on me than stuttering." We've also known several hermits; they had either speech defects or woman trouble.

There is also a curious mechanism called "displacement," which most of us use occasionally to reduce our anxiety. We start worrying about something else besides the real problem that is causing us such distress. The shift of focus seems to bring some relief, much as a hot water bottle on the cheek can ease a toothache. The scream of a little child in the night may reflect such a displacement, but perhaps a better example can be found in Andy.

Andy stuttered very severely when he came to us at the age of seven. He blinked his eyes, jerked and screwed up his mouth, and sometimes cried with frustration when he was unable even to begin a sentence. At times he spoke very well. But what struck us most about Andy was his furrowed brow. Whether he stuttered or not, he seemed to be constantly worried. His face always had an anxious expression. Finally we were able to get him to tell us what he was worrying about. Surprisingly, it was not about his stuttering or his parents' very evident concern about his speech. Andy said he was worrying about the moon hitting the sun. He said that if this happened, everything would blow up. He said that on those nights when there wasn't any moon, and both sun and moon were down under there someplace, that they might crash together. Andy said he could never sleep on those nights. His mother and father had told him this couldn't happen, but Andy said they had lied about Santa Claus; and how did they know, anyway, that it wouldn't happen? It took a lot of play therapy, speech therapy, and parent counseling before Andy was able to surrender his solar phobia and express his real anxiety, which concerned his speech.

We wish to conclude this section with a caution. Let us remember that some children with abnormal speech have no more anxiety than children who speak normally. All of us have some anxiety, probably need some. A bit of anxiety in the pot of life is like a bit of salt in a stew. It makes it tastier. But too much salt and too much anxiety ruin both. We have had to describe the anxiety-fraction of a speech handicap so that you will not add to it, perhaps so that you may relieve it. Those of us who come in contact with handicapped children or adults may unwittingly make their burdens heavier if we do not understand. But there are some fortunate persons with speech disorders who are lucky in their associates and ability to resist stress, who seem to manage to get along with a minimum of anxiety. They may find themselves loved and accepted. They may possess philosophies or compensating assets that make the speech problem minor in importance. Let us just give one example.

At thirty-two, a very talented singer developed cancer of the larynx, and it was removed surgically. She reacted to the challenge with courage, mastered esophageal speech, and began to specialize in the history of musical instruments, playing the lute, the Irish harp, and many other ancient stringed instruments. She said, "I would have been only a second-best vocalist, and I would have spent my life in self-love, self-exhibition, and frustration. Now I have many more friends and acquaintances. I have things to give. I hardly ever think of myself. It's a good thing I lost my voice."

So let us state our caution again. If there is excessive anxiety, recognize its face where you find it, no matter how it is disguised; but do not invent or imagine its presence if it is not there!

GUILT

Like anxiety, guilt also contributes a part of the invisible handicap that often accompanies abnormal speech. We have long been taught that the guilty are those who are punished. Intellectually we can understand that the converse of this proposition need not be true, that those who are punished are not always those who are guilty. But let affliction beset us, and we find ourselves in the ashes with Job of the Old Testament. "What have I done to deserve this evil?" We have known many persons deeply troubled by speech disorders and other ills, and most of them have asked this ancient question. Parents have asked it; little children have searched their souls for an answer. Here's an excerpt from an autobiography.

> Even when I was a little girl I remember being ashamed of my speech. And every time I opened my mouth, I shamed my mother. I can't tell you how awful I felt. If I talked, I did wrong. It was that simple. I kept thinking I must be awful bad to have to talk like that. I remember praying to God and asking him to forgive me for whatever it was I must have done. I remember trying hard to remember what it was, and not being able to find it.

It seems to be the fashion now to blame parents for many of the troubles of their children, for juvenile delinquency, for emotional conflicts, for defective speech. We can blame the school if Johnny cannot read, but few parents of a child who comes to school with unintelligible speech have escaped the blame of their neighbors. The father of a cleft-palate child often feels an urge to accuse the mother, and the mother the father, for something that is the fault of neither. When guilt enters a house, a home is in danger. Children who grow up in such an atmosphere of open or hidden recrimination are prone to blame themselves. Thus the emotional fraction of a speech disorder may grow.

Reactions to Guilt Feelings. Guilt is another evil that eats its container. In its milder forms of regret or embarrassment, most people can handle it with various degrees of discomfort. However, when shame and guilt are strong, they can become almost unbearable. To protect himself, the person may react with behavior that produces more penalty or more guilt. We have seen children deliberately soil themselves, throw temper tantrums, break things, steal things, even set fires so that they could get the punishment they felt their guilt deserved. After the punishment comes a little peace!

Other children punish themselves. We have watched stutterers use their stuttering to hurt themselves, using it in much the same way as the flagellants of the Middle Ages flogged and tortured their bodies for their sins. We have known children with repaired harelips and cleft palates who could not bear to watch themselves in a mirror even to observe the action of the tongue or soft palate. We have heard children cry and strike themselves when they heard their speech played back from a tape recorder. We who deal with such children must always be alert to this need for punishment lest they place the whip in our hands.

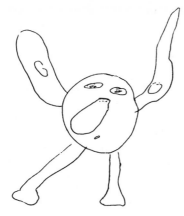

FIGURE 3: *Copy of a Crayon Drawing of Himself by a Cleft-Palate Child*. Note size of ears, nose, and mouth. His drawings of others in his family were very normal.

Here is what one adult with cerebral palsy painfully typed for us:

Sometimes when I lie in bed pretty relaxed I almost feel normal. In the quiet and the darkness I don't even feel myself twitching. I pretend I'm just like everybody else. But then in the morning I have to get up and face the monster in the mirror when I shave. I see what other people see, and I'm ashamed. I see the grey hairs on my mother's head and know I put them there. I eat but I know it isn't bread I can earn. Oh there are times when I get interested in something and forget what I am, but not when I talk. When I talk to someone, he doesn't have a face. He has a mirror for a face, and I see the monster again.

We who must help these people must also expect at times to find apathy and depression as reactions to the feelings of guilt. It is possible to ease the distress of guilt a little by becoming numb, by giving up, by refusing to try. Again, we may find individuals who escape some of their guilt by denying the reality of their crooked mouths or tangled tongues. They resist our efforts to help them because they refuse to accept the *fact* of abnormal speech. Somehow they feel that the moment they admit the existence of abnormality, they become responsible. And with responsibility comes the guilt they cannot bear. So they resist our efforts to help them. Finally, we meet persons who absolve themselves from guilt by projection, by blaming others for their affliction, by converting their guilt into hostility or anxiety. But this brings us to the next section.

HOSTILITY

Both penalty and frustration generate anger and aggression. We who are hurt, hate. We who are frustrated, rage. Here is an example to help you understand. It was written by an asphasic veteran who had been shot in the head.

> The worst feature of my brain injury was the frustration. I would know exactly what I wanted to say, but it would come out of my mouth differently. If I wanted to say "Please pass the cake," my mouth might say "Please part the ice," which didn't make sense to anyone else or even to my own ears. A hundred times a day this would happen. I'd find myself crying or cursing or frozen into some stiff posture or making some meaningless movements with my leg, and I knew that these were just my ways of trying to handle the complete feeling of inability that characterized my life.

Reactions to Hostility.   Hostility, like anxiety and guilt, ranges along a continuum all the way from momentary irritation through anger to intense hatred. Some children with severe speech problems show little hostility; yet we have known some with mild and minor disorders to show much. One child may have much anxiety or guilt but little hostility; another may reveal quite an opposite state of affairs. Some children just seem to roll with the punches and the frustrations and manage to get along with a minimum of emotional response. But often hostility and aggression are found, and so we must understand them.

HISTORY OF THE HANDICAPPED

There are times, when we survey the extent of human distress, that it seems that this dream of creating a better world is so unrealistic that it would be foolish to try to do anything to make it come true. Why seek to make one's own life meaningful in this way when there is such an immense amount of misfortune all about us? Why pick up a few beer cans when millions are discarded each day? Why try to help those who are less fortunate than we are when the powerful forces of our own culture keep generating more unhappiness? Is there any hope for mankind?

The history of the way society has treated the handicapped, sad and sorry as it is, may give us the glimmerings of that hope. Although we have some way to go before we can call ourselves civilized, the contrast between the present and past treatments of the retarded, the deaf, the blind, the crippled, the insane, the poor, and those who cannot talk normally shows very clearly that we have made gains. We find in this cultural history a hopeful progression from considering the handicapped persons as intolerable nuisances, then as objects of mirth, then as pitiful beggars, and now as challenging problems. Though these attitudes are still in evidence today, they are surely less prevalent.

Rejection.   Primitive society tolerated no weakness. Tribes struggled hard for survival, and those members who could not aid materially were quickly rejected. The younger men killed the leaders when they had lost their teeth or their energies had abated. The inhabitants of ancient India cast their cripples into the Ganges; the Spartans hurled theirs from a precipice. The Aztecs regularly sacrificed deformed persons in times of famine or when one of their leaders died. The Melanesians had a simple solution for the problem of the handicapped: they buried them alive. Among the earlier Romans, twins were considered so abnormal that one of them was always put to death, and frequently both were killed. They left their malformed children on the highways or in the forests. If the children survived, they were often picked up by those who always prey upon the handicapped and were carried to the market place to be trained as beggars. They were not valuable enough to be slaves.

The Bible clearly reflects these early rejection attitudes. Remember Job? The prevailing belief in Old Testament times was that man's physical state was determined by his good or bad relationship with his deity. Disabilities were regarded as divine punishment for sin. A normal person could invoke similar punishment merely by associating with those who had thus incurred the wrath of God. Consequently, the blind and the crippled wailed with the lepers outside the city wall.

During the Middle Ages the physically disabled were frequently considered to be possessed by evil spirits. They were confined to their own homes. They dared not walk to the market place lest they be stoned. Even in this century, elimination of the handicapped has been practiced. The Kaffir tribes in South Africa clubbed sickly or deformed children. The Nazis kept only the best of their civilian prisoners for slaves; the others died in the gas chamber.

In this country we would hang the man who killed his crippled son. We have come far in our journey toward civilization, but perhaps not far enough. Rejection takes many other forms. Spirits, too, can be killed. This is what one handicapped person has to say:

> We think the inhabitants of old Sparta cruel for putting to death the weak, those who would be unable to compete or to contribute much to their society; but were they, after all, much more inhuman than we who nurse the weakling, keep it alive, yet as much as possible keep it from normal persons, especially the children, for fear its contact will contaminate them; then throw it out to compete with normal adults? [2]

How many of those reading this book would unhesitatingly accept an invitation to a dance if it were tendered by a hunchback?

[2] R. V. McKnight, "A Self-analysis of a Case of Reading, Writing, and Speaking Disability," *Archives of Speech*, I (1936), 43.

Humor. It did not take the promoters long to discover that the handicapped provided a rewarding source of humor. One history of the subject states that before 1,000 B.C. the fool or buffoon became a necessary part of feast-making and "won the laughter of the guests by his idiocy or his deformity." In Homer's *Odyssey*, comic relief from tragedy was illustrated by the vain effort of the one-eyed Polyphemus to pursue his tormentors after they had blinded him. For a thousand years thereafter every court had its crippled buffoons, its dwarf jesters, its stuttering fools. Attila the Hun held banquets at which "a Moorish and Scythian buffoon successively excited the mirth of the rude spectators by their deformed figures, ridiculous dress, antic gestures, and absurd speech." Cages along the Appian Way held various grotesque human disabilities, including "Balbus Blaesus" the stutterer, who would attempt to talk when a coin was flung through the bars. In Shakespeare's *Timon of Athens,* Caphis says, "Here comes the fool; let's ha' some sport with 'im." Often this sport consisted of physical abuse or exposure of the twisted limb. These handicapped fools accepted and expected ridicule. At least it provided a means of survival, a livelihood, and it represented an advance in civilized living.

Gradually, the use of the handicapped to provoke mirth became less popular in continental Europe, and the more enterprising had to migrate to less culturally advanced areas to make a living. At one time Peter the Great had so many fools that he found it necessary to classify them for different occasions. When Cortez conquered Mexico he discovered deformed creatures of all kinds at the court of Montezuma. On the same continents today you may find them used to provoke laughter only in the circus sideshows, in the movies, on the radio, and in every schoolyard.

Pity. Religion is doubtless responsible for the development of true pity as a cultural reaction to the handicapped. James Joyce said that pity is the feeling which arrests the mind in the presence of whatsoever is grave and constant in human suffering and unites it with the human sufferer. It was this spontaneous feeling that prompted religious leaders to give the handicapped shelter and protection. Before 200 B.C. Asoka, a Buddhist, created a ministry for the care of unfortunates and appointed officers to supervise charitable works. Confucius said, "With whom should I associate but with suffering men?" Jesus preached compassion for all the disabled and made all men their brothers' keepers. In the seventh century after Jesus' death the Mohammedan religion proposed a society free from cruelty and social oppression and insisted on kindliness and consideration for all men. A few hundred years later Saint Francis of Assisi devoted his life to the care of the sick and the disabled. Following this, the "Mad Priest of Kent," John Ball, was so aroused by the plight of the crippled and needy left in the wake of the Black Death that he publicly pleaded their cause, often at the risk of his own life. With the rise of the middle class, true pity for the handicapped become much more commonplace. The oppression which the merchants and serfs had suffered left them more sympathetic to others who were ill used. The doctrine of the equality of man did much for the handicapped as well as for the economically down-trodden.

However, many crimes have been committed in the name of charity. The halt and the blind began to acquire commercial value as beggars. Legs and backs of little children were broken and twisted by their exploiters. Soon the commercialization of pity became so universal that it became a community nuisance. Alms became a conventional gesture to buy relief from the piteous whining that dominated every public place. True pity was lost in revulsion. Recognizing this unhappy trend, Hyperius of Ypres advocated that beggars be classified so that work could be provided according to their capacities. His own motives were humanitarian, but he cleverly won support for his cause by pointing out that other citizens "would be freed of clamor, of fear of outrage, or the sight of ugly bodies." His appeal was successful; and asylums and homes for the handicapped began to appear, if only to isolate the occupants so the public need not be reminded of their distress. Another motive which improved the position of the handicapped was the belief that one could purchase his way into heaven or out of hell by charity. The coin thrown to the cripple has been impelled by many motives. The longing for religious security, the heightening of one's own superiority by comparison with the unfortunate, the social prestige of philanthropy, and the desire to be freed from embarrassment have all contributed to the welfare of the handicapped. Pseudopity has accomplished much, but true compassion would have ended the tragedy.

PRESENT TREATMENT OF THE SPEECH HANDICAPPED

We have sketched the treatment accorded the handicapped at some length because the speech-defective person is diagnosed immediately as belonging to that unfortunate group. The moment the cleft-palate child or stutterer speaks he joins his brethren, the crippled, the deaf, the spastic, the blind, and perhaps the fool. He is different. He possesses an abnormality. A little child hesitates in his speech; his parents diagnose him as a stutterer; he reacts to his hesitations as though they were unpleasant; his playmates accept his evaluation or his parents' evaluation, and so he joins the unhappy tribe of the million stutterers who exist in this country today.

It may seem strange to learn that the primitive attitudes of rejection, humor, and pity are still very common reactions to the perception of speech defects today. Listen to these:

They got me inside a circle of them, and every time I tried to break out and go home, they pushed me back. "Make a speech. Make a speech." I tried to tell them I had to get my groceries home. My mother had to have them for supper, but the men would just laugh all the harder and push me back. They told me to say different things if I wanted to get out, things like "She sells sea shells" and dirty words. I was crying and I got mad and swore at them, and then they let me go but I can hear them yet.

I asked the girl for a dance and had a hard time getting it out. She flushed, then blurted out, "Well, I'm not that hard up yet."

I can take almost anything but that pitying glance. It's sort of as if I have a cup in my hand every time I talk and people feel they ought to put some pennies in it. I can't explain it, but when they look away or down at their feet I feel like something unclean. I can't help it that my operation tore loose, and I talk through my nose, but I can't even explain it to them.

We no longer keep our "Balbus Blaesuses" in cages, but a current radio program features a "comedian" whose main humorous appeal is based upon his substitution of *w* for *l* and *r*. The song about "K-K-K-Katy" is still being sung although "Stuttering in the Starlight" and "You-you-you tell 'em that I-I-I stutter" have been forgotten. Cartoons and comic strips do not fail to exploit the impediments of speech.

Nevertheless we end this chapter on a hopeful note. Throughout our society we discern a need for change. We are beginning to reduce exploitation and pollution. We no longer accept selfishness as the basic law of human interaction. We are beginning to care for those less fortunate than we are, realizing that the unhappiness of others diminishes our own good fortune. We cannot continue to live in a world polluted by misery, injustice, and cruelty. We must do what we can.

REFERENCES

Articles

1. Boone, D. R. "Treatment of Functional Aphonia in a Child and an Adult." *Journal of Speech and Hearing Disorders,* XXX (1965), 69–74.
   Describe the voice problems of these two individuals and tell how they were treated.
2. Celler, J. "Helpless, Not Hopeless." *Mental Hygiene,* LX (1956), 535–50.
   This article has meant much to some of our handicapped patients. Why?
3. Duncan, M. "Emotional Aspects of the Communciation Problem in Cerebral Palsy." *Cerebral Palsy Review,* LXXVI (1955), 19–23.
   What emotional problems are described?
4. Emerick, L. "A Clinical Success: Mark; and a Clinical Failure: Sherrie." In Fraser, M., ed., *Stuttering, Successes and Failures in Therapy* (Memphis, Tenn.: Speech Foundation of America, 1968). Pp. 21–39.
   What were the emotional problems existing in these two cases, and how did they affect the success and failure of treatment?
5. ———. *The Parent Interview.* Danville, Ill.: Interstate, 1969.
   What basic principles are involved in interviewing?
6. Heffron, M. "Council of Adult Stutterers." *Journal of Rehabilitation,* XXXV (1969), 35–36.
   Describe how this group functions.
7. Johnson, W. "I Was a Despairing Stutterer." *Saturday Evening Post* (January 5, 1957), 26–27.
   Why did he despair, and how did he come out?
8. Kowalsky, M. H. "Integration of a Severely Hard of Hearing Child in a Normal First-Grade Program: A Case Study." *Journal of Speech and Hearing Disorders,* XXVII (1962), 349–57.
   How did they manage to get this child to make the adjustment to school?
9. McKibben, S. "The Spastic Situation." *Journal of Speech and Hearing Disorders,* VIII (1943), 147–53.
   According to the author, who is herself a spastic, what were the major problems encountered?
10. Matis, E. E. "Psychotherapeutic Tools for Parents." *Journal of Speech and Hearing Disorders,* XXVI (1961), 164–70.
    Recount some examples of the ways the parents profited from the psychotherapy?
11. Murphy, A. T. and Fitzsimons, R. M. *Stuttering and Personality Dynamics.* New York: The Ronald Press Company, 1960.
    Read Chapter 5 and state the authors' view of the relationship between anxiety and stuttering.
12. Pedrey, C. "Letter to the Editor." *Journal of Speech and Hearing Disorders,* XV (1950), 266–69.
    Tell how this stuttering convict was treated for his disorder when he was a boy.
13. Slutsky, H. "Maternal Reaction and Adjustment to the Birth and Care

of Cleft-Palate Children." *Cleft Palate Journal,* VII (1967), 425–29.
What are the common reactions of mothers to their cleft-palate children, and how should they be dealt with?

14. Travis, L. E. "The Unspeakable Feelings of People with Special Reference to Stuttering." Chapter 19 in L. E. Travis, ed., *Handbook of Speech Pathology* (New York: Appleton-Century-Crofts, 1957).
List these unspeakable feelings.

15. Van Riper, C. "Case Study of a Secondary Stutterer." In Berg, I. A. and Pennington, L. A., eds., *An Introduction to Clinical Psychology,* 3d ed. (New York: The Ronald Press Company, 1966). Pp. 354–61.
Why did this case require both speech therapy and psychotherapy?

16. ———. "Success and Failure in Speech Therapy." *Journal of Speech and Hearing Disorders,* XXXI (1966), 276–79.
What is this author's basic philosophy of living and working?

17. Weiner, P. S. "The Emotionally Disturbed Child in the Speech Clinic: Some Considerations." *Journal of Speech and Hearing Disorders,* XXXIII (1968), 158–66.
Should the speech therapist work with children like John, Ruth, Tim, Bill, and Dan?

18. Wolpe, Z. S. "Play Therapy, Psychodrama, and Parent Counseling." In Travis, L. E., ed., *Handbook of Speech Pathology* (New York: Appleton-Century-Crofts, 1957).
Describe the methods suggested for dealing with the emotional problems of speech handicapped children.

Texts

19. Brown, C. and Van Riper, C. *Speech and Man.* Englewood Cliffs, N.J.: Prentice-Hall, Inc., 1966.
This book seeks to acquaint the reader with the tremendous importance of speech in defining the self, and in thinking, feeling, and communicating.

20. Lukens, K. and Panter, C. *Thursday's Child Has Far to Go.* Englewood Cliffs, N.J.: Prentice-Hall, Inc., 1969.
The inspiring story of a handicapped person who had many obstacles to face.

21. McDonald, E. T. *Understanding Those Feelings.* Pittsburgh: Stanwix House, 1962.
One of the best books available for helping clinicians and their cases understand their emotional hang-ups. The section on counseling parents of handicapped children is especially valuable.

22. Ritchie, D. *Stroke.* New York: Doubleday & Company, Inc., 1961.
This is a very readable description of the tragedy which ensues when a stroke deprives its victim of language. The author was a correspondent for the British Broadcasting Company. A moving story of a man seeking the language he has lost.

23. Wedberg, C. F. *The Stutterer Speaks.* Boston, Expression Co., 1937.
A stutterer's tale of his own suffering and eventual triumph.

2

The Disorders of Speech

Unlike some of the other afflictions that contribute to human unhappiness, the disorders of communication can be reduced or eliminated by appropriate therapy. Some problems such as poverty or a befouled environment require vast and concerted energies of many people all working together for many years. Any participant in these worthy causes finds it hard to discern his personal impact, but in speech therapy the results of one's concern and work are soon evident. We can help these persons who do not talk normally. We can aid them to overcome their speech handicaps. To do so, however, we must understand their problems; and our first task is to know what they are. We begin by listing a few of their names.

Spasmophemia, rhotacism, uranoscolalia, lambdalalia. Do not worry. We do not intend to inflict such a heavy burden of polysyllabic jawbreakers upon your tender memory. Translated, in sequence, these terms refer to stuttering, defective *r* sounds, cleft-palate speech, and defective *l* sounds. Excessive nasality, lisping, delayed speech characterized by jargon all have long jawbone names. And there are others, for this is not a complete list by any means. We start this chapter with this esoteric chanting only to make the point that there are many speech disorders. We must learn how to identify them.

A few letters may help to vivify the need for such identifying information.

Dear Sir: I am a country schoolteacher in a two-room school. In my room there is a little boy in the third grade with a kind of funny voice. I mean he doesn't talk like other children. He can't say some of the words right that he knows just as well as I do. I have tried to correct

27

him on the word "scissors" which is hard for him, but he just can't get it out right. Is this stammering or just baby-talk, and how can I cure him? Please send me some tongue exercises or something. He is a sweet little child and needs some help.

Here is another:

I want you should help me. My boy he dont talk right. He gets tangeled up in his nose and it sounds funny. When can I bring him.

And another:

I have a bad habit in talking that makes my talk so other people can't understand me although I know what I'm saying. They yell at me as if I'm deaf and dumb, but I can hear good. I just can't talk good.

One more:

I have an impediment or something in my mouth. Sometimes I talk all right but not always. I open my mouth and the words won't come out right.

These examples should demonstrate not only the necessity for further investigation and analysis but also the need for information as to the common patterns of abnormal speech. In this chapter we present the symptom pictures of the various speech disorders. Once we know these we can hope to begin our differential diagnosis.

But first we must face another problem well known to the physician too: "Does this person actually have anything wrong with him?" There are thousands upon thousands of variations in normal speech. If there were not, we could never recognize our friends by their voices. Even the same person seldom says the same word twice in identical fashion. When is a speech difference a speech defect? How do we judge?

These questions are not academic. Misdiagnosis has caused untold misery. A mother who did not know that few children master their *str* and *spl* blends before the age of five, grew anxious about her three-year-old's mistakes on those sounds, and then she corrected him so frequently, made so many visits to elocution teachers, faith healers, and physicians, and punished him so severely that finally the child stopped talking altogether and remained mute for three years. Another child with delayed speech was misdiagnosed as being deaf and feeble-minded. We found her, at sixteen, using sign language and unable to understand except when she lip-read, this despite the fact that her audiogram revealed normal hearing and a performance test a normal IQ. Many a normal child has been turned into a severe stutterer by having the normal hesitation and repetitions of early speech labeled and penalized as stuttering until finally he came to accept the label and began to avoid speech or to struggle with his utterance. Many a child has been treated as a lisper when his *s* and *z* sounds were well within the limits tolerated by anyone except the hypercritical parent or teacher who committed the crime. So let us define a speech defect.

Definition: Speech is defective when it deviates so far from the speech of other people that it calls attention to itself, interferes with communication, or causes its possessor to be maladjusted.

We can condense this definition into three adjectives. Speech is defective when it is *conspicuous, unintelligible,* or *unpleasant.* The first adjective refers to the fact that abnormal speech is different enough to be noted. It varies too far from the norm. A child of three who says "wabbit" for "rabbit" has no speech defect, but the adult of fifty who uses that pronunciation would have one because it would be a real deviation from the pronunciation of other adults. If you said *deze, doze,* and *dem* for *these, those,* and *them* in a hobo jungle, none of the other vagrants would notice. If you used the same sounds in a talk to a P.T.A. meeting a good many ears would prickle. Many of us force the airstream down too broad a tongue groove to produce the high-pitched *s* sound characteristic of our English speech. Because we do so does not necessarily mean that we have lateral lisps. Only when our *s* is so slushy and low in pitch that it calls attention to itself can we be said to have that type of speech defect.

How wide a variation is required before we should be concerned about a speech difference? Only the cultural norms can answer this question. Among the Pilagra Indians no attention is ever paid to baby-talk or peculiar speech until the child is at least seven years of age. Many Indian tribes do not even have a word for stuttering, although many of their membership no doubt have hesitant speech. According to the famous anthropologist Sapir, who worked among the Nootka, repetitive and hesitant speech seems to be more common than fluent rhythmic speech in this tribe of Indians. One would have to stutter badly indeed to have a speech defect in such a culture. In England the dropping of an *h* or the flatting of a vowel would cause instant social penalty in upper class society, whereas the same behavior would be quite unnoticeable in Australia. Excessive assimilation nasality would not be noticed by a Tennessee mountaineer, but the same voice quality in an Eastern girls' school would send its owner to the speech clinic. A speech defect, then, is one which is so different from the normal speech of the social group that it is highly conspicuous. The individual who refers a case to the speech therapist should evaluate its context accordingly.

The second part of the definition refers to intelligibility. When a speech difference interferes with communication it tends to be labeled as defective.

When you listen, not to what a stranger says, but to his peculiar voice or hesitations or distorted consonants, communication is broken. If his face suddenly jumps around as he struggles to utter an ordinary word, all communicative content is lost in amusement or amazement. Many stutterers habitually lower their eyes to escape the shock of observing the expression of incredulity and surprise on the faces of their auditors. Cleft-palate adults have been known to pretend to be deaf and dumb and to beg for a pencil so that their communication could be accomplished without interruption.

If, as one of our eighteen-year-old cases illustrated, you heard someone reciting "Poh koh an tebbuh yee adoh ow pohpadduh baw poh uhpah dih kawinaw a new naytuh" you might find it very hard to understand him—unless you knew he was saying the first lines of Lincoln's "Gettysburg Address." Speech is defective when it is difficult to understand, when its intelligibility is poor.

That communication is impaired when a person loses his voice (aphonia) is obvious. The person whose larynx has been removed is pretty helpless until he learns to swallow air and speak on the expelled burp. But even then, the monotone is difficult to listen to or to understand. The cleft-palate child's teacher finds great difficulty in fathoming what he is trying to recite. A falsetto voice distracts attention from what is being said. The more conspicuous the vocal abnormality, the more unintelligible the speech becomes.

Many a stutterer has had to ask for a paper and pencil in order to make his simplest wants known. The words emerge from such contortions and broken garblings of utterance that frequently both the stutterer and the listener give up.

A speech defect, then, is one which calls attention to itself and interferes with communication.

The final part of our definition deals with the maladjustment and emotional handicap which the speech defective adds to his disability. Sometimes this maladjustment is the dominant feature of the disorder. We worked with a woman who claimed to have stuttered actually only once in her life—during a high-school graduation speech. Her speech was certainly not fluent, since it was marked by numerous hesitations, pauses, and avoidances of certain words. She was badly handicapped socially and vocationally. Her listeners were constantly puzzled and confused by her peculiar speech behavior. And yet she had actually "stuttered" only once. This case, of course, is an extreme instance of the importance of maladjustment in producing a speech defect. Usually, the abnormality of rhythm, voice, or articulation is sufficiently bizarre to provoke so many social penalities that maladjustment is almost inevitable.

CLASSIFICATION OF SPEECH DISORDERS

There are many ways in which we could classify the various speech disorders, but if we look at the behavior itself we find that they seem to fall into four major categories: *articulation, time, voice,* and *symbolization* (language). This fourfold classification, it should be understood, refers to the *outstanding* features of the behavior shown. Thus even though his stuttering causes certain sounds to be distorted, we place the stutterer in the second category because the major feature of his disorder is the broken timing of his utterance. The person with aphasia often shows articulation errors, broken rhythm, inability to produce voice; but the outstanding feature of aphasia is the inability to handle symbolic meanings and language. Therefore, we would place aphasia under disorders of symbolization or language. Certain individuals show more than one of these disorders. A child with severe cerebral palsy, for example, may show all four.

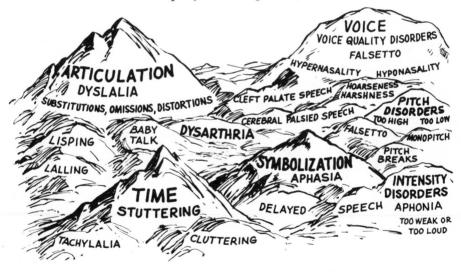

FIGURE 4: *The Field of Speech Pathology*

ARTICULATION

To introduce this section, let us present a handful of word pictures of some persons who have disorders of articulation. These are not typical cases; they merely illustrate the variety.

Robert was in the third grade when we first met him. No one called him "Bobby." He was a loner, preferring to stay in his seat at recess, and when forced to leave, stood shyly at the school entrance watching the other children. They did not penalize him; they just ignored him. Although of normal intelligence and doing well in arithmetic, he had marked disabilities in reading and spelling; and the teacher felt that this was probably due to his many defective sounds. With some difficulty it was possible to understand what he said when he did offer a few words, but often a word or phrase would be completely unintelligible. When asked to repeat, he would say it over and over again in a sad little voice, and always in the same fashion. In analyzing a fair sample of his speech we found that he consistently produced all the vowel sounds correctly and also the *m, n, p, b, w, t, d*, and *f* sounds. Most of the other sounds were either omitted or replaced with these sounds, although on a few words such as "can" and "gum" we heard him say the *k* and the *g* very normally. His mother reported that he had not really begun to talk until the year before he entered kindergarten, and the school records indicated that he had not improved in the four years since he entered school. We enrolled him in the clinic, enlisted the aid of his teacher and his parents, and gave him intensive speech therapy for an hour each day. By the end of six months he was speaking almost normally, and a year later showed no sign of any articulatory problem. He had also made great gains in reading and spelling. But what was even more important, he began to participate in the play activities of his schoolmates and changed from being an isolate to a member of their groups.

Mrs. M. was referred to us by her dentist whom she had threatened to sue for malpractice. She was a big belligerent woman, a high-school teacher of speech who spoke in highly conscious, pear-shaped tones. She gestured with the hand supine, the hand prone, and the ictus. Mrs. M. also had conducted an interview program over the local TV station once a week but had recently been replaced. She felt that this had occurred because of the change in her speech subsequent to the fitting of an upper dental plate. Our examination revealed that her sibilants, the *s, z*, and *sh* sounds, were distorted by a very obvious, high-pitched whistle. The dentist informed us that he had varied the appliance in every way possible to alter this unpleasant whistling and had brought in consultants from his own field to help, but without success. He had hoped that as she became accustomed to the denture, the whistle would disappear; but it had now persisted for three months and, if anything, was getting worse. It was evident that Mrs. M. had become morbidly conscious of these whistled sibilants; and so, in our trial therapy, we piped in masking noise through earphones as we asked her to attempt *s* sounds while anchoring the tip of her tongue against her lower teeth. The whistle disappeared immediately, and we tape-recorded Mrs. M.'s speech to show her that it did so. She was delighted and worked hard to eliminate the abnormality, and within a month was speaking normally again. We suspect that prior to the fitting of the denture she had habitually used this lower tongue position to produce the sibilants and had developed the whistle by constantly exploring tongue contacts with the unfamiliar appliance in her mouth.

We do not wish to leave the impression that disorders of articulation present little difficulty to the therapist. Some of them have been our toughest cases. Somehow we remember our failures much more vividly than we do our successes. They haunt us. What did we do wrongly or what did we fail to do? One of them was Joe.

Joe was in the fifth grade when we first worked with him. Only one of his sounds was defective—the vowel r sound as in *fur*. He was able to make the consonantal r perfectly, articulating it correctly whenever it occurred as the initial consonant of a syllable. He could say "run," "radio," or any other word beginning with r without error. Even the consonant blends, *pr, tr, gr,* etc., were uttered normally. But when the r occurred as a vowel as in *church,* he said "chutch." He said "theatuh," "mothuh," "guhl." When the r was part of a diphthong as in *ar, or, ir,* not only was the r distorted but the preceding vowel was often misarticulated. Instead of "far," he said "foah," and in these distorted diphthongs we heard sounds that we had never heard before. We worked hard with Joe and initially felt that the prognosis was good, that we could probably effect a transition from the consonantal to the vowel r with ease. We failed completely. He tried and we tried with all our might. We used every technique known to us. We vainly explored every possible reason for the persistence of the errors. We tried different therapists. They failed. When Joe was a senior in high school we tried again with the same result. We still wonder what else we might have done.

As we have seen from our scrutiny of the preceding examples, the basic problem shown by a person with a disorder of articulation is that he has failed to master the speech sounds of his language. Each of these three persons could be characterized as having a *phonemic* disorder rather than one of voice or of fluency or of symbolization. Although they differed one from the other in the pattern of their phonemic errors, they all showed one or more of the following types: (1) substitution of one standard English phoneme for another; (2) a distortion of a standard sound; (3) an omission of a sound that should be present; or (4) an addition or insertion of an irrelevant sound. These are the kinds of articulatory errors which these people show. Most young children during the course of their speech development show all of these at one time or another; but some children persist in their usage, having failed to perceive the contrasting features of the correct sound as compared with the defective one, or having been unable to achieve its correct production.

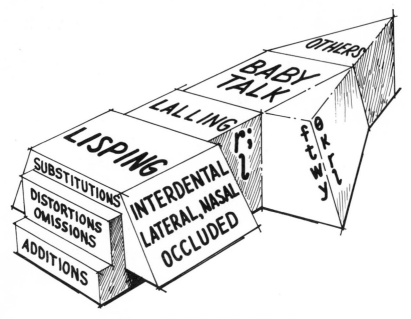

FIGURE 5: *Articulation Disorders*

Articulatory errors often appear in clusters, and some of these clusters have acquired common names. *Lisping* is one such cluster. It consists of defective sibilant sounds such as the *s* and *z*, the *sh* [ʃ], and *zh* [ʒ], and others that are characterized by the friction of air escaping through a narrow opening. Names have also been given to subvarieties of the lisp. Thus we have the *interdental* or *frontal* lisp in which the voiced or unvoiced *th* sounds are substituted for the *s* and *z* respectively: "Thum people like thum thingth and other people like other thingth but ath for me, I like thpitting. I can even thpit in thirclth and thpiralth," said one of our lispers and proceeded to do so. Another common variety of lisp is the *lateral* lisp in which the sibilants are distorted. The *s* and *z*, and even the *ch* [tʃ], *j* [dʒ], and *th* sounds are spoken mushily. When older people are first fitted with dentures, they tend to show some of this lateral omission of air, and so do college students when intoxicated. Some little children learn this sort of a sibilant and never master the correct ones. There are also other lisps: the occluded type in which the *s* may be prefaced by a short *t* sound or the *z* by a *d*. Such a person would say, "TSally had a dzipper that wouldn't open." In cleft-palate speakers we often find nasal lisps in which the airstream is emitted through the nose instead of through the teeth. Nasal lispers snort their sibilants.

Another term which is fortunately fading from the speech therapist's professional vocabulary is *lalling*. It refers to a cluster of errors, primarily upon the *r* and *l* sounds, in which the tongue tip fails to lift sufficiently to produce the contact or contour necessary for correct production. If you will anchor your tongue tip below your bottom teeth and refuse to lift it as you say, "Lulu was a lallapalooza of a laller" you will recognize the kind of speech which some still prefer to call lalling.

You doubtless have heard the term *baby-talk*, which was dignified by the synonymous phrase "infantile perseveration" some years ago. The term does not have a precise referent, but usually it means that the person seems to be using the kinds of substitutions, distortions, and omissions common in early childhood. "Muvver, the doddie (doggie) want to dow owdoh" might represent the kind of speech which the lay person would call baby-talk.

Actually these names do not denote different types of disorders. They are not mutually exclusive. Lallers often lisp, and lispers talk baby-talk, and all of them show oral inaccuracy. The important feature of all articulatory disorders is the presence of defective and incorrect sounds. The forty-year-old farmer who wept when he heard his voice on a recording of a children's rhyme did so because of the defective and incorrect sounds he had produced. A six-year-old said this:

> Tinko Tinko itto tah,
> How I wondah wheh you ah,
> Up abuh duh woh soh high
> Yike a diamon' in duh kye.

As the above selection indicates, most articulatory cases have more than one error and are not always consistent in their substitutions, omissions, insertions, or distortions. This is not always the case, however. Thum lingual lithperth merely thubthitute a *th* for the *eth* thound. Othershshkwirt the airshtream over the shide of the tongue and are shed to have a lateral lishp. Others thnort the thnound (nasal lisp). Many children have been known to buy an "ites tream toda" or an all-day "tucker."

It would be impossible to portray the acoustic characteristics of some of the distortions used by articulatory cases, even if we used the phonetic alphabet. Seldom does an adult substitute a true *w* for the *r* as he attempts such a phrase as "around the rock." He usually produces a sound "something like a *w* and something like the velar *r* made with the back of the tongue elevated and the tip depressed." In some lateral lisping, the sound produced is more of a salivary unvoiced *l* instead of the *s*, a sloppy slurping sound which disgusts not only its hearers but its speaker too.

Many of the omissions heard in articulation cases are merely weakly stressed consonants. In a noisy room, an eighteen-year-old boy in describing a winter scene would seem to say, "The 'ky and 'no in wintuh." The missing sounds, however, were evident in quiet surroundings and were perfectly formed; but their duration was so brief that any noise seemed to mask their presence. Many cases, however, do entirely omit sounds they cannot produce. Additions of linking sounds are frequently found in blends ("the buhlue-guhreen color of spuhruce trees"); and when a child adds *ee* to every final *r* sound, as one of our cases did, the peculiarity is very noticeable.

To many persons, articulatory defects seem relatively unimportant. But severe articulation cases find the demands of modern life very difficult. We knew a woman who could not produce the *s*, *l*, and *r* sounds and yet who had to buy a railroad ticket to Robeline, Louisiana. She did it with pencil and paper. A man with the same difficulty became a farmer's hired hand after he graduated from college rather than suffer the penalties of a more verbal existence. Many children are said to outgrow their defective consonant sounds. Actually, they overcome them through blundering methods of self-help, and far too many of them never manage the feat. One man, aged sixty-five, asked us bitterly when we thought he would outgrow his baby-talk.

Some of these articulation cases have a great deal of difficulty communicating. Mothers cannot understand their own children. Teachers and classmates fail to comprehend speech when it is too full of phonemic errors. Try to translate this familiar nursery rhyme:

Ha ta buh, Hah ta buh,
Wuhnuh peh, two uh peh,
Ha ta buh.

Tippo Tymuh meh a pyemuh,
Doh too peh,
Ted Tippo Tymuh to duh pyemuh
Yeh me tee oo weh.

Many children who are severely handicapped by unintelligibile speech also find it very difficult to express their emotions except by screaming or acting out their conflicts. Most of us relieve ourselves of our emotional evils by using others as our verbal handkerchiefs or wastebaskets. We talk it out. But when a child runs to his mother crying "Wobbuh toh ma tietihtoh" and she cannot understand that Robert stole his tricycle, all he can do is to fling himself into a tantrum. The same frustration results from his inability to use speech for self-exhibition. Often penalized or frustrated when he tries to talk, he soon finds it better to keep quiet, to use gestures, or to get attention in other ways. Many people tend to regard articulatory errors as being cute or relatively unimportant. Some of the most handicapped people we have ever known were those who could not speak clearly enough to be understood.

DISORDERS OF TIME OR PROSODY

One of the dimensions of speech is *time*. We speak sequentially. Sound follows sound; syllable follows syllable. When speech is defective in the timing of its utterance we speak of disorders of time or rhythm. This rhythmic characteristic of speech is, of course, not evenly spaced or regular except in sing-song or some types of chanting. Nevertheless, the syllables of a sentence are definitely patterned in time. The sounds of a word, the words of a phrase, must fit into a set pattern if speech is to be normal. Again we find a range of permissible variation. Some of us speak very rapidly; others very slowly. Some of us are remarkably fluent and some of us have speech which is full of um's and er's, hesitations and repetitions. Only when the timing of our sounds and syllables is so far off the standard that our speech is conspicuous, unpleasant, or unintelligible do we have a disorder of time. In stuttering we have such a disorder.

Stuttering. It is difficult to find typical illustrations for this disorder since it is characterized by a high degree of variability. Nevertheless we present some examples from our practice.

William was brought to us by his concerned parents. They were especially worried because the father had stuttered as a child and a grandfather and uncle had been stutterers. When he was introduced to us, he said, "I'm nnnnot Wuh-Wuh-Wuh-Wuh-W-W-William. I-I-I-I'm Billy. Thuh-Thuh-that's my name." He seemed to be unaware of his repetitions and showed no reluctance to talk. Indeed he jabbered easily and constantly. Billy was an extrovertive, outgoing child, and a very active one. We had to do most of our analysis of the problem on the wing as he explored every corner of our office, opening the drawers, playing with our instruments, even going through the pockets of our overcoat in the closet. All this was accompanied by a verbal commentary on what he was doing or perceiving and much of what he said either to us or to himself was full of short syllabic repetitions or the prolongations of sounds. Only rarely would he say an entire phrase or short sentence without them. He just burbled, bubbled, and bounced without any signs of frustration. His parents said that this was the way he talked most of the time except when saying his prayers. Then he was fluent. Although many children show some of this sort of disfluency between the second and fourth years as they master speech, Billy had much more than the normal amount. He almost seemed to be speaking a stuttering language. What concerned us more was that the number of syllabic repetitions per word averaged four or five, whereas in normally speaking children they seldom exceed two per word. Moreover, Billy was using the "schwa" or neutral vowel ("uh") on many of his repetitions. He was not saying "bo-bo-bo-boat" but "buh-buh-buh-boat." He was also prolonging certain sounds. Once he said, "fffffffor," with the *f* being prolonged for over two seconds. Finally, these "stutterings" did not seem to reflect variations in communicative stress. They were too consistent. We accepted him for treatment.

Peter was an eleven-year-old stutterer. Speaking, to him, was hard labor. Although he stuttered on other words also, it was on the first words of his utterances that he had the most trouble. He would open his mouth and nothing would come out. You could see him forcing and struggling. His face was contorted. Sometimes he would just give up and tears came to his eyes. Not all of his blockings were of this type however. On certain words he would drawl out the vowel ("Caaaaaaan"), and the pitch would rise. On others he would repeat a syllable compulsively many times, and these syllables too would show the same fire-siren effect. When relaxed or distracted Peter could be very fluent, the stuttering occurring in volleys; yet he did not seem to avoid speaking nor did he attempt to disguise his trouble. The more he stuttered, the more he seemed to feel a need to talk. He was hurt and frustrated by his stuttering and was highly aware of it when it happened, but he showed no signs of fear.

Cynthia was sixteen, a very attractive girl, popular with her classmates and the boys, an excellent student. Outwardly she stuttered very little so far as repetitions or complete blockings were concerned. She talked very fast, but her speech was full of postponement tricks, avoidances, and disguise reactions. She feared certain sounds and words and would substitute synonyms for those she though she might stutter on, or pretend to think or cough or revise her sentences or say "ah-ah-ah-ah" or "well" or "Oh, you know" to gain time or hide her stuttering. She was very skillful in using these disguise reactions in her ordinary, casual speech. When she had to read aloud however, as she did in French class, some severe repetitive stuttering was very evident. It also showed up when she had to introduce herself or someone else. Although outwardly she was a gay, almost scatterbrained girl, this was a facade. She worried greatly about her stuttering and was very despondent in private. Her word, sound, and situation fears were very intense. She was very ashamed to be a stutterer.

In considering this disorder, let us observe its various aspects. The stutterer shows breaks in the usual time sequence of utterance. The usual flow is interrupted. There are conspicuous oscillations and fixations, repetitions and prolongations of sounds and syllables. There are gaps of silence that call attention to themselves. If you ask a stutterer a question, the answer may not be forthcoming at the proper time. The stutterer's speech sometimes seems to have holes in it. Some sounds are held too long. Syllables seem to echo themselves repeatedly and compulsively. Odd contortions and struggles occur which interfere with communication. The stutterer may show marked signs of fear or embarrassment. He fits our definition because his speech behavior deviates from the speech of other people in such a way that it attracts attention. All of us hesitate and repeat ourselves, but the stutterer hesitates and repeats himself differently than we do, and more often.

One of the interesting features of stuttering is that it seems to be a disorder more of communication than of speech. Most stutterers can sing without difficulty. Most of them speak perfectly when alone. Usually, it is only when they are talking to a listener that the difficulty becomes apparent. Stuttering varies with emotional stress and increases in situations invested with fear or shame. When very secure and relaxed, stutterers often are very fluent. In extreme cases even the thinking processes seem to be affected—but only when they are thinking aloud, and again in the presence of a listener.

Stuttering takes many forms; it presents many faces. The only consistent behavior is the repetition and prolongation of syllables, sounds, or speech postures. It changes as it develops, for stuttering usually grows and gets worse if untreated.

Initially, and for some time thereafter, the child's speech is broken by an excessive amount of repetitions of syllables and sounds or, less frequently, by the prolongation of a sound. He does not seem to be aware of his difficulty. He does not struggle or avoid speaking. He does not seem to be embarrassed at all. Indeed he seems almost totally unconscious of his repetitive utterance. He just bubbles along, trying his best to communicate. An excerpt from a parent's letter may illustrate this early stuttering:

> I would appreciate some advice about my daughter. She is almost three years old, and has always been precocious in speech. Four weeks ago she recovered from a severe attack of whooping cough, and it was immediately after that when she began to show some trouble with her

speech. One morning she came downstairs and asked for orange juice, and it sounded like this: "Wh-wh-wh-where's my orange juice?" Since

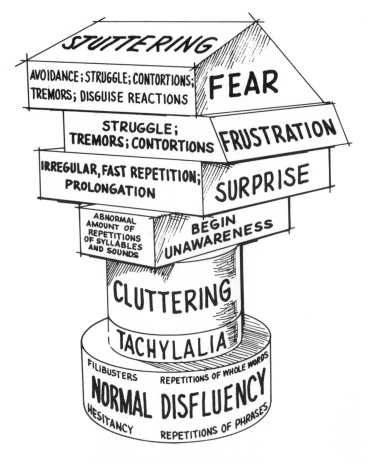

FIGURE 6: *Disorders of Time*

then, she has repeated twice, and sometimes eight or nine times. It doesn't seem to bother her, but I'm worried about it as it gets a lot worse when she asks questions or when she is tired, and I'm afraid other children will start laughing at her. One of her playmates has already imitated her several times. No one else in our family has any trouble talking. What do you think we should do? Up to now we have just been ignoring it and hoping it will go away.

Unfortunately, stuttering does not always remain so effortless. The child begins to react to his broken communication by surprise and then frustration. The former effortless repetitions and prolongations become irregular, faster, and more tense. As the child becomes aware of his stuttering and is frustrated by it, he begins to struggle. Finally, he becomes afraid of certain speaking situations and of certain words and sounds. Once this occurs, stuttering tends to become self-perpetuating, self-reinforcing. The more he fears, the more he stutters, and the more he stutters, the more he fears. He becomes caught in a vicious circle.

In the older stutterer, stuttering occurs in many forms, since different individuals react to their speech interruptions in different ways. One German authority carefully described ninety-nine different varieties of stuttering (each christened with beautiful Greek and Latin verbiage), and we are sure that there must be many more. Stutterers have been known to grunt or spit or pound themselves or protrude their tongues or speak on inhalation or waltz or jump or merely stare glassily when in the throes of what they call a "spasm" or a "block." The late Irvin S. Cobb described a certain Captain Joe Fowler who manifested his stuttering through the use of profanity. Captain Joe was able to speak very well under ordinary circumstances; but when he got angry or excited, his speech stopped entirely, and he was able to get started again only through the use of a stereotyped bit of cursing. Some of the imitations of stuttering heard in the movies and on radio may seem grotesque, yet the reality may be even more unusual.

Some stutterers develop an almost complete inability to make a direct speech attempt upon a feared word. They approach it, back away, say "a-a-a-a" or "um-um-um," go back to the beginning of the sentence and try again and again, until finally they give up communication altogether. Many stutterers become so adept at substituting synonyms for their difficult words, and disguising the interruptions which do occur, that they are able to pose as normal speakers. We have known seven severe stutterers whose spouses first discovered their speech impediments after the wedding ceremony. Stutterers have preached and taught school and become successful traveling salesmen without ever betraying their infirmity, but they are not happy individuals. The nervous strain and vigilance necessary to avoid and disguise their symptoms often create stresses so severe as to produce profound emotional breakdowns.

Cluttering.   Another disorder in which the time sequence is disturbed is called cluttering. It is frequently confused with stuttering because it too shows many repetitions. However, the major features of cluttering are first, the excessive speed of speaking; second, the disorganized sentence structure; and third, the slurred or omitted syllables and sounds. The clutterer can speak perfectly when he speaks very slowly, but it's almost impossible for him to do so except for short periods. They truly have "tangled tongues."

The speech is cluttered speech; it is disorganized, pell-mell speech, sputtered speech. The true clutterer has no seeming awareness of his excessive speed or garbled utterance. He is always surprised when others cannot understand him. He has no fears or shames. He does not struggle or avoid. Some clutterers become stutterers as well; most do not. Clutterers speak by spurts, and their speech organs pile up like keys on a typewriter when a novice stenographer tries for more speed than her skill permits. An old text in speech correction has this description: ". . . a torrent of half-articulated words, following each other like peas running out of a spout"; but the torrent is also irregularly interrupted in its flow. People constantly ask the clutterer to repeat. They are empathically irritated by his uneven volleys of hasty syllables. They find themselves interrupting during his panting pauses and then in turn being interrupted by a new overwhelming rush of jumbled words.

Voice Disorders (Dysphonias)

Our first illustrative voice case is Miss J., a kindergarten teacher who shouldn't have been a kindergarten teacher. If she once had loved little children, that affection had long gone. She screamed at the kids, tried vainly to establish order in the chaos which prevailed in her room, and at the end of each afternoon was so fatigued she had to go to bed as soon as she came home from school. We got to know her well, for every March for several years she would get aphonia (lose her voice) and come to us for treatment. There were no growths (nodules) on her vocal folds, nor any organic pathology of significance, though her throat was usually inflamed. She could only speak in a strained whisper. The symptoms, of course, were convenient in that she could not teach. March is a long way from either Christmas or summer vacation. Most of our therapy was palliative (time-gaining) and consisted of various exercises in breathing and soft phonation. Finally we were able to persuade her to get the psychological counseling which had been our main goal all along. With this and our help in getting her a position as a receptionist in a medical clinic, her voice returned, this time permanently as our five-year follow-up revealed. We felt we had done a good deal, not only to alleviate her own misery, but also that of many small children.

Another voice case, Nancy, had a voice that was very nasal and also so harsh as to repel anyone who had to listen to her for any length of time. She was not very attractive in face, figure, or personality. She had never dated in all her nineteen years and was a very unhappy person. Her mother, who brought her to the clinic, was an attractive woman of forty, but we noted immediately that she had the same sort of voice quality. Examination revealed no organic pathology, though at times Nancy sounded almost as nasal as a person with a cleft palate. We even probed and used transillumination to see if a submucous cleft existed, but there was none. None of her consonants was accompanied by nasal airflow. The soft palate seemed to be functioning adequately in whispering; but when she produced vocalized vowel sounds, it and the walls of the throat showed little movement. Tests of her hearing revealed a moderate hearing loss in the low frequencies. When we played back to her a tape of her voice with amplification, Nancy was shocked and appalled. She had never known how she sounded. It would take too long to describe her therapy. It required the fitting of a hearing aid and over a year of clinical sessions twice weekly in which we taught her to speak more softly, more breathily, and at a lower pitch. We separated her from her mother by helping her get a college scholarship. We arranged it so that she was placed in a dormitory suite with several of our majors in speech pathology, who took her under their wing, reinforced her new voice, improved her grooming, and in general created a new personality. Speech therapy involves more than the mouth or throat.

Speech is made up of noises and tones. In articulation we add noises and modify the tones. But the tones themselves may be defective; they may vary too far from the norm to be acceptable. When we scrutinize the tones of speech we find that they themselves have three subdimensions. The *loudness* of the speech tones is one of these subdimensions; *pitch* is another; and voice *quality* is the third. In each of these we may find abnormality, and there are voices which may be defective in all three dimensions.

Disorders of Pitch. The normal range of pitch variations depends upon sex, age, and several other factors. The voices of men are generally lower in average pitch than those of women. A deep-voiced male would have no voice disorder; the woman who speaks with a bass voice is conspicuous. A six-year-old boy with a high-pitched treble voice would incur no penalty from society; a thirty-year-old man would find raised eyebrows if he began to speak in such tones. Under conditions of great excitement, many of us have voices which crack or show pitch breaks. But when an adult shows these same pitch breaks upward into the falsetto when he orders a hamburger or says goodbye, we suspect the abnormal. Again, there are times when it is appropriate to speak with a minimum of inflection, but a person who consistently talks on a monopitch will find his listener either irritated or asleep. In deciding whether a person has a pitch disorder we must always use the normal yardstick.

The above discussion has anticipated our listing of the pitch disorders. They are as follows: *too-high pitch, too-low pitch, monotone* or *monopitch, pitch breaks,* and *stereotyped inflections.*

The following description was uttered by a two-hundred-pound football player in his high, piping, shrill, child's voice:

> Yes, I was one of those boy sopranos and my music teacher loved me. I soloed in all the cantatas and programs and sang in the choir and glee clubs, and they never let my voice change. I socked a guy the other day who wisecracked about it, but I'm still a boy soprano at twenty-two. I'm getting so I'm afraid to open my mouth. Strangers start looking for a Charlie McCarthy somewhere. I got to get over it, and quick. Why, I can't even swear but some guy who's been saying the same words looks shocked.

A high-pitched voice in a male is definitely a handicap, communicative, economic, and social.

When a woman's voice is pitched very low and carries a certain type of male inflection, it certainly calls attention to itself and causes maladjustment. The following sentence, spoken by a casual acquaintance and overheard by the girl to whom it referred, practically wrecked her entire security: "Every time I hear her talk I look around to see if it's the bearded lady of the circus."

On every campus some professor possesses that enemy of education, a monotonous voice. A true monotone is comparatively rare, yet it dominates any conversation by its difference. To hear a person laugh on a single note

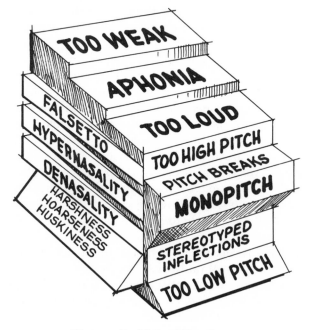

FIGURE 7: *Voice Disorders*

is enough to stir the scalp. Questions asked in a true monotone seem curiously devoid of life. Fortunately most cases of monotonous voice are not so extreme. Many of them could be described as the "poker voice"— even as a face without expression is termed a "poker face." Inflections are present, but for fear of revealing insecurity or inadequacy they are reduced to a minimum.

By stereotyped inflections we refer to the voice which calls attention to itself through its pitch patterning. The sing-song voice, the voice that ends every phrase or sentence with a falling inflection, the "schoolma'am's voice" with its emphatic dogmatic inflections, are all types of variation which, *when extreme*, may be considered speech defects.

Pitch Breaks. These may be upward or downward, usually the former. The adolescent boy, learning to use his adult voice, often experiences them. Often they can be very traumatizing. To have your voice suddenly flip-flop upward into a falsetto or child's voice is to lose control of the self. When you want to speak you don't wish to yodel. Often individuals who fear this experience use a monopitch or too low or too high a pitch level to keep the flip-flopping from occurring. Pitch breaks wreck communication; they define the speaker as one who cannot control himself or who is very emotional. They often interfere with the person's ability to think on his feet since he must forever be monitoring his voice. They may sound funny to others, but we have not found them so.

Disorders of Voice Intensity. Almost in parallel with the disorders of pitch are those of intensity. We have *too loud* a voice, *too weak* or soft a voice, no voice at all (*aphonia*), peculiar *stereotyped patterns of loudness* or emphasis, and voices which are *tremulous*, as in old age or in certain forms of cerebral palsy.

The intensity disorders need little illustration. Many of us have experienced *aphonia,* after prolonged abuse of voice through screaming or when laryngitis has caused us to "lose" our voice. People who earn their living by their mouths—among them, singers, train announcers, clergymen, and schoolteachers—are subject to aphonia, hysterical or otherwise. Most very soft or weak voices are due to insecurity or hearing loss. The extremely loud—to the point of irritation—voices are often due to personality problems or defective hearing. The *strident* voice combines excessive intensity with a harsh voice quality to pierce the ears and rasp the sensibilities of its victims. One of the most difficult voices to correct is that which is marked by sudden bursts of loudness or by the "trailing off into nothingness" at the end of each phrase. Both irritate their listeners.

It is obvious that a voice which is too soft or weak will handicap the person when he must speak under conditions of masking noise or to large audiences. Anyone who has lost his voice for a period of days will tell you that his existence changed markedly during that time. Aphonia may be due to organic reasons such as growths on the vocal folds or to emotional causes. Hearing loss may produce either too loud a voice or one too soft or one which blasts at inappropriate times. So can anger. The ears of others gauge our personalities by scanning our voices. One of the items they scan is our vocal intensity since often it indicates how we feel about ourselves.

Disorders of Voice Quality. The normal range of voice qualities is immense. There are almost as many different voices as faces in this world of ours. The quality of the voice depends on the patterning of the overtones and their variable intensities. The differing sizes and shapes of the many resonating cavities within different human heads account for the uniqueness which permits us to identify each other by listening to these tones. Indeed it almost seems incredible that we can do so since each of us is capable of producing voices of many differing qualities. We can speak nasally or harshly or huskily almost at will. Why we settle upon the voices we finally use habitually is often a mystery. Some of us adopt the voices of those with whom we identify most closely. Others use the voice which best reflects the way we feel about ourselves and others. Most of us seem unaware of these voice qualities of ours and are surprised when we hear them played back from a tape recorder. Some of us are shocked.

Among those who are shocked are those whose voices are *hypernasal, denasal, strident* (harsh), *falsetto, breathy* (husky), or *hoarse*. Those are the abnormal voice qualities sufficiently distinct to be labeled.

That the disorders of voice quality are difficult to describe is indicated not only by the names which we listed earlier in our classification but also by the names we omitted. Voices have been called *thick, thin, heavy, sweet, round, brilliant, hard, metallic,* and *rich,* as well as *poor.* The terms we have used are not much better, but at least they do not confuse auditory perceptions with those of taste or touch. The science of experimental phonetics has not yet been able to provide a better classification for variations in timbre.

The quality of *excessive nasality* (hypernasality, rhinolalia *aperta*) is easily recognized. Its possessor not only seems to speak his *m, n,* and ŋ sounds through his nose, but also many of the vowels and voiced continuants such as *r, v,* and *z*. When combined with certain inflection patterns it has been described as a "whining" voice. In certain sections of the country a variety of hypernasality is dialectal, and of course in this setting it would not be a speech defect. In *assimilation nasality* only the sounds preceding or following the *m, n,* and *z* sounds are excessively nasalized; but these can occur frequently enough to provoke audience irritation.

In *hyponasality* (denasality, adenoidal voice, rhinolalia *clausa*) the speaker does not or cannot utter the nasal sounds through the nose. The voice quality is deadened and muffled, as though its owner had a perpetual cold. The *m* resembles a blend of *m* and *b* spoken simultaneously, and the other nasals have similar cognates. Often habituated during the presence of adenoidal growths in early life, it persists long after the adenoids have been removed. People listening to denasal voices find themselves swallowing and clearing their throats and consumed by the urge to get out of range.

Other voice quality disorders are occasionally noted by the teacher doing speech correction in the public school. Many boys' voices become husky and hoarse during the two or three years prior to voice change and become clear again after that event. Overstrain due to prolonged yelling, screeching, or shouting can cause this quality in any of us. Perhaps the *strident, hoarse, husky,* and *breathy* qualities of voice indicate a two-factor continuum involving (1) breath expenditure and (2) muscular strain. The strident voice shows a preponderance of tension in the muscles that squeeze the pharynx, while the breathy voice represents a minimum of strain and a maximum of breath expenditure.

The words *throaty* and *pectoral* as adjectives to describe voice quality are probably identical save for the sex of the person concerned. Throaty voices in the female are paralleled by the voice of hollow, booming, pectoral timbre in the male. Both involve lower pitch levels, rounded mouth openings, and retracted chins. Pectoral voice has been called the "rain-barrel voice." There are echoes in it. It reverberates like song in the bathtub. It was formerly much used by preachers and politicians and by undertakers and insecure high-school teachers. These terms, *throaty* and *pectoral* or *guttural,* are not terms commonly employed by speech therapists, perhaps because they probably are low-pitched falsetto voices. Usually *falsettos* are high in pitch and are produced by a complicated and different type of vocal cord vibration than that normally used. An adult who can speak only in *his* falsetto voice (for all of us have them) is truly handicapped.

SYMBOLIZATION DISORDERS

The problem of *dysphasia* (the general term for all disorders of symbolic formulation and expression) is rarely met in public-school speech correction. Occasionally it occurs in mild form as a pronounced reading, writing, and speaking disability. In the speech clinic we often are required to help aphasics, and the end of World War II required the services of a good many speech correctionists to teach those who had received head and brain injuries. Children who have had meningitis or jaundice, and some adults who have suffered a paralytic stroke, often demonstrate the symptoms of aphasia. Such persons find it difficult to use or comprehend linguistic symbols, whether they be written or spoken. In the motoexpressive type of aphasia, the case may say "bum-bum-bum" for "cigarette," and "bum" for "shoe." Another aphasic may grope for words in attempting to say "pencil," but say "eraser" or "pen" or "stick" instead. Yet he knows his errors the instant they are spoken. In the receptive type of aphasia the difficulty lies in the perception. R. V. McKnight describes her own aphasic reaction to the word "your" as f llows:

> I mentally heard it, but it had no meaning. I felt that it was related to the word "you," but I could not figure out the relationship between the two. I continued to puzzle over this until the speaker had finished his lecture and sat down. . . . More generally, when I do not recognize the meaning, I do not recognize the sound. The word is a jumble of letters.

Children who have such difficulties are often mistakenly diagnosed as hard-of-hearing or feeble-minded. Some cases of delayed onset or slow development of speech are probably due to aphasia.

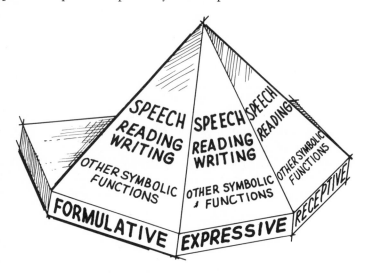

Figure 8: *Symbolization Disorders: Aphasia, Language*

The child with *delayed speech* may, or may not, belong in the category of symbolization disorders. Injuries to the brain have often, in young children, interrupted speech development or retarded it. The differential diagnosis of "congenital aphasia" is always difficult, as we shall see in later chapters. It is also certain that many children who are mute or speak in an unintelligible jargon or gibberish have been called "brain-injured" when they were entirely normal individuals who just had not been taught to talk. Some parents learn their child's language instead of teaching them the adult tongue. Delayed speech often approximates the pattern of a very severe articulation disorder, and some cases so diagnosed probably belong in this category.

Multiple Speech Disorders

We have been discussing the four major types of speech disorders, those of rhythm, articulation, voice, and symbolization as though they were always distinctive entities. It is obvious that a given speaker might have deficiencies in more than one of these dimensions of speech. We have said that lallers may lisp; they may also possess an infantile voice. Clutterers certainly often have both a disorder of rhythm and one of slurred articulation. The aphasic often misarticulates certain of his speech sounds. It is always necessary to scan each one of our cases in terms of all four of these dimensions if we are to decide our point of attack upon the problem. Illustrating this need are certain disorders which almost always have multiple features of abnormality.

Cleft-Palate Speech. People whose speech has been affected by their cleft lips or palates often show articulation errors such as nasally emitted consonants. Their voices usually are hypernasal, though some denasality also often occurs. Finally, the rhythm of the speech may be faltering and labored due to the nasal leakage of air that makes it difficult to utter phrases or sentences on a single breath. They pause to breathe at the wrong times.

Foreign Accent. This is another disorder that involves both articulation and voice. Speakers of a foreign tongue use sound substitutions and distortions, and they also use inflection patterns unfamiliar to our ears. The rising inflection at the conclusion of the phrase as spoken by a Scandinavian speaking English may serve as an illustration. In treating such a disorder we organize our therapy so as to attack both phases of the problem.

Deaf and Hard-of-Hearing Speech. These individuals also show multiple disorders. The congenitally deaf are deficient in language and symbolization; their voices are oddly abnormal in pitch, intensity, and quality; their rhythms are unusual; they make many articulation errors. Depending upon the degree of involvement, those persons who are hard of hearing may also show similar disabilities.

Cerebral Palsy. This handicapping problem is due to a brain injury that affects the coordination of the muscles. Some of the cerebral palsied find it difficult or even impossible to walk or feed themselves. Some of them find speaking very hard. We have worked with cerebral palsied children who had aphonia, pitch breaks, weak voices, tremulous voices. As though those were not enough, they also found it almost impossible to twist their tongues into the proper postures necessary to produce many of the speech sounds. Some of them gasped and faltered in their flow of speech. Some were aphasic as well. A few of them spoke perfectly.

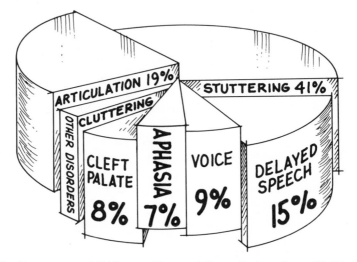

FIGURE 9: *Percentage of Different Types of Cases Referred to WMU Speech Clinic in a Ten-Year Period.* (Hearing cases are not shown.)

We hope that we have made it clear that speech has four dimensions and that abnormality may be found in any one or any combination of the four.

REFERENCES

1. Blackman, R. S. and Battin, R. "Case Study of Delayed Language." *Journal of Speech and Hearing Disorders,* XXII (1957), 381–84.
   Describe this case and the factors which seemed to have contributed to the delay.
2. Blake, J. N. "A Therapeutic Construct for Two Seven-Year-Old Non-verbal Boys." *Journal of Speech and Hearing Disorders,* XXXIV (1969), 363–69.
   What was the therapy plan for these boys?
3. Blakeley, R. "The Child with Cleft Lip and Palate." *Hearing News,* XXXIV (1964), 18–20.
   Summarize the basic information in this article.
4. Boone, D. R. *An Adult Has Aphasia.* Danville, Ill.: Interstate, 1965.
   What is the nature of the problem in aphasia?
5. Burton, M. L. H. "The Story of Mark." In C. Van Riper, ed., *Speech Therapy: A Book of Readings.* Englewood Cliffs, N.J.: Prentice-Hall, Inc., 1953, pp. 36–40.
   Retell this tragic yet triumphant tale.
6. Carrow, M. A. "Case Study of Delayed Language." *Journal of Speech and Hearing Disorders,* XXII (1957), 381–84.
   Describe the communicative problem in this case.
7. Cohen, J. "Development of a Blind Spastic Child: A Case Study." *Exceptional Children,* XXXII (1966), 291–94.
   How was this multiply handicapped child enabled to make such a good adjustment?
8. Dalrymple, L. H. "Our Child Had a Cleft Palate." *Hygeia,* XXVII (1949), 186–87.
   Retell this tale of tragedy and triumph.
9. Du Bard, E. "A 'Deaf' Child Who Did Not Learn." *Volta Review,* LXIV (1962), 589–92.
   How did they discover that this child was not deaf?
10. Earle, H. "The Comeback Battle of Clifton Utley." *Today's Health* (February, 1959), 45–46.
    What does it mean to lose and then regain your speech?
11. ———. "An Analysis of an Exceptional Case of Retarded Speech." *Journal of Speech and Hearing Disorders,* XIX (1954), 239–43.
    If a child is blind and has cerebral palsy, how can he be helped?
12. Egland, G. O. *Speech and Language Problems.* Englewood Cliffs, N.J.: Prentice-Hall, Inc., 1970.
    Read pp. 98–109 and describe the kinds of articulatory disorders presented by the author.
13. Goda, S. "Stuttering Manifestations Following Spinal Meningitis." *Journal of Speech and Hearing Disorders,* XXVI (1961), 392–93.
    Was the stuttering due to the disease or the change in the person's life? Present your argument.
14. Gregory, H. H. "Speech Clinic Helps the Adult Stutterer." *Rehabilitation Record,* V (1964), 9–12.
    Outline the kind of treatment offered in this clinic.

15. Halpern, H. "A Case Report of Elective Mutism." *Journal of Communication Disorders,* II (1969), 69–71.
    What did the speech therapist do to help this child?
16. McWilliams, B. J. "The Language Handicapped Child and Education." *Exceptional Children,* XXXII (1965), 221–28.
    Describe the kind of clinically oriented teaching needed by these children.
17. Panagos, J. "Help a Boy Pronounce [r]." *Western Speech,* XXXIV (1970), 33–37.
    Describe how the speech therapist taught him the [r] sound.
18. Porter, F. "Speech Correction in an Orphanage." *Journal of Speech Dis-Disorders.* X (1945), 241–49.
    What kinds of speech problems did the clinician find in this setting?
19. Rose, R. H. "A Physician's Account of His Own Aphasia." *Journal of Speech Disorders,* XIII (1948), 244–305.
    How did this man regain the ability to use language again?
20. Schell, R. E., Stark, J., and Giddan, J. J. "Development of Language Behavior in an Autistic Child." *Journal of Speech and Hearing Disorders,* XXXII (1967), 51–64.
    How did the therapists work with this child?
21. Sheehan, J. G., Cortese, P. A., and Hadley, R. G. "Guilt, Shame, and Tension in Graphic Projections of Stuttering." *Journal of Speech and Hearing Disorders,* XXVII (1962), 129–39.
    What did the pictures reveal about the stutterers?
22. Shryock, H. "Speech Without a Larnyx." *Hygeia,* XXV, (1947), 789–92.
    How does one learn to talk without a larynx, and what effects other than speech are the result of its surgical removal?
23. Smith, M. E. "A Clinician's Story." *Quarterly Journal of Speech,* XIII (1948), 268–72.
    Describe some of the problems she encountered.
24. Wolski, W. and Wiley, J. "Functional Aphonia in a Fourteen-Year-Old Boy: A Case Report." *Journal of Speech and Hearing Disorders,* XXX (1965), 71–75.
    How was voice therapy combined with psychotherapy in this case?
25. Wylie, D. "Tommy Tunes In." *Exceptional Children,* XXXII (1965), 259–61.
    How did the teacher help this brain-injured child to improve his verbal communication?

3

The Development of Speech

Many of the speech disorders we described in our last chapter begin very early in life and represent the person's failure to learn or acquire the standard speech that we must possess if we are to take our place in this very verbal world. As we shall see, learning to speak normally is not as easy as one might think. Learning to walk, to play the piano, or to write and spell are very simple achievements in comparison. Intricate coordinations must be mastered; meanings must be coded and decoded; a very complex set of rules for linking words together must be comprehended. Among many other things, the child must be a linguist, a semanticist, and a virtuoso.

THE BEGINNINGS OF SPEECH

Many of us would say that speech begins with the birth cry, although few of us would agree with Schopenhauer, the vinegar-penned old philosopher, who claimed it was a protest against having to enter this miserable world. By outrageously placing a buzzing doorbell against the mother's abdomen, researchers found they could cause an increase in the movements of the foetus, thus indicating that the unborn baby may hear. Even more incredible, there seems to be some evidence that a few infants have vocalized while still in the uterus.[1]

All three of this author's babies, fortunately, were mercifully silent during the months before birth, but they more than made up for it thereafter. We heard their birth cries, however, noting that these were produced

[1] P. F. Ostwald, "The Sounds of Human Behavior," *Logos*, III (1960), 21.

on inhalation, and wryly wondered if they would turn out to be Hottentots, whose language consists primarily of inhalatory sounds. Most of the early vocalization of all babies seems to be reflexive in nature, whether it be on inhalation or exhalation or, more commonly, both. This seems to be true for both crying and comfort sounds. They talk in and out like donkeys. We have heard such sounds in the struggling speech attempts of adult stutterers and aphasics. We have heard lispers who sucked air inward for their *s* sounds. Some of our cerebral palsied friends have never learned to speak on exhalation alone. The baby, like these cases, has a lot of untangling and learning to do in mastering speech.

The skills involved in speech begin to be acquired as soon as the child is born and are seldom perfectly mastered, even during a lifetime. Much of the speech learning during the first six months is relatively independent of the stimulation given by the child's parents. Even in the crying and wailing of infants the short, sharp inhalation and prolonged exhalation so fundamental to true speech are being practiced. Lip, jaw, and tongue movements involved in the production of all the speech sounds in all human languages are repeatedly performed. The early awareness of these movements and their accompanying sounds provides the foundation for speech readiness. Throughout the first years of life there are many ways in which parents can help or hinder the development of speech. Their knowledge or ignorance determines whether the child will learn to talk because of his parents' efforts or in spite of them. Their application of principles, so obvious that we wonder why they should ever be violated, will determine whether the child's speech will be an asset or a handicap. Time after time the speech correctionist tries to trace the cause of a stutter or an articulatory defect, only to lose it in the vague parental memories of childhood. It is vitally important for the student of speech pathology to know how speech develops.

Crying Versus Comfort Sounds. The first reflexive sounds are the shrill, nasal wails of a struggling child in discomfort. As Lewis writes, "At first these are the only sounds that a child makes. He cries when he is uncomfortable; otherwise he is silent." [2] For the first month most of the child's vocalization consists of this wailing.

Even during the first month, the vocalizations vary from child to child. One infant may coo and laugh when taken from the breast; another may whimper; and still another may kick and scream. Research indicates that even at this period there are more vowels and consonants used in noncrying vocalizations than in whimpering, and more sounds used in whimpering than in ordinary crying.

---

[2] M. M. Lewis, *How Children Learn to Speak* (London: George G. Harrap Company, Ltd., 1957), p. 15.

Whenever we interview the mother of a child with a severe articulation disorder or a child who has not acquired any intelligible speech, we routinely ask her if the child cried a lot more than her other babies during the first months of his life. (We never ask the father this; he is bound to say yes.) The answer may be the starting point of the trail to important information concerning the child's physical condition, family conflicts, or even maternal rejection. But we also know that a child who spends all his time in crying will not have the practice time for experimenting with other sounds, with other movements of the mouth and body.[3]

Many parents seek to prevent all crying, although a certain amount of it does exercise the child's vocal and respiratory coordinations as well as its parents' patience. They jounce their baby up and down, juggle it back and forth, or rock it, pat it, and whirl it until it is dizzy enough to end its crying through unconsciousness. Other parents resolutely ignore their newborn's howls because of a mistaken fear that they might spoil the child. These babies may cry away so many of their waking hours that their speech-sound repertoire will be necessarily limited. As we have seen, fewer sounds are used in crying than in noncrying speech. Again, many parents interrupt their children's automatic vocalization by embracing them or conversing with them. They should let the vocal play period complete itself. During this first period the muscular development of the tongue may be delayed and abnormally high palatal arches may be produced by bottle feeding with improper nipples. These organic conditions may delay speech development.

The noncrying sounds are composed of grunts, gurgles, and sighs, and include most of the front vowels, the consonants *k*, *l*, *g*, and the glottal catch. These particular consonants involve contacts and tongue movements similar to those used in swallowing. All of these sounds are accompanied by movements of the arms, legs, or trunk. They sometimes occur during the act of sucking or immediately after feeding. Compared to later vocalizations, the noncrying sounds produced by a healthy baby during the first month are relatively infrequent. More crying is done than whimpering, and more whimpering noises are produced than noncrying ones. Perhaps it was this fact which led one scientific father, faithfully and no doubt solemnly, to record his baby's wails, first phonographically and then in the phonetic alphabet. After a profound mathematical analysis of the records, he concluded that the wails increased in pitch. Most night-walking fathers would agree that the wails also increase in loudness and meanness.

[3] C. A. Aldrich, C. Sung, and C. Knop, in their article, "The Crying of Newly Born Infants," *Journal Pediatrics*, XXVII (1945), 89–96, state that the average crying time spent by babies less than eight days old was 117 minutes per day. Peak periods of crying occurred at 6 P.M. and at midnight. They attributed 35 percent of the crying to hunger, 28 percent to dirty or wet diapers, and the rest to unknown causes, which the present author interprets as meaning just for the hell of it. Moreover, his own babies preferred the 5:30 A.M. hour to any other.

The comfort sounds, although nonpurposive, are the ancestors of true speech, and somehow most parents seem to know it. When they occur, the mother comes close and bathes the child with the sounds of love. This may be more important than one might think. There seems to be a curious phenomenon called *imprinting* at work. Scientists have found that an animal's response to certain sounds seems to be imprinted shortly after birth. For example, Hess and others have performed experiments such as one where freshly hatched ducklings were given a mechanical decoy which said "gock, gock, gock," and the ducklings from that time on followed and came to the mechanical "gock" of the decoy in preference to a real duck's honking.[4] Of course, humans are not ducks, and we do not know much about human imprinting.

But we do know that orphanage babies begin to talk later and have more speech defects than babies whose parents care for them. A baby needs a mother's voice if it is to talk, and it is important that the mother's voice have love in it. Even parakeets will not talk unless they are fed and spoken to lovingly. This is why in interviewing parents we are interested in discovering whether the baby was unwanted or illegitimate, in discovering how soon the mother had to go back to work, in knowing what sort of a person took care of the infant while she was gone. We also ask about feeding problems. Some babies have a tough time getting enough milk or keeping it down. They cry more and coo less. A tired, frantic mother may forget that babies, like husbands, talk most after they've been fed. This is the time for bathing the babe in pleasant sound, partly his own and partly the mother's.

The feeding-speaking situation will always be important for many reasons. Consider the nipple on the baby's bottle. Very often, in taking case histories of lallers, we find the mothers mentioning that the child had great difficulty in getting enough milk, that he was a "slow feeder," and that they had to widen the opening in the nipple. To us, this is very significant, for when a baby sucks, he does not suck with the lips alone. The tongue tip is thrust forward and upward in the squeezing action. He needs to learn this coordination so basic to many speech sounds. Some babies never get a chance to learn it; it's all they can do to keep from drowning, and they keep the back of the tongue high to survive. Many cleft-palate children retain this rear elevation of the tongue in speech, and some authorities feel that much of the excessive nasality is due to it. There are others who feel that the design of the ordinary rubber nipple is very poor and contributes to later malcoordination of the tongue and to the habituation of the "infantile swallow." This latter term refers to a form of swallowing in which the lips are pursed and the tongue is thrust forward. In the

[4] E. H. Hess, "Imprinting," *Science*, CXXX (1959), 133–41.

normal swallow, these two behaviors do not occur. When a child continues to use this "infantile" form of swallowing—and he swallows on the average about twice each minute—certain tongue-thrust habits are created which have been said to produce such dental abnormalities as protruding teeth or an open bite, or such speech defects as a lisp.[5] The matter is still, however, in dispute.

Private and Social Babbling. Babbling usually begins about eight weeks after birth. It consists of odd little vowels, usually the *ee, ih, uh,* and others made in the front of the mouth, a few *m, b,* and *g* consonant sounds, and snorts, gurgles, and grunts, all combined with squeals and sighs and a few Bronx cheers for good measure. It is a delightful fairy language. There are times when the baby uses it when others are around, bathing him, waving huge fingers in front of his eyes, talking nonsense to him. Then it can be shared and enjoyed by all. But there are other times when the baby needs to play with his toes and his mouth, privately.

A good share of this vocal play is carried on when the child is alone, and it disappears when someone attracts his attention.

> One child played with her babbling each morning after awakening, usually beginning with a whispered "eenuh" and repeating it with increasing effort until she spoke the syllable aloud, whereupon she would laugh and chortle as she said it over and over. The moment she heard a noise in the parents' bedroom this babbling would cease and crying would begin.

The parents who joyfully rush in and ruin this speech rehearsal are failing to appreciate its significance in the learning of speech. The child must simultaneously feel and hear the sound repeatedly if it is ever to emerge as an identity. Imitation is essentially a device to perpetuate a stimulus, and babbling is self-imitation of the purest variety. When the babbling period is interrupted or delayed through illness, the appearance of true speech is often similarly retarded. Deaf babies begin to babble at a normal time; but since they can not hear the sounds they produce, they probably lose interest and hence have much less true vocal play than the hearing child. Mirrors suspended above the cribs of deaf babies have increased the babbling through visual self-stimulation.

About the fifth or sixth month, when the infant can fixate an object with his eyes, grab a toy and maneuver it into his mouth, or hoist his hind end up to crawl, there appears a new kind of babbling which we call *vocal play.*

Vocal Play. The child begins to use his vocalization (with more

---

[5] S. T. Fletcher, R. L. Casteel, and D. P. Bradley, "Tongue Thrust Swallow, Speech Articulation, and Age," *Journal Speech and Hearing Disorders,* XXVI (1961), 201–8.

vowels than consonants) for getting attention, supporting rejection, and expressing demands. Frequently he will look at an object and cry at the same time. He voices his eagerness and protest. He is using his primitive speech both to express himself and to modify the behavior of others. This stage is also marked by the appearance of syllable repetition, or the doubling of sounds, in his vocal play. He singles out a certain double syllable such as *da-da* and frequently practices it to the exclusion of all other combinations. Sometimes a single combination will be practiced for several weeks at a time, though it is more usual to find the child changing to something new every few days and reviewing some of his former vocal achievements at odd intervals. True disyllables (*ba-da*) come relatively late in the first year, and the infant rejects them when the parent attempts to use them as stimulation.

At this time the child will often "answer back." Make a noise and he makes a noise. The two noises are usually dissimilar, but it is obvious that he is responding. In his vocal play, most of the vowels are still the ones made in the front or middle of the mouth, but a few *oo* and *oh* sounds (which are back vowels) can be detected in the child's vocal play. There are also more consonants to be heard, the *d*, *t*, *n*, and *l* having appeared; but it's still hard to separate them out of the flow of unsorted utterance unless you have long, sharp ears. Some private babbling continues throughout these months, but now the child seems to take more pleasure in public practice. He's listening to himself but also listening to you. He is talking to himself but also sometimes to you. This is *socialized vocalization.*

We must not conclude this section without pointing out some implications which babbling and vocal play have for speech therapy. Svend Smith, a Danish speech therapist, has devised a set of rhythms based on the bongo drum chants of South African natives, and he has his patients utter strange and unfamiliar cries in unison with the rhythmic beat. We too have used his methods, and often find that children and even adults can follow our own chanting as it progresses from these strange cries into standard sounds of English. We find that they can make sounds which previously they were unable to produce. Often we use the baby's comfort sounds or the repeated syllables of vocal play in these chants. The rhythm helps to create the freedom to try new sounds. Some children become so tense when attempting a sound which they have never successfully produced, that they cannot possibly find the new coordinations. Babbling and vocal play can free them from this tension. To vary our production of sound, we must feel some of the same freedom that the baby experiences when babbling or doing vocal play. In this regard, it is interesting to note that in England and elsewhere on the continent, a speech therapy session often begins with a period of relaxation. We know of no better way to relax than by free babbling, especially when the therapist is babbling freely too. Perhaps we are returning to an earlier period when learning to speak was fun.

Inflected Vocal Play. Although some squeals and changes in pitch and loudness have previously occurred in the babbling, it is not until about the eighth month that inflections become prominent. It is then that the vocal play takes on the tonal characteristics of adult speech. We now find the baby using inflections that sound like questions, commands, surprise, ponderous statements of fact, all in a delightful gibberish that has no meaning. We hear not only the inflections and sounds of English but those of the Oriental languages as well. No baby can be sure he will end up speaking English. So he practices a bit of Chinese now and then. We have tried hard to imitate some of these sounds and inflections and have failed. The baby can often duplicate whole strings of these strange beads of sound.

The private babbling and social vocal play continue strongly during this period from eight months to a year. The repertoire of sounds increases. There is a marked gain in back vowels and front consonants. Crying time diminishes, though few fathers would believe it. They begin to get interested in their sons and daughters about this stage, however. The infant is becoming human. He'll bang a cup; he'll smile back at the old man. He'll reach out to be picked up. He begins to understand what "No!" means. But most important of all, he begins to *sound* as though he is talking.

We have previously spoken of various stages of development, but it should be made very clear that, although most children go through these stages in the order given, the activity in any one stage does not cease as soon as the characteristics of the next stage appear. Grunts and wails, babbling, socialized vocalization, and inflection practice all begin at about the times stated, but they continue throughout the entire period of speech development.

It is during this period that the baby begins to use more of the back vowels (u, ʊ, o, ɔ) in his babbling. According to Irwin and Curry, 92 percent of all vowels uttered by babies are the front vowels as compared to the 49 percent figure for adult speech.[6] They say, "It is evident that a fundamental process of development in early speech consists of the mastery of the back vowels." It is interesting that when we work with adult articulation cases, we prefer syllables such as *see* and *ray* and *lee* to those involving the back vowels like *soo* and *low*. Front vowels seem to be more easily mastered.

The baby, through his vocal gymnastics, gradually masters the coordinations necessary to meaningful speech. But it must be emphasized that when he is repeating *da-da* and *ma-ma* at this stage, he is not designating his parents. His arm movements have much more meaning than those

[6] O. C. Irwin, and T. Curry, "Vowel Elements in the Crying of Infants Under Ten Days of Age," *Child Development*, XII (1941), 99–109.

of his mouth. It is during these months that the ratio of babbling to crying greatly increases. Comprehension of parental gestures shows marked growth. The child now responds to the parent's stimulation, not automatically, but with more discrimination. His imitation is more hesitant, but it also seems more purposive. It begins to resemble the parent's utterance. If the father interrupts the child's chain of *papapapapapapapapa* by saying *papa*, the child is less likely than before to say *wah* or *gu* and more likely to whisper *puh* or repeat the two syllables *puhpuh*. During this period, simple musical tones, songs, or lullabies are especially good stimulation. The parent should observe the child's inflections and rhythms and attempt to duplicate them. This is the material that should be used for stimulation at this period, not a long harangue on why mother loves her little token of heaven.

This period, too, has a message for those who wish to help the child with abnormal speech. We see that new sounds are not acquired solely in meaningful words; they appear singly, or doubly in syllables, and nonsense syllables at that. We note that they occur in the context of pleasurable contacts with others who share them. They are to be played with, not demanded. We have known many children who could make a perfectly good *r* sound in isolated words like *church*, yet who failed to say this sound when it occurred on a falling inflection as in the word *father*. Speech therapy should not be done in monotonous drill. The baby tells us that the way to acquire new sounds is to use them expressively and socially.

THE FIRST WORDS

Sometime between the tenth month and the eighteenth, the normal child learns to say his first true words. Comprehension shows a great spurt of development at this time. The baby suddenly becomes a very human being. He learns to walk and to talk and to feed himself, three of the most fundamental of all human functions. He's quite a fellow indeed. Let us see how he masters his first words.

The Autism Theory. Experiments in teaching birds to talk led O. H. Mowrer, a famous American psychologist, to formulate what is known as the autism theory of speech acquisition.[7] He found that his birds would reproduce human words only if these words were spoken by the trainer while the birds were being fondled or fed. After this had happened often enough, the word itself could apparently produce pleasurable feelings in the bird. Since myna birds and parakeets produce a lot of variable sounds, it is almost inevitable that a few of these sounds might resemble the

[7] O. H. Mowrer, "On the Psychology of 'Talking Birds'—A Contribution to Language and Personality Theory," in *Learning Theory and Personality Dynamics* (New York: The Ronald Press Company, 1950).

human word that produced such pleasant feelings. Thus when the bird hears itself making these similar sounds it feels again the pleasantness of fondling and being fed. So it repeats them, and the closer the bird's chirp-word comes to resemble the human word, the more pleasant the bird feels. By properly rewarding these progressive approximations, we can facilitate the process. However, finally the bird will find that "Polly-wants-a-cracker" or "To-hell-with-Iowa" [8] is pleasant enough to be self-rewarding. The word "autism" refers to the self-rewarding aspect of the process. At any rate, these phrases seem to sound almost as good to the bird as a piece of suet tastes.

When this theory is applied to the child's learning of his first words, it seems to make a lot of sense. Certainly, the mother says "Mama" or "baby" a thousand times while feeding, bathing, or fondling the child. Also it is certain that the baby will find *mama mama* or *bubbababeeba* sometime in his babbling and vocal play. If these utterances flood him with pleasant feelings, he will repeat them more often than syllables such as "gugg" which have no special pleasant memories attached to them. It is also true that the closer the child comes to the standard words, the more reward he will get from the mother. There still remains the problem of giving meaning to utterance, and this is explained in terms of the context. "Mama" is used when the mama is present; "baby" is used when he sees himself in a mirror or plays with his body. This theory raises some objections, but it seems to be the best explanation we have yet been able to formulate.

The Imitation Theory. This theory has been formulated in several ways, some of which are circular and nonexplanatory. Certainly there seems to be no primary instinct of imitation at work. If by imitation we mean that the baby suddenly begins to reproduce exactly what he sees or hears, the facts do not support the theory. Nevertheless, during the last months of the first year, most children seem to make some attempts to reproduce movements which they witness, but rarely are these movements exact. Imitation, as used in the larger sense to denote attempted reproduction, seems to be motivated by the desire to perpetuate the stimuli that intrigue one's interest. It is the child's way of maintaining his interest. The child's memory span is very weak and short, and to compensate for this deficiency he seeks to perpetuate the stimulus by repeating it. This accounts for the doubling and repetition of syllables in the vocal play and for the persistence with which he pounds the rattle on the table.

When the process of speech imitation is studied, we discover that

---

[8] One of the author's graduate students taught a parakeet to say this most reprehensible phrase, knowing well that the author had received his doctorate at that excellent institution. The author is presently engaged in teaching the bird to stutter when it says it, having found it impossible to extinguish the phrase, or, for that matter, the bird.

it begins when the parent starts to imitate the child. This may sound paradoxical, but its truth will be apparent when the situation is defined. During vocal play the child happens to be repeating the syllable *ma*. The hearing of the sound interests him, and so he repeats it again. Suddenly the sight of his mother interrupts his response to his own stimulation, and he lapses into silence. But the mother, unaware of the perfection of her technique, says to him, "Mama? Did you want mama?" and immediately the interesting stimulus is there again. Wishing it to continue, he makes the same vocal coordinations he made when alone, and again the same interesting sounds are heard, *mamaamaama*. Whereupon the mother rushes to the phone to tell her husband that the child has spoken his first word.

Only when the child uses the word as a definite tool of communication with such a meaning as "Mother, come here," or "Mother, lift me up!" can we say with certainty that he has acquired his first word. Nevertheless, the process of word acquisition has been described. The first step in teaching a child to talk should be the imitation of the sounds being made by the child during his vocal play. This should be preceded, if possible, by the parental imitation of other movements, such as pounding the table. If the child can be stimulated to return to his own former pounding by watching the parent pound, half the battle is won, for the first requisite is gained: the perpetuation of a stimulus given by another person. In imitating the speech of the child, the parent should seek to interrupt the child's activity before it is completed. For example, if the child is saying *da-da-da* over and over, it is wise to interject the parental *da-da* as soon as the child's first *da* has been produced. This will produce the most favorable conditions for getting the child to return to his own former activity, and usually he will maintain it much longer and much more loudly than he usually does. At first only a few sounds should be used in this way, preferably those that later can be used to represent the people doing the training. Thus the child will acquire *mama* in a situation which always represents her presence, and it is wise for her to say the word whenever she picks the child up. Thus the child will come to associate the interesting sound with the person, and it will thereby come to have meaning.

The child should be given such training until he responds consistently with eager repetition whenever the parent has interrupted vocal play by imitating his vocalizations. After that it is wise for the parent to utilize the silence periods, which occur during the babbling, as intervals of strong stimulation with the sounds previously used by the child. For example, the child has been babbling and suddenly becomes silent. The parent then attracts his attention and repeats *mamama* (or any other syllable which the child has been practicing). If the child will respond to this stimulation by attempted repetition, a second step in word acquisition has been taken. After considerable training involving the practice of both steps, the parent having been careful to pick the appropriate times, the child will suddenly surprise everyone by using the word very meaningfully, perhaps accompanying it with the gesture of reaching. In similar fashion, other early words may be taught.

In one sense, it may be said that the first words are acquired through stabilization. Out of all the vocal tangle of sounds produced by the baby, certain monosyllables or repeated syllables appear as familiar entities. They already have meaning for the child since they have expressed his needs or bodily conditions. He has played with them on so many pleasant occasions that they are old friends. He knows them well. Now, these same syllables become associated with certain conventional gestures (*bye-bye*) or consistent objects (*mama*) which appear repeatedly in his daily life. The first words have been his for a long time. They merely get a stabilized adult meaning.

> One parent, whom we studied with some interest, tried by every device of conditioning known to educated idiots to have his boy say the word "Ralph" (the father's name) as his first meaningful word. He worked with the boy for hours. When the first word did arrive (fourteen months late) it was "teetee" and referred to a cat.

Even as certain gestures such as reaching become stabilized from the wild undifferentiated arm-swinging of the infant, so, too, do the first words from their early matrix of vocal play.

Gesture is very important in stabilizing the first words. Sometimes it is almost too powerful.

> We observed one child who had the following history. At nine months the mother stretched out her arms to the child whenever the latter asked through gestures to be taken up. At nine months, eight days, the child would imitate the mother by reaching out bimanually whenever the mother did so. The mother then began to say "mama" whenever she used the gesture. At 9:14, the child would say it with the mother as they stretched out their arms. At 9:16, the child said "mamama" as she responded to the mother's silent gesture of reaching. On the same day she also said "mama" as she reached for her cup. At 9:19 she said "mama" to the father when he reached out to take her. Long after she could say "Daddy" imitatively and spontaneously, the gesture of reaching was always accompanied by "mama."

Fortunately, the effect of the accompanying gesture is seldom so persevering. Phonetic and intonation patterns of adult vocalization usually accompany the gesture and are perceived by the child as a whole. He responds not merely to the warning shake of the parent's head but to his own imitative head wagging and to the peremptory tone of the phrase "No, No!" and, if these fail, to the swat on his bottom as well. Even the mother's turning of her head or body as she recognizes and says "Daddy" is a meaningful gesture. Comprehension of speech for the baby consists of his interpretation of gesture, intonation of patterns, and the presence of syllables which he has previously practiced. Those gestures spontaneously used by the child are much better than any that parents could think up. If you interrupt his hand-waving by your own similar gesture, and say "bye-bye" and then take him outdoors, the word will be learned fairly easily. But if you try to teach him to kiss his father's picture and say "Daddy" at the same time, the work will be long and hard and perhaps useless.

These first words of the child may sound very much like those of adult speech, but they differ greatly in meaning. Some of them are no doubt "abracadabra" words. The child says "mama" and magically she appears. Other early words are mere signs of recognition or acquaintance-ship. "Ba" may mean, "I know you. You're a ball. You're that round smooth thing I throw and bounce." He utters it with the same, smug self-satisfaction that our friends manifest when, hearing a familiar musical phrase, they pat their egos and murmur, "Brahms, of course!"

Again we find some important clues which can be used in helping the child who does not talk or who talks defectively. Speech is not acquired through demand or command. A recent study shows that most parents use demands and commands for speech as their preferred method in helping their children who have difficulties in mastering normal speech.[9] "Say this . . . Say that . . ." are the common phrases heard by such children. "Say it again . . . Say it right!" These are the phrases that ring in a little child's ears. Few speech therapists use such primitive methods. They know that good speech will come if they can create the proper conditions, and the proper conditions are much like those used by parents in teaching the baby to say his first real words.

Reinforcement Theory. Another explanation of how the child develops his first words is based upon learning theory. Since most students who read this book will already have had courses in psychology, we will not present the principles of reinforcement here. Studies of myna birds, cats, and dogs have shown that it is possible to increase the amount of vocal behavior in these creatures by conditioning.[10] We ourselves, through

    [9] R. L. Shelton, W. B. Arndt, and J. Miller, "Learning Principles and Teaching of Speech and Language," *Journal Speech and Hearing Disorders*, XXVI (1961), 368–76.
    [10] J. H. Grosslight, P. C. Harrison, and C. M. Weiser, "Reinforcement Control of Vocal Responses in the Mynah Bird (*Growla religiosa*), *Psychological Record*, XII (1962), 193–201. M. E. Molliver, "Operant Control of Vocal Behavior in the Cat," *Journal of Experimental Analysis of Behavior*, VI (1963), 197–202. K. Salzinger, and M. B. Waller, "The Operant Control of Vocalization in the Dog," *Journal of Experimental Analysis of Behavior*, V (1962), 383–89.

contingent reinforcement, once shaped the squawks of two myna birds from India until one of them said a very clear "Hello!" The other, to our dismay, under exactly the same schedule of reinforcement, ended up with "Allah"; and we could do nothing to change the utterance further. Probably a Pakistani bird!

Human infants have also been the subjects of conditioning experiments. Rheingold and his associates used some operant procedures, first getting a baserate or baseline of the number of vocalizations, and following each one by "a broad smile, three 'tsk' sounds, and a light touch to the infant's abdomen." [11] (Can't you see them at work?) However, they found that the babies increased their vocalizations when these reinforcements were present; and when they were removed, the number decreased to the former level. There are other studies in this vein. Weissberg, Todd, and their co-workers have demonstrated that social reinforcers of this sort do indeed increase the three-month-old baby's utterances, a finding that will come as no surprise to most mothers.[12] These workers also showed that pleasant sounds alone are not sufficient to increase vocalization, because when tape recordings were used instead and no person was visible to the baby, no increase was found. Unlike parakeets that can learn to increase their whistles, songs, or words by hearing commercial phonographic recordings, the child evidently needs the presence of a responding adult.

These experiments, however, do not explain why the babies vocalize in the first place. Perhaps the need to yell or coo or babble is built into the very substance of the human being, much as dogs are born to bark or cows are born to moo. Winitz however adds the concept that these early vocalizations of the infant human may also be viewed as anticipatory goal responses.[13] The hungry baby, he believes, makes his mouth move in anticipation of sucking and feeding; and perhaps later on he may babble in the hope that soon his mother will come to babble to him. Anyone who has had to listen to a hungry, yelling baby might easily believe this about the crying; but it's a bit difficult to be sure that the baby is responding more to the hope of food than to the spasms in his belly. We just don't know very much about the hopes and expectations of infants.

Winitz also describes a second stage of speech development in which secondary reinforcement plays a dominant role:

The mother's vocalizations precede and accompany the administration

[11] H. L. Rheingold, J. L. Gewirtz, and H. W. Ross, "Social Conditioning of Vocalizations in the Infant," *Journal of Comparative Physiological Psychology*, LII (1959), 68–73.

[12] P. Weisberg, "Social and Nonsocial Conditioning of Infant Vocalizations," *Child Development*, XXXIV (1963), 377–88. G. A. Todd, and B. Palmer, "Social Reinforcement of Infant Babbling," *Child Development*, XXXIX (1968), 591–96.

[13] H. Winitz, *Articulatory Acquisition and Behavior* (New York: Appleton-Century-Crofts, 1969), pp. 36–37.

of food (primary reinforcement). In most instances the child will turn his head (instrumental response) in order to obtain the food. Sometimes, however, the mother will vocalize and the child will turn his head, but no food will be given (partial reinforcement). In time the mother's vocalizations follow other infant acts, such as looking at the parent, controlled by body movement, and smiles. However, the mother will not always vocalize when the child responds.

Because an infant's vocalizations resemble his mother's vocalizations they "acquire" secondary reinforcing properties as the mother's vocalizations transfer to the child's vocalizations. Maternal vocalizations, of course, occur almost continuously prior to and during the care of an infant. Quite understandably, the infant's own vocalizations thereby acquire secondary reinforcing properties. In addition, the mother's vocalizations continue to be paired with the administration of food as well as with other primary reinforcing acts, thereby preventing extinction of the child's vocalizations [Winitz, p. 44].

It is therefore probable that the specific child's sounds and syllables which more nearly resemble those of the parent's speech will inevitably acquire more secondary reinforcement than those which do not. Moreover, the parents will probably respond more enthusiastically and immediately if the child says "mamama" than if he says "mfoo" or "unk." Certainly when the one-year-old produces something that sounds enough like "milk" ("muk," "mik," "miuk") and observes that his mother runs for that lovely bottle, we can see how such a specific utterance would be strengthened. Thereafter, we suspect, through differential reinforcement, those variations which come closer to the standard word as opposed to those which do not will be uttered more often. The shaping process thereby set into operation may result finally in a close resemblance to the adult word.

Motor Theory of Perception.   None of these explanations is entirely convincing in explaining how the first words are really produced. Many a child will suddenly say a word he has never said before and has not been taught. One of our daughter's first words was "pretty" referring to a flower. There had been no babbling which had resembled it. It had not been shaped by progressive approximations. No one had asked her to say it. It was not imitated at that moment. Doubtless she had heard the word with reference to flowers, but how had she learned it? One possible explanation has been offered by Liberman, who hypothesizes that auditory perception is based upon covert articulation.[14] We have always been impressed by how carefully the child watched our face when we were saying words to her, almost as though she were hard of hearing. Perhaps, as she listened, she was rehearsing our words to herself, forming the sounds as

[14] A. M. Liberman, F. S. Cooper, D. P. Shankweiler, and M. Studdert–Kennedy, "Perception of the Speech Code," *Psychological Review*, LXXIV (1967), 431–61.

though lipreading, and had acquired the word in this fashion. This mystery within a mystery has yet to be unwrapped.

SPEECH DEVELOPMENT IN THE LAST HALF OF THE SECOND YEAR

At eighteen months, the child is toddling about the room and pushing chairs and toys from one position to another. He climbs without discrimination. He spills with a spoon but manages to feed himself after a fashion. His handedness is pretty well established. Extremely active, he seldom plays with any one object or activity very long. As fond of music as before, he now prefers marches to lullabies except before bedtime. When angry, he screams, kicks, or holds his breath, but this mass activity is not focused or directed against any particular person. He initiates games such as "Peekaboo" and seems to take great pleasure in "making" adults cooperate. A large empty box is his dearest toy. He usually plays beside other children rather than with them, and he plays better alone. He relies on adults for assistance and attention but shies away from strangers. He should never be asked to speak to them at this age.

At eighteen months the child's speech activity consists of a *few meaningful words*, a little solitary *vocal play*, some *echolalia*, and a great deal of what we shall call *jargon*. Again, let us repeat that we are discussing the mythical average child. The average child has acquired from ten to twenty meaningful words with which to manipulate his elders and express his needs. He not only has names for members of his family but for many other things. Some typical examples are: [mo] for *snow*; [ɔgɔn] for *all gone*; [baɪbaɪ] for *bye-bye*; [aɪt] for *light*; [kækə] for *cracker*; [pɑp] for *pot*. Many of these are used as one-word sentences, and they are very general in their reference. [kækə] can refer to *cracker* or *bread* or even to the fact that the dog is chewing a bone. Many parents lose a great deal of pleasure by not trying to solve these little crossword puzzles of infancy.

Parents of our acquaintance put the problem to us in these words: "Why does our eighteen-month-old daughter refer to both the cat and a champagne bottle by the same word *dih* [dɪ]?" At the time we could not answer, but during the child's third year the word *dih* changed to *ding* [dɪŋ], then to *dink* [dɪŋk], and finally to *drink*. The child had been fascinated by the sight of the cat drinking its milk.

Occasionally the use of one word will spread to include a great many unrelated objects. The child feels little of his parents' confusion when he uses the word *behbuh* [bɛbə] to mean first "baby," then "bib," then "bread and butter." In this instance, the referential spread was no doubt due to the phonetic similarity of all these words. Had the parent taught them at different times or with different intonation or stress, the spread would not have been so great. Soldiers and others who suffer damage to the brain show these same symptoms.

Many early words are generalizations because they are so few and must serve a child so often. When a child who learns the word *puppy* as the designation for his varying perceptions of dogdom is suddenly confronted by a pony, he must needs make *puppy* do for both until he gets a new term. One child used the sound *fffff* as a generalized word for flowers. We also use a similar generic term. But he used *fffff* for perfume, for cigarette smoke, and for the figures on the wall paper. As the child comes to discriminate between objects, he needs terms to fix the contrasts involved. As long as ponies and dogs are merely big creatures with four legs on the corners and a hairy coat, they require but one word, and *puppy* is adequate. But when he realizes that ponies neigh, and he can ride on them, and they are bigger and eat carrots and never sleep by the fireplace—then a new word is needed, and it is acquired.

How, then, do children acquire these new words? The answer seems to be that at the moment when the child is undergoing some new experience in perception, or has an urgent desire to manipulate some new object in order to know it better, the adult intervenes, supplying a new word. If the child perceives this vocalization as part of the total experience, and at the same time produces the word through imitation, he finds he has a more efficient tool than the old generalized word. As the process repeats itself, the child comes to realize the greater expressiveness of conventional language forms. The whole process is, of course, also influenced by other factors: by the child's growing discrimination, by the strength and constancy of adult intervention at the crucial moments, and even by the natural responsiveness of the child.

These first words are used by the child even in his play. He yells "bell-bell-bell" (or a reasonable facsimile thereof) to himself as he rings it. He repeatedly labels the eyes, nose, and ears, not only of the mother who taught him but of his dog or doll, and he pokes them in the labeling. The early words are still accompanied by gesture or pertinent activity. He needs the parents' gestures in order to comprehend their utterances, and so he gestures and speaks in his turn. Only about one-fourth of his speech attempts on these words can be understood by strangers. Each family seems to elect one of its members as interpreter. Nevertheless these first ten or twenty words of the eighteen-month-old child are a wonderful achievement. His manner shows that he knows it even if you do not. One child beat his chest and war-whooped whenever he used a new word successfully.

Jargon. The largest share of the average eighteen-month-old child's speech is *jargon*. This unintelligible jabber is probably more important for speech development than people realize. It is the lineal descendant of vocal play, but it differs from the earlier babbling in its rich variety and its seeming purposiveness. The child seems to be talking to other people or to his toys, rather than playing with the sounds themselves. He seldom repeats the same syllable.

> One boy, aged nineteen months, was observed banging a teddy bear with a hammer and between wallops addressing his victim as follows: "Gubba! Dadda bo-bo!" (Another hammering.) "Show gubba mahda." (Hammers again.) "Ashlee? Baá!" (Throws teddy bear over his shoulder.) In phonetics, the discourse was transcribed: gʌbə dædə bobo . . . ʃo gʌbə mɑdɑ . . . æʃli . . . bɑ . . .

> Often this conversational jargon includes words he has mastered. Reaching out his dish for more ice cream he said, "ɛːɛ adə mamə i ɪ nænə aɪ kim ʃlæ?" The words which we have underlined are certainly understandable, and perhaps [nænə] refers to "banana," a favorite food, but the other syllables are difficult to interpret. And most of the child's jargon is even less intelligible.

As Gesell phrases it, "At eighteen months her jargon was beguiling. She would talk confidentially for minutes at a single stretch, uttering not a single enunciated word but conveying much emotional content." [15] As this quotation hints, jargon is probably the child's practice of fluency. Most young children swim in a river of fastflowing meaningless adult jargon. Why should they not imitate their elders in fluency even as they copy their speech sounds and inflections? Certainly the gap between the few halting words of the child and the ceaseless ebb and flow of adult speech is very wide. Jargon is the bridge. It reaches its peak at eighteen months, dropping out rapidly, and it is usually gone by two years. A few children never use any jargon. When words fail, they gesture or cry or remain silent. Most babies are like adults. They must talk whether what they say makes sense or not.

Vocal Play and Echolalia. The babbling play of infancy still appears, usually when the child is in bed or alone. He plays with repeated syllables or prolonged sibilant sounds. His new teeth enable him to produce new whistling sounds, and so he must practice them. Often you can hear him whispering to himself and working up to the crescendo of vocalization. Prolonging sounds with his finger in mouth, or fumbling rhythmically with lips, he discovers again (and not for the last time) how fascinating he is. Jargon is his vocal response to a vocal world. Vocal play is his private rehearsal.

[15] A. Gesell, *The Psychology of Early Growth Including Norms for Infant Behavior and a Method of Genetic Analysis* (New York: The Macmillan Company, 1938).

Echolalia appears very markedly in some children during this period, and it probably occurs in all children occasionally. By this term we mean the parrotlike echoing of words he hears. Occasionally whole phrases and sentences will be repeated so faithfully that the parent fairly jumps. In one instance a year-and-a-half-old girl almost wrecked a church service by saying, "and ever and ever amen!" fourteen times in the middle of the preacher's sermon. She had only spoken a few words prior to this event, and she never uttered the phrase again for years. Parents frequently use echolalia to teach their children nursery rhymes, most of which are first learned backward. The parent says, "The cow jumped over the moon." "Moo," says the child automatically. Soon the parent begins to hesitate before the last word, and the child fills in.

Echolalia occurs almost instantly and unconsciously as if in a dream. The child's attention is elsewhere. Feeble-minded adults show a great deal of echolalia, as do aphasics and some psychotics. Any fairly normal person who has ever held a conversation with one of these echolalics will never forget the experience:

Are you ten years old?
Ten years old?
Yes.
Yes.
I mean . . .
I mean . . .
When is your birthday?
Birthday?
Yes.—Oh let it go!
Let it go.

There madness lies. But in little children echolalia is a normal stage of development, and sensibly they pass through it in a hurry. It is seldom observed in the normal child after two and a half years.

Speech at Two Years. By the time the child reaches his second birthday he should be talking. Speech has become a tool as well as a safety valve or warning siren. He is saying things like: "Where Kitty?" "Ball all gone." "Want cookie." "Kiss baby." "Go bye-bye car." "Shut door." "Big horsie cry." "Put 'bacco in pipe."

Simple and compound sentences are often heard. The jargon is almost gone. His articulation is faulty; his speech rhythms are broken; his voice control ranges from loud to louder, but he has learned to talk. He may still turn out to have any of the speech defects, but he isn't mute. Not by a good many decibels, he isn't.

In summary, we may say again that children *learn* to talk. Their parents do the teaching, and it is usually very poor. Because of the widespread ignorance concerning speech development and the teaching of talking, many children: (1) fail to practice their speech sounds in vocal play; (2) do not learn how to imitate sounds; (3) do not learn that sounds can be meaningful and useful tools; (4) do not practice or profit from their jargon; (5) resort to gesture and other substitute behavior rather than develop a growing vocabulary, and therefore (6) they lay the foundation for defective speech.

LATER SPEECH DEVELOPMENT

The third and fourth years of life are especially important in the development of speech, for it is during these years that most of the speech disorders might be said to begin. Certainly it is then that articulatory errors become fixed, stuttering starts, and voices begin to assume characteristics which may last throughout the person's life.

The young child has much to learn in the months that surround his third birthday. Prohibitions become important in his life, and he becomes negative in turn. Bursting with energy, he meets frustrations everywhere. He must learn to become a social being, whether he wants to or not. The world of words becomes vastly important to the three-year-old. Through speech he finds expression for his emotion. By means of talking, he manipulates his associates and satisfies his needs. He has great need for fluency and precision of utterance.

The few infantile words that he learned during his first two years cannot possibly serve his growing needs. He now needs to express relationships and qualifications. He needs plurals and gender. He becomes conscious of the past and the future, and these demand new verb forms. The whole problem of English syntax presents itself as a challenge to the three-year-old. At the same time, his needs for a larger vocabulary are increasing. "What's that? What's that?" is a game which every parent learns to play, on the answering end. The three-year-old is into everything strange. He tests and tries everything, including the patience of his associates. These explorations yield him many moments of confusion when something never before seen has no name to identify its impact. Thus one three-year-old, who had shown precocious speech development with few if any breaks in fluency, suddenly observed a parachute descent and cried out "ε-ε-ʌ-ʌ-ε -bʌ (gesture of pointing and excited breathing), -bʌd-bʌd-goʊ-bum." At the time, her normal speech was being recorded, and therefore the transcript was accurate. Her usual speech was rhythmic and fluent. It is interesting also that she showed a return to earlier phraseology: "go boom" for the "fall down" which she had been using for over a year. Under the pressure of haste, the unfamiliarity of the experience, the confusion of *airplane* [ɛɚ] and *bird* [bʌd], both of which were probably felt to be inadequate, the child's fluency broke down and she showed hesitant speech similar to that of stuttering.

MASTERING THE RULES OF THE LANGUAGE

Building Sentences. About eighteen months of age, many children begin to join words together in a meaningful fashion. This is probably the most important discovery the child will ever make, yes, even though he becomes the first man to walk on Mars. It is probably the most important one the human species ever made, for it enabled this two-legged race of mammals to exploit the immense potentials of symbolization. To have to speak only in single-word utterances would be as limiting as using one toe to play an arpeggio on the piano.

One of the fascinating aspects about language acquisition is that, within an interval of two and a half years, most children learn an incredible number of the complex rules for combining words. The achievement is so huge that many linguists have felt some inborn predisposition for perceiving these patterns must exist.

These first word combinations are not at all random; they are patterned from the first. By collecting and analyzing a large number of the child's utterances, one finds that his words may be grouped into several categories. We find two classes of these words in his early verbalizations: "pivot" words, which are characteristically used to initiate the primitive sentence and serve much the same purpose as do the function words of adult speech; and "open class" or "operator" words, which carry the important meanings in much the same way as do the content words of grownups. Our grandson, Jimmy, at one year and ten months, had these two basic sets of words in his repertoire, and at one time or another, he combined most of those in the left hand column with those on the right. The pivot words were usually used first in the sequence.

Pivot Words	*Open Class Words*
here, more, big, that,	milk, cup, car, plane,
bye-bye, see	Jimmy, shoe, bottle,
	Mummy, ball, doggie, bed,
	eye (and about fourteen others).

Thus he would say such combinations as "bye-bye plane" or (when getting up from his nap) "bye-bye bed," an utterance which he had never heard his parents use. He would say "more milk," but he also said "more shoe" when he wanted the other one put on; and this too could not have been learned through any sort of imitation. Never did he combine any two of the pivot words to make an utterance; although some linking of the open class of words was shown when he said "milk cup" as he pushed away the bottle and pointed, indicating that he wanted to drink his milk from a cup. All these two-word linkings were uttered on a single breath.

Within a month Jimmy showed clearly that he had discovered how noun phrases and verb phrases could be constructed: "my cup," "that shoe," "that car," "big milk." In naming pictures he would use the article "a" or the demonstrative "that" before each of them. No longer would he merely say "cow" or "house." It was always "a cow" or "that house." If we forgot to put in the prefatory word, he would become enraged and say, "No, no! 'a' cow," and correct us. He wasn't going to have his newly learned rule violated. If we said "big cow," that was all right, but no more single words for him! Something similar also occurred with verbs, though this came later. Verb phrases consist of the combination of an antecedent verb with a noun or a noun phrase. Jimmy's first one was "bang cup," but within a week he was saying not only "pay pono" (play piano) and "wah miuk" (want milk) but also "weed a booh" (read a book) and, showing us that he could do so, "frow duh bih bah" (throw the big ball), thus combining the verb with a noun phrase.

For almost two months, Jimmy stayed at this level of speaking in noun phrases and verb phrases, making many gains in vocabulary and practicing many different applications of the rules he had discovered. The noun phrases were then expanded: "Daddy big shoe." Verbs were followed by noun phrases as well as single nouns. He would say such things as "Jimmy want big ball" and even "Doggie eat Jimmy toast," thus indicating some sense of the possessive. Some of these verb phrases soon showed expansion by linking adverbs or prepositional phrases with the verb: "Fall down," "Go now in big car." It was fascinating to see him experimenting with these noun and verb phrase combinations. That he was not merely repeating phrases that he had heard his parents use, but actually and deliberately linking the words together is shown by some of these utterances: "Here bye-bye" (I've got to go now), "Go Mummy bed," and "No that button." These were not imitations of parental speech. They were the result of his attempts to construct a grammar, to relate words appropriately and meaningfully.

Then one day we heard the first true kernel sentences. "Jimmy want coat." "Jimmy go car." "Big ball fall down." He had found a new way of combining. Noun phrases could be joined to verb phrases. Subjects could have predicates. He didn't know these terms, but he had the idea. Whee! When he said one of these new combinations, he would run around in circles, shriek with pleasure, and collapse on the floor in ecstacy.[16]

---

[16] So did his grandfather.

For some time Jimmy seemed to be practicing these kernel sentence combinations. Even in his one-word sentences he had long been able to use intonations which were questioning or commanding or negating, as well as declaring. Now he began to use them in his primitive sentences along with some new words such as "what" and "where." We heard such utterances as "Daddy go work house?" (interrogative); "Jimmy dink milk" (declarative); "Jimmy no dink milk!" (imperative). He also began to lengthen his word strings through the use of conjunctions. "Daddy eat ice cream and Mommy eat and Jimmy eat ice cream."

This is as far as Jimmy has come at the time of this writing, but we know what lies ahead. He will have to master what the linguists call transformations. He must discover that he can take the kernel sentences and manipulate them in many ways. The major operations will involve first additions, then deletion and substitution and permutation. He will have to master the rules of verb tense and number, to explore the use of the very valuable auxiliary verbs, to make sense out of plurals and other suffixes. Though he lives to be a hundred, he will never make so great an achievement as that involved in learning the complexities of his language.

Mastering Correct Articulation.   Besides acquiring his vocabulary and learning to join his words together appropriately, the child must also learn to articulate his sounds and pronounce his words correctly. This, too, is not an easy task. At first he shows an inability to grasp the distinctive features of phonemes that sound quite similar. "Goggy" and "doggy" do not differ much in the ears of a two-year-old. One plosive seems similar to another; one fricative resembles several others. How does he learn the differences in the sounds of the words he hears in the speech of adults? He never hears his parents using "rings" except in the context of fingers, whereas they talk about "wings" when talking about birds. Unfortunately all the words of English do not possess such contrasting pairs. If they did, we suspect that children would develop correct articulation very early and almost universally. If the name for spinach were "tandy," no child would ever use that expression for "candy" more than once or twice.

Parents often wish to know how well their child is doing in mastering the speech sounds. All we can offer are averages, and these often are unfair. Girls acquire the difficult consonants earlier than boys. Children from homes in the higher socioeconomic bracket speak more clearly than those from economically poorer homes. There are many factors which may influence a specific child's progress, and so we hesitate to provide any norms. We do so only with the caution that you use these averages as averages and not as yardsticks.

Generally speaking, we can say that the research indicates that children of three years should have mastered most of the vowels, diphthongs, and the

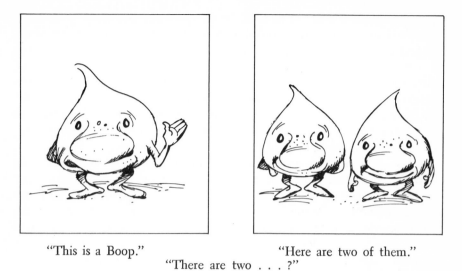

"This is a Boop."   "Here are two of them."
"There are two . . . ?"

FIGURE 10: *Testing the Child's Comprehension of Pluralization.* Modified from J. Berko, "The Child's Learning of English Morphology."

p, b, m, w, t, d, n, and *h* consonants; should be speaking in short sentences; and should have a vocabulary of about nine hundred words. Many of the other consonants may be heard at times; but their use is not consistent, and errors of omission, substitution, and distortion occur. However, over 90 percent of the three-year-old's speech should be readily understood. By five years of age all of his speech should be understandable; and the *k, g, f,* and *v* sounds should be used with fair consistency except in the blends (*gr, cl, st,* etc.). Then during the sixth year the *l* sound, the *s* and *z,* the *sh* and *ch,* and occasionally the *r,* which seems often to be very difficult, begin to show themselves regularly. Most of the research indicates that the average child should be speaking standard English by the time he enters first grade or about the time of his seventh birthday. Let us say again that these are averages, that there are always some children developing faster and others more slowly than these norms who must be considered normal.

But there are also children who vary so far from the norm that they need help. Indeed, we feel that every child should be helped by his parents to learn to talk. If the mother would stimulate the child with isolated and nonsense sounds in verbal play, the child would find it easier to master those sounds. Many children have to master their alphabet of sound the hard way, by catching the sounds on the wing. They need easier models. They need to hear what these sounds are like. In our next chapter we will describe ways of teaching the alphabet of sound, and tell you how to help a child recognize that words have heads and tails, and show you how a parent should set models for self-correction. If parents had this information, we feel, many articulatory disorders could be prevented.

Attaining Fluency. If we may return for a moment to the crucial third and fourth years, we will find the child learning to be fluent, learning to keep the utterance flowing. The basic need here is to provide good models for the child, models that are within his reach. Many children go through a temporary period of hesitant speech at this time, which, we feel, presents a danger that might be avoided if parents knew what to do.

Just as he imitates his father's pipe-smoking or his mother's sweeping with extreme fidelity, so, too, will he imitate their inflections and voice quality *and* attempt to imitate their fluency. It is in this last item that much of our trouble with stuttering begins. Children of this age do not have the vocabulary to keep their fluency up to adult standards. The adults about them speak to one another and to the children themselves in compound-complex sentences, in paragraphs that flow one after the other in endless series. If they pause, it is for so short an instant that the child cannot get his speech under way. Grownups often penalize interrupting children, but they will interrupt the child's speech with impunity. They finish the child's sentences before he has been able to get them half said. They interrupt to correct a plural or a pronoun or a past participle, and often seize the opportunity to rush on with their own flow of verbalization. When a child tries to adopt an adult fluency pattern of which he is not capable, or if he is bombarded by many of these parental interruptions, he will have hesitant speech. Anyone who has tried to speak a half-learned foreign language with a fluent native will understand what little children undergo. The average parent does not realize what has happened until the child's speech fails to develop normally.

If this childish urge to speak as fluently as his parents when he has neither the vocabulary nor the necessary skills can precipitate stuttering, we should try to decrease its intensity. Whenever frustration is produced by having an aspiration level far above the person's performance level, we should try to reduce the former. In the case of the child learning to talk, the problem can be solved fairly simply. If the parents will speak to the child, using short phrases and sentences, using simple words whose meaning he can comprehend, using the simplest of syntax, the child will never need to feel speech frustration. He can achieve these fluency patterns without too much difficulty. We have been able, clinically, to free many children from primary stuttering by merely getting their parents to speak more simply. As an example let us quote from a parent's report:

Each evening, as you suggested, we have been holding a family conference and confessing to each other our errors in handling Ruth.

Among other things, we found ourselves constantly talking over her head. Today, for instance, I said to her, "Ruth, do you suppose you could go to the bathroom and bring down some of the dirty towels and washcloths? Mama's going to wash." She looked at me intently, then went upstairs and came down with some soap, and said, "Woothy wa-wa-wa-wash bath bath . . . ," and she stuttered pretty badly. So I thanked her for the soap and said, "Ruthy go upstairs. Bring Mama washcloth, please." Her face lit up, and she ran upstairs and down again in a hurry, bringing me the washcloth and a towel too. Then she said, "Woothy bwing wash coth. Nice girl." I begin to see what you mean by speaking more simply.

One need not talk baby-talk in order to speak more simply. We must merely give our children fluency models within their performance ability.

If we are to prevent speech defects, we must prevail upon parents to change their present policy of sporadic correction and *laissez-faire*. They must learn how to help the child master the difficult skills with which he is confronted in adult speech. They must learn how to keep from making speech-learning difficult. They must not do all the wrong things so blithely.

Acquiring Vocabulary.   Most parents are eager enough to help the child to get his first twenty or thirty new words. Some parents are even too ambitious at first; they try to teach such words as "Dorothy" or "Semantha." But their teaching urge soon subsides. The child seems to be picking up a few words as he needs them. Why not let him continue to grow at his own pace? Our answer does not deny the function of maturation in vocabulary growth. We merely say that parents should give a little common-sense help at moments when a child needs a new word, a label for a new experience. When parents notice a child hesitating or correcting himself when faced with a new experience, they should become verbal dictionaries, providing *not only the needed new word, but a definition in terms of the child's own vocabulary.* For example:

John was pointing to something on the shelf he wanted. "Johnny want . . . um . . . Johnny want pretty pretty ball . . . Johnny wanta pretty . . . um . . ." The object was a round glass vase with a square opening on top. I immediately took it down and said, "No ball, Johnny. Vase! Vase!" I put my finger into the opening and let him imitate me. Then we got a flower and he put it in the opening after I had filled it partially with water. I said, "Vase is a flower cup. Flower cup, vase! See pretty vase! (I prolonged the *v* sound slightly.) Flower drink water in vase, in pretty vase. Johnny, say 'Vase!' " (He obeyed without hesitation or error.) Each day that week, I asked him to put a new flower in the vase, and by the end of that time he was using the word with assurance. I've found one thing though; you must speak rather slowly when teaching a new word. Use plenty of pauses and patience.

Besides this type of spontaneous vocabulary teaching, it is possible to play little games at home in which the child imitates an older child or parent as they "touch and say" different objects. Children invent these games for themselves.

> "March and Say" was a favorite game of twins whom we observed. One would pick up a toy telephone, run to the door of the playroom, and ask his mother, "What dat?" "Telephone," she would answer, and then both twins would hold the object and march around the room chanting "tɛpoʊn tɛpoʊn" until it ended in a fight for possession. Then the dominant twin would pick up another object, ask its name, and march and chant its name over and over.

In all of these naming games, the child should always point to, feel, or sense the object referred to as vividly as possible. The mere sight or sound of the object is not enough for early vocabulary acquisition. It is also wise to avoid cognate terms. One of our children for years called the cap on a bottle a "hat" because of early confusion.

Scrapbooks are better than the ordinary run of children's books for vocabulary teaching because pictures of objects closer to the child's experience may be pasted in. The ordinary "Alphabet Book" is a monstrosity so far as the teaching of talking is concerned. Nursery rhymes are almost as bad. Let the child listen to "Goosey Goosey Gander, whither dost thou wander" if he enjoys the rhymes, but do not encourage him to say the rhymes. The teaching of talking should be confined to meaningful speech, not gibberish. The three-year-old child has enough of a burden without trying to make sense of nonsense. When using the pictures in the scrapbooks, it is wise to do more than ask the child to name them. When pointing to a ball, the parents should say, "What's that?" "Ball." "Johnny throw ball. Bounce, bounce, bounce" (gestures). Build up associations in terms of the functions of the objects. Teach phrases as well as single words. "Cookie" can always be taught as "eat cookie." This policy may also help the child to remember to keep it out of his hair.

REFERENCES

Articles

1. Berko, J. "The Child's Learning of English Morphology." *Word*, XIV (1958), 150–77.
   What are the author's main conclusions about how children learn words? What are "wugs?"
2. Brown, R. and Fraser, C. "The Acquisition of Syntax." In Bellugi, U. and Brown, R., eds., *The Acquisition of Language* (Monographs of the Society for Research in Child Development, Nos. 92, 29, 1964).
   How were the authors able to discover how children develop their grammatical systems?
3. Carrow, Sister M.A. "The Development of Auditory Comprehension of Language Structure in Children." *Journal of Speech and Hearing Disorders*, XXXIII (1968), 99–111.
   Describe the test used by the author to assess comprehension.
4. Deutsch, M. "The Role of Social Class in Language Development and Cognition." *American Journal of Orthopsychiatry*, XXXV (1965), 78–88.
   What behaviors are there in social interaction between parents and child in lower-class homes that can account for retarded language development in the children of these homes?
5. Fodor, J. A. "How to Learn to Talk: Some Simple Ways." In Smith, F. and Miller, G. A., eds., *The Genesis of Language* (Cambridge, Mass.: Massachusetts Institute of Technology Press, 1966).
   What are these simple ways?
6. Greene, M. C. *Learning to Talk*. New York: Harper & Row, Publishers, 1960.
   Read pages 1–76 and summarize this material.
7. Irwin, O. C. "Speech Development in the Young Child: II. Some Factors Related to the Speech Development of the Infant and Young Child." *Journal of Speech and Hearing Disorders*, XVII (1952), 269–79.
   What are the differences in the frequencies and kinds of sounds used by normal and brain-damaged children?
8. Lenneberg, E. H. "Understanding Language Without Ability to Speak." *Journal of Abnormal and Social Psychology*, LXV (1962), 419–25.
   Describe this boy and summarize the author's discussion of the relationship between speaking and comprehending.
9. Leopold, W. "The Study of Child Language and Infant Bilingualism." *Word*, IV (1948), 1–17.
   What effect, if any, is there when two languages are taught to the infant?
10. Lovaas, O. I., Berberich, J. D., Perloff, B. F., and Schaeffer, B. "Acquisition of Imitative Speech in Schizophrenic Children." *Science*, CLI (1966), 705–7.
    How did they get these two children to imitate speech?
11. McConnel, F., Horton, K. B., and Smith, B. R. "Language Development and Cultural Disadvantagement." *Exceptional Child*, XXXV (1969), 597–606.
    Describe the plan and results of the three-year project.

12. Menyuk, P. "Syntactic Structures in the Language of Children." *Child Development*, XXXIV (1963), 407–22.
How do children learn the rules of language for combining words into sentences?

13. Metraux, R. W. "Speech Profiles of the Preschool Child 18 to 54 Months." *Journal of Speech and Hearing Disorders*, XV (1950), 37–53.
Summarize the developmental trends in articulation and fluency as shown by these profiles.

14. Mowrer, O. H. "Hearing and Speaking: An Analysis of Language Learning." *Journal of Speech and Hearing Disorders*, XXIII (1958), 143–52.
How do talking birds illustrate the basic principles of language learning?

15. Murphy, A. T. and Fitzsimmons, R. M. *Stuttering and Personality Dynamics*. New York: The Ronald Press Company, 1960.
Read Chapter 3 and tell how these authors view the development of speech?

16. Mykelbust, H. R. "Babbling and Echolalia." *Journal of Speech and Hearing Disorders*, XXII (1957), 356–60.
Sketch the author's view of speech development in terms of imitative identification and internalization, and tell how babbling and echolalia may indicate pathology.

17. Poole, I. "Genetic Development of Articulation of Consonant Sounds in Speech." *Elementary English Review*, XI (1934), 159–61.
Summarize her norms of articulation development.

18. Schreiber, F. R. "How to Talk with Children." *Today's Speech*, XI (1963), 6–9.
How should the mother talk to the child to develop vocabulary?

19. Winitz, H. "The Development of Speech and Language in the Normal Child." In Rieber, R. W. and Brubaker, R. S., eds., *Speech Pathology* (Philadelphia: J. B. Lippincott Co., 1966).
What usefulness does linguistics have for helping a child learn to acquire speech and language?

Texts

20. Bellugi, U. and Brown R. *The Acquisition of Language*. Monographs of the Society for Research in Child Development, No. 92, Volume 29, 1964.
This small volume contains some excellent papers on the acquisition of language. The contributions of modern linguistic theory are illustrated clearly.

21. Lewis, M. M. *Infant Speech: A Study of Language*. New York: Humanities Press, 1951.
A fascinating play-by-play account of the development of speech from earliest infancy.

22. ———. *Language, Thought and Personality*. New York: Basic Books, Inc., Publishers, 1963.
Part One of this book tells how speech develops in the infant, how language and thinking follow a parallel course of development, and finally how language shapes the personality and determines social relationships.

23. Morley, M. E. *The Development and Disorders of Speech*. 2d ed. London: Livingstone, 1965.
This book reports a longitudinal investigation of speech and language development and their disorders.

24. Templin, M. C. *Certain Language Skills in Children: Their Development and Interrelationships.* Minneapolis: University of Minnesota Press, 1957. This book presents the results of a longitudinal investigation of speech and language development.
25. Van Riper, C. *Teaching Your Child to Talk.* New York: Harper & Row, Publishers, 1950.
A book written primarily for parents of a first-born child so that they can understand and enjoy the development of speech.
26. Winitz, H. *Articulatory Acquisition and Behavior.* New York: Appleton-Century-Crofts, 1969.
Pages 1–49 of this text present an excellent review of the research on speech development and the theories concerning language acquisition.
27. Wood, N. *Delayed Speech and Language Development.* Englewood Cliffs, N.J.: Prentice-Hall, Inc., 1964.
This book surveys the essential information on speech and language development, presents the usual causes of delay, and describes how to examine and evaluate the problems due to that delay.

4

Delayed Speech and Language

Our last chapter dealt with how a child learns his language and thereby joins the human race. In this one we consider that group of tragically handicapped persons who, for one reason or another, have not been able to decipher the code in its entirety—as all of us must do if we are to communicate effectively. We have seen what a complicated code it is, and we should not be surprised to find that some children have real trouble mastering it.

It should be stressed immediately that there is a marked contrast between these language-deficient children and those who have trouble saying their sounds correctly, those who stutter, or those who have strange voices. The latter have learned the language. They know the code. The lisper, the cleft-palate speaker, and the stutterer have plenty of blemishes and difficulties in their speech; but they have no problems in comprehending, or in formulating their thoughts into appropriate words or sentences. The children of this chapter have a language problem as the basis of their speech problem. Our task with a lisper is to remove the flaws in a tool he already can use; but when we work with a child with delayed language, we have to help him build the tool and teach him how to use it. Even though these children may make many errors in articulation or seem unduly hesitant, we do not work on sounds or fluency. Their disorder is one of symbolization. We must help them acquire a vocabulary and learn how to link the words together appropriately and meaningfully. In doing this, we should never forget that linguistic competence and comprehension come first. Somehow these children must perceive that speech is patterned. Somehow they must discern the features of the language system.

Viewed superficially, these children seem merely to be speech deficient, but when closely scrutinized, the majority of them are seen to possess linguistic deficits that make it impossible for them to express themselves verbally in a normal manner. They simply do not comprehend how utterance is organized. This comprehension (or as Noam Chomsky phrases it, "this competence") is always the prime requisite for expression or performance. Even though a mother may tell us that her son understands everything said to him, we often find major deficiencies in speech perception—impairments in auditory memory span; in comprehending sequences of words and sounds; in discriminating between opposites, singulars, and plurals, or present and future tense; and many of the other grammatical features so essential for the communication of verbal meaning. Sometimes the child understands a parental command by "reading" the gestures or vocal inflections. We remember one mother who insisted her son always understood the negative "No!", but when we had her say it without shaking her head from side to side it was obvious that he did not understand the *word* at all.

This is not to say that all children with delayed language and speech cannot understand anything that is said to them. Many of them comprehend more than might be expected. Lenneberg studied an eight-year-old, completely speechless boy who was able to follow such complicated commands as "Take the block and put it on the bottle." [1] Nevertheless, it seems clear that most children with delayed speech are also delayed in language acquisition. Some of them do not even have any usable words when they come to us and are essentially nonverbal, yet finally we can help them as this case study by Schlanger indicates:

> Dick is a post-encephalitic child with no motor or hearing defect. He was first seen at 4.8 years of age. An occasional grunt, used indiscriminately comprised his total verbal output. No imitative oral responses could be elicited. Communicative contact was pointedly evaded, and he was extremely hyperactive. Gestures were infrequently used to indicate what he wanted. The prognosis made by physicians was that he would never develop the use of speech. At 6.8 years he was imitating sounds and producing word approximations. Spontaneous speech was limited to one-word sentences, but symbol meaning was clear only when the subject was known to the listener. Responsiveness and contact were improving. At 8.2 years he was able to imitate most of the consonant sounds; spontaneous speech was frequently understandable, although still limited in output. Phrases and sentences such as "open the door," "your green car," "boy drink milk," objects and picture-naming, and ready responses to greetings were indicative of a much improved communication adjustment. [2]

[1] E. H. Lenneberg, "Case Report: Understanding Language Without Ability to Speak," *Journal of Abnormal and Social Behavior*, LXV (1962), 419–25.

[2] B. B. Schlanger, "A Longitudinal Study of Speech and Language Development of Brain-damaged Retarded Children," *Journal of Speech and Hearing Disorders*, XXIV (1959), 358–59.

Here is another child who could only grunt and gesture:

> Don was five years old, physically normal, and his parents were com-
> pletely convinced of his intelligence. His hearing was good and so
> were his coordinations. He seemed to comprehend speech very well
> and could follow directions with ease. Possibly because of an early
> isolation on a farm with few playmates, he had few friends and pre-
> ferred to play alone. He was well behaved, and his lack of speech and
> of interest in socialization seemed to be his only real difference. His
> parents had become quite anxious about his delay in learning to talk
> but seemed to love him. He was an only child. With this brief intro-
> duction, let us give you the observer's report. The observer watched
> the child and his parents through a one-way mirror and heard him
> over a hidden intercommunication system.
>
> Father told Don to take off his hat and coat and to hang them on
> the rack. Boy did this without hesitation, then returned to the play
> table and looked at toys. Father told him to help himself. He worked
> the little pump, and when the little ball came out of the spout he
> smiled, looked at the father and said, "uhn, uhn, uhn, uhn" and
> pointed to the ball. Father told Don to put ball back into upper hole
> of pump. Don did, then pumped handle, but ball was stuck. Looked
> at father who was not paying attention. Took pump to father and
> said, "oo." Father shook pump and ball came out. Don put ball back
> and shook pump. Ball did not come out so he put it down and put
> his thumb in his mouth. Father withdrew it without comment. Don
> said, "no," and put thumb back in mouth. Father said, "Cut it out,
> you hear me?" Don obeyed but held thumb in other hand. Father
> opened picture-book and said, "See cow? Say cow." Don looked but
> did not respond. Father said, "Say cow. Try it anyway." Don said,
> "uhn."
>
> This was typical of the entire half-hour of observation. The only
> recognizable word was "No." The boy used monosyllables to get
> attention and then conveyed his meaning with gestures. If he could
> not make himself understood, he just gave up, waited quietly, or
> turned to something else.

Blake describes two seven-year-old boys, Jim and Ted, neither of
whom had usable speech. We describe them here to show the marked variability in these problems of delayed language. Ted had been diagnosed as
having been brain damaged; Jim had congenital heart disease. They differed markedly in personality, Ted being extremely hyperactive and aggressive, while Jim was shy and well controlled.

At the beginning of therapy they both seemed to comprehend some
spoken language fairly well, as demonstrated by the ability to follow

simple instructions, understand simple gestures, play with and relate to objects, and by their response to other informal tests. Neither had adequate voicing in his attempted vocalizations. Ted's vocal quality was hoarse and extremely breathy, whereas Jim's vocalization attempts were whispered. Neither child was classified as verbal. Ted's main attempt at vocalization at the beginning of therapy was a rhythmical oronasal production of "k-k-k, k-k-k, k-k-k." He did attempt an approximation of *mama* which was vocalized as [a-a], with no attempt at labial (lip) closure or valving at the lips for the [m]. The word *daddy* was also approximated as [æ-i]. The words *yes* and *no* were vocalized as [hʌ] with the appropriate head gesture for each. This was the observable extent of Ted's intelligible vocabulary.

Jim's mother described him as a child who seemed to understand what was said to him but who made very little or no attempt to verbalize on his own. His only intelligible vocabulary approximation was observed (and confirmed by his mother) to be a whispered production of "mama." [3]

These two boys might appear to the casual observer as being hopelessly lost. We know that once the most favorable age of readiness for the acquisition of language has been passed—it is usually felt to be during the second to fifth years—the prognosis is poor. Nevertheless, Blake's experience and that of many of us who have worked intensively with these children may provide hope. Here is what he reports:

> Both Ted and Jim have developed functional speech far beyond the expectations of their parents and the clinician. Their vocabularies are continuing to grow, and they use sentences with as many as seven or eight words now. They use functional speech in appropriate context and show promise of developing more complex speech and language skills. After one year of therapy, which has included two 30-minute sessions of language stimulation per week, Ted and Jim speak in sentences with an average length of four words [pp. 368–69].

Not all of these children are so restricted in their verbal utterance. Some of them vocalize almost constantly, but speak a gibberish which no one can understand. It resembles the jargon which many young normal children use. The utterances are full of inflections and are accompanied by gestures so that one almost believes that they are truly trying to communicate, but we have analyzed many of their vocalizations and have been unable to find any consistency which might indicate a self-language.

[3] J. N. Blake, "A Therapeutic Construct for Two Seven-Year-Old Nonverbal Boys," *Journal of Speech and Hearing Disorders*, XXXIV (1969), 362–69.

One of the children we examined vocalized every minute of her stay with us. She was a restless, wandering child whose attention constantly shifted. As she picked up one toy, threw it down, ran to the window, tapped at the pane, shook her skirt, sucked her thumb, laughed at her reflection in the mirror, and performed a hundred other consecutive activities, she accompanied each with a constant flow of unintelligible jabber. By using a hidden microphone, we were able to record some samples of her speech. The speech sample together with the object of her attention ran like this:

"Yugga boo booda . . . iganna min . . ." [jʌgə bu budə igæ nə min]. Picked up the toy automobile and threw it down. "Annakuh innuhpohee . . . tseeguh . . . tseekuh . . ." [ænakə inəpohi tsigʌ tsikə]. Looked out window and tapped at pane.

In this case we were unable to recognize any mutilations of familiar words, though in most cases of delayed speech careful analysis will isolate a few words, consistently used, which bear some resemblance to their conventional cognates. Both of these general types of delayed speech can result from fixation at an infantile level of speech development. They can also occur regressively as the result of a sudden accident, illness, or emotional shock, even when the previous speech development has been excellent. Both mutism and unintelligibility are relative terms, since noises are made by all mutes, and even in the worst jargon faint resemblances to meaningful words are occasionally found. The problem of delayed speech, however, is more than that of a severe articulation defect. These children are also handicappped linguistically and semantically. They often do not comprehend the language of others, nor are they particularly interested in vocal symbols even when they can understand them. The longer they go without receiving help in attaining a normal method of communication, the more they tend to ignore the speech of others. Jerry and Larry were fraternal twins with normal speech development in their first year. They had begun to speak in one-word sentences when Larry became ill and was hospitalized for six months, during which Jerry learned to speak in sentences, but Larry regressed to grunts and babbling. Speech therapy was begun at once, and the parents cooperated fully, but Larry stayed behind Jerry's speech level until they were in the third grade. Neither emotional factors nor residual effects of the illness seemed to have caused the delay. Instead, it seemed that Larry had by-passed the critical period of speech readiness.

Much more frequently found than any of the kinds of problems we have described are those in which the children do have some useful language and can communicate to some extent, but where it is clear that marked emotional problems or linguistic deficits are present. Wood describes a hyperactive and possibly schizophrenic boy named Paul with various perceptual difficulties.

> Paul had developed speech, but failed to communicate ideas through speech. He usually talked at inappropriate times and on inappropriate subjects. He might begin with a specific idea, which he apparently wished to discuss, but his speech would wander away from the subject and he would include things which had occurred in the past, or objects which he had seen in his surroundings, or people's names which he seemed to remember suddenly. His conversation sounded something like this: "I saw a dog—ah—the chalk mama put to the desk—ah—on the picture pinned there—have you seen the car? My name is Paul. I am eight years old. Goodbye.[4]

Although this speech indicates some comprehension of the rules of the language; yet in the sentence "the chalk mama put *to* the desk," we note just one small indication of deficit. In the following description, we find the telegrammic speech of early language development. Many of the function words are absent. The British girl who spoke this passage was eight years old. Hers was a disorder of language, not of speech.

> I went to Reading. See, see bus. Long time. Went swimming. Mummy. Me. And the black man by. Mummy job. Down a stream. Quiet. Married. Long way. Very long way. Church. When I went there, fell I did. And I went soon, soon. Know her, she bride. Went to Reading, bus. Went to seaside. Not. Only next. Next. See the bridge. Way to holidays.[5]

Many children with delayed language are not so impaired, but the flavor of the telegram with its omitted words is always present. The syntax is limited. Some of these children have not mastered the use of question words, the appropriate pronouns, plurals, or the use of verb tense. Others can use noun or verb phrases, but fail to combine them into subject-predicate sentences. Here is a sample of the speech of a five-year-old boy who was denied entrance into kindergarten because of his language deficiency:

> Me go. [Pause.] Outdoor. Mama in car now. Firsty [thirsty]. Dink Tommy cup. No dink now. Go Mama now. Tommy bed. [Was he trying to tell us he was tired?] Car. Car now. Dink mama car now. [He wanted to go home.]

[4] N. Wood, *Delayed Speech and Language Development* (Englewood Cliffs, N.J.: Prentice-Hall, Inc., 1964), p. 109.

[5] C. E. Renfrew, "Speech Problems of Backward Children," *Speech Pathology and Therapy*, II (1959), 35.

Jenifer, a girl the same age as Tommy, spoke much better, but she too showed language difficulties. She was telling us what she was doing with our playhouse:

> Here the kitchen and stove is there and Jenny cook stove eggs for breakfast. Um and Jenny go sleep here by bed. See! Oooh, bathtub. Soap no um in in a bathtub? [Questioning inflection.] You get soap for wash feet? Me like bathtub. Spash [splash] on water all over.

The amount of language delay varies markedly from one child to another, and it is necessary to analyze both the comprehension and the production of speech if we are to help the child. If he has no words at all, we must help him gain these. If he has trouble distinguishing present from past tenses of verbs, or uses *me* instead of *I*, we work to facilitate his understanding of these differences. Each child presents his own unique set of language deficiencies.

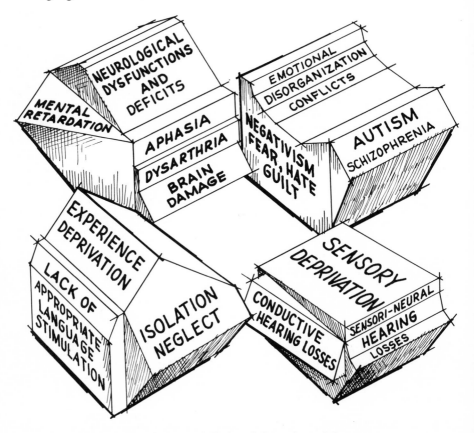

FIGURE 11: *Causes of Delayed Speech and Language.*

CAUSES OF DELAYED SPEECH AND LANGUAGE

The causes of delayed speech and language fall into four main categories: (1) sensory deprivation, such as that due to a hearing loss; this makes it very difficult for the child to scan the speech of those around him for the vocabulary and the linking rules he must acquire if he is to learn the language; (2) neurological dysfunctions or deficits, such as those shown in cerebral palsy, minimal brain damage, aphasia, and mental retardation; (3) emotional disorganization as illustrated by childhood schizophrenia, autism, or such milder problems as negativism; and (4) experience deprivation, wherein a child is raised under environmental circumstances that provide little opportunity for the learning of language and actively interfere with its mastery. It is very difficult to determine the actual cause of the delay in some of these children since our diagnostic instruments are crude, and several of these factors may be simultaneously present. As Menyuk says, "Even the application of a diagnostic label such as deaf, aphasic, mentally retarded, etc., does not guarantee that we have isolated the factors which have determined the child's lack of "linguistic behavior." [6]

Sensory Deprivation. Output must always follow input in the development of language. If a child cannot hear the words and sentences of his parents and playmates, or hears them distortedly and faintly, he will have a very hard time in acquiring his word tools and in deciphering the rules of the linguistic code that makes speech possible. Even adults who learned speech early and have used it adequately all their lives begin to find a decay in the precision and intelligibility of their utterance when they become deafened. Consonants become fuzzy, the vowels distorted. We need a monitoring ear to speak a language without abnormality. One can readily see how difficult it must be for the child who does not hear well. The sounds of speech may be faint or missing or unintelligible. It would be like learning to speak Chinese with your fingers in your ears. You might give up; you might even manage to learn a little, but it wouldn't be very good Chinese. Children who are born deaf seldom, if ever, acquire a normal voice or natural speech sounds despite the best of teaching. Some of them can master enough intelligible speech to get along.

However, not all children who have impaired hearing are deaf; some may merely have hearing losses. By hearing loss we mean that some usable hearing still exists. The person can hear certain sounds at a certain loudness level. He may hear some of what you say. He may be able to hear sounds

[6] P. Menyuk, *Sentences Children Use* (Cambridge, Mass.: M.I.T. Press, 1969), p. 13.

which are low in pitch yet fail to hear the high-frequency sounds. He may be able to hear pretty well by bone conduction, although when sounds come through the air they seem muffled and distorted.

There are two major kinds of hearing losses: conductive and perceptive. By the first, the conductive, we mean that the loss is caused by some defect in the outer or middle ear. There may be wax in the ear canal; there may be fixation of one of the tiny bone transmitters in the middle ear behind the eardrum. There are many possible reasons for conductive loss, but the important thing to remember is that the lower and middle frequency tones are usually heard as being more muffled or fainter than they should be. Children with conductive loss usually learn to speak, though a little retardation may occur. They often, however, show many severe articulation errors of substitution and omission.

The other type of hearing loss is perceptive. It may be due to an injured or malfunctioning cochlea in the inner ear, or to a damaged acoustic nerve, or to injury to the brain itself. Of the two types of hearing loss, this is usually the more serious for speech learning or maintenance, because it introduces distortion as well as muffling of sound. The reason for this is that the hearing loss is not equal for different frequencies of sound. Most children with perceptive loss have a harder time hearing the high-pitched sounds than they do those lower in pitch. Sounds such as *s, th, f, ch,* and *t* are some of the high-frequency sounds. If you had a perceptive loss, these would be faint or unheard at the same time that the vowels and the *m, n,* and a few other consonants would be quite loud enough. If you could not hear the announcer on the television because you had such a perceptive loss, turning up the volume wouldn't help you much because the low sounds would seem to be blasted out so much louder proportionally. The tiny high-pitched overtones would still be lost. A person with a high-frequency loss can never hear normal speech as it really is. What he is able to hear will be a distorted facsimile. Engineers have invented filters to cut out all the high-frequency sounds of speech. When we listen to recordings played through such filters, we are lucky to understand barely forty percent of what we hear, and even then we have to guess.

But even more important is the difficulty that children with auditory disorders experience in figuring out the structure of language itself. The child with normal hearing is provided with a wealth of speech samples from which he can find the combination rules that are acceptable; the deaf child is impoverished. However, even when taught very carefully in a highly favorable environment, the profoundly deaf child seldom seems able to overcome completely the handicap of his sensory deprivation. He is usually four or five years behind his hearing peers, even in the activity of silent reading. His written language is not only sparse but is characterized by many errors which show that he has not mastered the rules of the language, as evidenced by some sentences spoken by a boy who was about to graduate from high school and who had been deaf from birth:

> Which best game you played? Are you brave or coward? He hit you like bee's sting. Want to play bridge game? Don't park between this signs. Joe can one blow lick anybody. As well as I better leave now although there aren't any space left.

Deprived of the auditory experience of his own speech attempts and those of others, many children who do not hear often lose heart and make little effort to communicate except on the most primitive levels. Why try to talk when other people do not seem to understand? Why try to understand when others present only the picture of silent, moving lips. Confused and frustrated, they often retreat into a restricted, isolated as well as silent world. Finally, because these children have been severely limited in language growth and have had to rely primarily upon visual and tactual concepts, they tend to have great difficulty with abstractions. Their concepts tend to deal with the concrete. They have trouble with most relationships that cannot be seen or felt, and language involves many of these.

Neurological Dysfunctions and Deficits. Anyone who has ever viewed the impact of brain damage on an adult who has long been able to comprehend and speak normally and then suddenly becomes aphasic will have no trouble understanding that children who suffer such damage may also have difficulty in mastering the complexities of language.

Some children get off to a bad start on the road of life by having birth injuries. Others start well but fall victim to severe illnesses or accidents along the way. When the brain is damaged by any of these traumata, there is always the possibility of speech delay. If the central nervous system is damaged, we may find a general mental deficiency causing delay in most functions, but, in other instances, we may find instead the awkward coordinations of cerebral palsy or the inability to use meaningful symbols as in aphasia. In other injuries, a central hearing loss may be the result. There are also some less conspicuous aftermaths of brain damage—hyperactivity, irritability, inability to tolerate stress, perceptual difficulties—all of which may make it difficult for the child to learn to talk. To learn to speak, we must hear; we must be able to coordinate our muscles; we must be able to handle symbols; we must have good auditory perception. Brain injury can affect any or all of these items.

Dysarthria. This term refers to distorted speech caused by injuries of the central nervous system which make the coordinations needed for speech very difficult. Tongues may be clumsy; the lips may flutter tremulously, the jaw may fail to move on time or move sidewise; the larynx may be wrenched out of place; the chest may be expanding as in inhalation at the very time the child is trying to talk. The degree of involvement may be either widespread or almost hidden to all but the expert eye. We have worked with individuals whose only dysarthria was in the utterance of the tongue-tip sounds. Some cerebral palsied individuals find the task of coordination so difficult they never learn to speak.

Aphasia.   The term aphasia refers to the loss of speech, and so it may seem inappropriate to use it in children who have never developed speech. Some speech therapists prefer to use the term "developmental aphasia" instead. As we have seen in Chapter 2, aphasia refers to disorders of symbolization, to disorders of language rather than speech. It may include disabilities in reading, writing, gesturing, calculating, drawing, as well as in speaking. The basic problem revolves about the use of symbols. So far as speech is concerned, these children find difficulty in formulating their thoughts in words, in expressing them verbally, or in comprehending what others are saying. It's hard for them to send messages or, less frequently, to receive them. Formulating, expressing, comprehending, these are the functions which trouble the person who is aphasic. Some aphasic children have more difficulty with visual symbols; others, more trouble with symbols involving sounds. Some who cannot read (alexia) can write or copy the symbols they see on the printed page. Others can read but cannot write (agraphia). There are many varied disabilities lumped under the name of aphasia, but we hope that we have made our point—that aphasia refers to the difficulty in using symbols meaningfully; it is a disorder due to brain damage.

There is no doubt that aphasia can occur in children who have had speech and then lost it as a result of brain injury. We have worked with many such children. Here is one.

> Walter had been speaking very well, indeed much better than most children his age, when the automobile accident occurred on his fifth birthday. Thrown from the wrecked car, his head had struck a concrete abutment, and he was unconscious for over a week. When he was able to leave the hospital, he was almost mute although occasionally a snatch of jargon would pass his lips. He had difficulty recognizing his parents and sister but a gleam of recognition came when the family dog nuzzled him once they were home. His first word was "Tiber" which he used for the dog's name (which was Tiger). Even his gestures were confused at first. He shook his head sideways for yes and vertically for no. He had forgotten how to cut with the scissors or to hold a crayon. Emotionally, he now appeared very unstable. He cried a lot and had uncontrollable outbursts of temper. It was difficult for him to follow directions or to remember. Occasionally he would come out with swear words his parents had never heard him speak. Gradually the speech returned, aided by our patient tutoring and the parent counseling that was so necessary. At the present time, four years later,

he is speaking very well but has a marked reading, writing, and spelling disability.

There exists some argument among certain speech pathologists concerning the concept of congenital or developmental aphasia. These terms refer to disabilities in the *learning* of symbols or language as contrasted with the *loss* of ability previously learned which is what we find in true aphasia. Our own position, based upon our clinical experience, is that such congenital or developmental aphasias do exist. These aphasic children present different problems than those whose delay in speech is functional or due to mental retardation or hearing loss, although they may not become apparent until after some speaking has been learned. They may have gaps in their comprehension; intermittently appearing almost deaf; they may show inabilities in finding or uttering words which they have often used before. They confuse opposites, saying *hot* for *cold*; they use associated words instead of the ones they should use. One of our cases who could always name a chair when he saw its picture, could not say anything but "sit" when he desired to talk about it.

You want to sit down in that little chair?
Yes . . . No-no-no! Me want baby sit. . . .
You want the little chair?
No, no, no, no. Me no, no. Want baby bear, no, big man sit, sit down.

We gave him the big chair that he wanted and noted the repeated perseverations, the confusions of opposites, the use of the rhyming word *bear* for *chair* and, once more, the use of the action verb *sit* for the noun *chair*. We do not find this sort of thing when we teach the nonbrain-damaged child to talk.

The aphasic child also often shows difficulties in perception, not only of sounds but also visual forms. They may make a cross when trying to draw the square in front of them. They show inversals or reversals of letters and words: *d* for *b* or *p*; *tac* for *cat*. Sometimes they get them badly scrambled not only in writing but in speaking. One of our aphasic children kept saying his own name, Tommy, as "Ommty," and he called his father "Addad." The auditory memory span—the ability to retain sequences of sounds—is often very short. We must speak to such a child in short sentences and give him enough lag to let the meaning filter in. Some of these children get the necessary delay for comprehension by using echolalia, repeating exactly and automatically what others say to them until they can scan the meaning and respond appropriately. We also see them try out words silently, in pantomime, before speaking them, to make sure they are correct. They obviously hunt for words, and produce some which have a few odd articulation errors in them: *nap* for *cap* or *chig* for *pig*. At times in the middle of very clear speech a single jargon word will appear: "I plush my eraser in school." (He meant "lost.") The aphasic child often shows a telegrammic form of speech, omitting all the little words. "Tuck [truck] go fall hill down boom." Prepositions such as *under* or *in* or *of* seem to be very difficult, no doubt because they are abstractions involving relationships.

Wood has a good passage which testifies to this confusion:

> If one word were selected to describe children with aphasia that word would be *confused*. Dennis was a good example of this particular kind of confusion. He was unable to follow simple commands or directions, unable to match colors, unable to assemble puzzles or form boards adequately, unable to sort objects into common groups, and generally unable to perform adequately on any task which required organization. Dennis was distractable on many occasions, particularly when unpredicted movements or light changes occurred. On rare occasions he seemed to respond to sounds in his environment, but these responses were inconsistent and infrequent. Either his expression was one of questioning, with furrowed brows and an intense look, or, completely to the contrary, his expression might be totally blank, as if a veil had dropped between him and all that surrounded him. He had periodic temper tantrums, frequently unrelated to any of the activities which were going on about him at the time. His temper tantrums and emotional outbursts seemed to be related to his inability to communicate and to his general disorganization. He gave the impression that he knew what he wanted to do and what he wanted to say, but that he was at a total loss to find his way out of the communicative maze he was in, all of which increased his confusion and disorganization.[7]

When we examine these children we find a wide range of behaviors and deficits. Dennis, in the passage above, is far from typical. We tried to find from our own case records an example which would be more representative, but we could not. The variation is just too great. Wood's impressions of Dennis are useful primarily because they show clearly how hard it would be for a confused and disorganized child to learn his language. Or perhaps "unorganized" would be a better adjective since, to a large degree, it is through our ability to use language that we organize the reality about us.

The Minimally Brain-Damaged Child.   There are some children who have no history of cerebral injury nor any discernible neurologic signs

---

[7] N. E. Wood, *Delayed Speech and Language Development* (Englewood Cliffs, N.J.: Prentice-Hall, Inc., 1964), pp. 112–13.

that indicate brain pathology and yet who show many of the same behaviors and difficulties in acquiring language which the aphasic children
demonstrate. No truly satisfactory term for them has yet been accepted,
but generally they are classified as "brain-injured," "perceptually handicapped," "minimally brain-damaged" children. The diagnosis is based upon
an analysis of the child's behavior rather than upon electroencephalo-
graphic examination or any of the other methods used by neurologists to
reveal true impairment. These children do not seem to have hearing
losses; they are not mentally retarded; they do not resemble the emotionally disturbed. Their labeling and their diagnosis is therefore based
upon inference and presumption; but since these children exist and present
real problems to parents and teachers, some term to classify them had to
be found.

This is the general picture they present: (1) they clearly have an
inadequate ability to regulate or control themselves, as shown by hyperactivity, great distractability, perseveration, violent shifts in emotionality,
incoordination, and impulsivity. (2) They show an inadequacy in being
able to integrate sensory information as demonstrated by perceptual difficulties involving awareness, discrimination, figure-ground relationships,
sequencing, retention and recall, and many other similar deficits. They also
show difficulties in forming concepts, in categorizing and classifying, in
handling abstractions. (3) They have disturbed self-concepts and disturbances in laterality and in self-identification. They have small tolerance
for frustration, little sense of past or future. They are often controlling,
negativistic, and very hard to live with, for they do not perceive the needs
of others. They do not relate well.

Not all these children fail to acquire language, but it should be
obvious from their characteristics that they do so with difficulty; and some
of those who do learn to speak continue to show marked disability later
on when faced with the other language skills of reading and writing. There
are also some whose lack of self-control, inability to integrate, or inadequate
sense of self are just too overwhelming to enable them to learn the language system. Perhaps the many frustrations experienced by an intelligent
brain-damaged child who tries to live meaningfully in a world full of
words often make him seem hyperactive and excessively irritable. In
working with these children you often have to do speech therapy on the
wing. They are squirrelly, on the move constantly. It's hard for them to sit
still, to concentrate, to be patient. Their frustration tolerance may be
abnormally low, but we suspect it is only that they are overloaded with
frustration. Occasionally they may go beserk, and show what in the adult
aphasic is termed the "catastrophic response." One such boy, who had been
working at his table quietly, suddenly began to scream, ran around wildly,
tearing his clothes and shuddering. It was not a seizure. We held him

firmly but soothingly for a while until he calmed; then he went back to his work. If these children find it harder to inhibit emotional displays than the normal child, we must understand and help.

Can they be taught to talk? Or read or write, or understand speech? We feel that the answer is yes, although we have had enough failures with some children to say the word hesitantly. It's so hard to get through to a child who cannot talk, who sometimes cannot understand. Somehow it's harder for a therapist to remember his successes than his failures. Perhaps the best way to put it is to say that many of these children can be taught to talk and do all the other things if given the proper help at the proper time.

Emotional Problems. All of us have difficulty putting our deepest emotions into words, and perhaps only the poet manages to do so. Some unfortunate children experience almost constant storms of emotion, and it is easy to understand why they would have trouble learning to talk. When we speak we enter into a relationship with our listener; if most of our unpleasant emotions center in that listener, we find it hard to talk to him. Emotionally disturbed children cannot find the words to express the surges of unpleasantness that flood their beings. Perhaps their private world of protective fantasy has few words in it. When there are no words for communicating the incommunicable and when one fears or hates his listeners, why try to speak the unspeakable?

The range of problems encountered in this category is wide. In it we find children who are psychotic or autistic at one extreme, and children who are emotionally immature or negative at the other. They do not learn to talk because, perhaps, they fear the communicative relationships which speaking demands or because their flood of inner emotional static prevents them from hearing the models they need. Some of these children live in a world of their own. Others find their *lack* of speech a powerful tool for controlling others. There are children who find the awaiting world of adult life too unpleasant a prospect after they hear their parents screaming at each other, and so they prefer to remain infants all their days. What better way than to refuse to talk? Why should a child wish to put something into his mouth if it is unpleasant or painful? Why should a child speak if speaking puts him in contact with someone he fears or hates? Speaking is revealing; there are children who cannot bear the exposure.

Childhood Schizophrenia. The child with this type of mental illness may show normal language development until the ages of two or three and probably does not belong in the category of delayed language. However, he is truly delayed in using the language competence he has achieved to communicate and relate to others. When overheard, the verbalizations are bizarre. Here is one sample:

Big train . . . under bed . . . [screams]. . . . I eat um up . . . and go toidy [toilet] . . . hurt hurt . . . [screams] . . . choo-choo-choo-choo . . . was dirty . . . I big house . . . green house and red and black and blue and . . . Mama, you go bed now.

All of this speech was uttered while playing with a truck on the floor. These children live in a private world, one often full of terrors perhaps, but yet better than the intolerable world of reality.

Rubin, Bar, and Dwyer give this account of another case:

An older girl, with excellent language but poor articulation, which she wasn't interested in modifying, was preoccupied by birds. The clinician here had not only to restrict the topic to feathered creatures but to enter actively into the girl's fantasies about birds before she cooperated eagerly with his attempts to improve her articulation.

This concentration upon certain restricted language themes is characteristic of this population when they do talk to other people.[8]

Some of them show very little verbal output. They are so mute that they often are thought to be deaf. Mykelbust feels that this mutism is one of the key signs of emotional disorder.[9] Their refusal to speak is compulsive rather than voluntary. In the histories of some of our cases of delayed speech we find that at one time they had begun to talk not only in single words but also in kernel sentences. Then something happened, a shock, an accident, a frightening experience, a separation from the mother, a stay at the hospital—and the child stopped talking.

Austra was a Latvian girl of seven who had experienced many of the terrors of displacement and bombing raids. She came to us two years after her father had finally managed to get to the safety of the United States. Her mother and brother and two sisters had been killed. Austra seemed to comprehend everything we said to her and her performance on the Wechsler Intelligence Test was superior but she talked only in grunts and gestures. The father told us that she had spoken very well until the age of three. She seemed to be a very happy child. Her father put the matter succinctly: "Austra has forgotten, but her mouth remembers." It took a lot of doing, but Austra learned to talk and is now in college.

[8] H. Rubin, A. Bar, and J. H. Dwyer, "An Experimental Speech and Language Program for Psychotic Children," *Journal of Speech and Hearing Disorders*, XXXII (1967), 242–48.

[9] H. Mykelbust, *Auditory Disorders in Children* (New York: Grune and Stratton, 1954).

Autism. The schizophrenic child often talks more to himself than to other people, but will communicate with them at times, though his speech often reflects his obsessions. The autistic child—a very strange child—resists verbal interaction with others. He won't answer questions and he rarely asks one. If he does reply to a demand it is a perfunctory reply, often an exact but monotonous repetition of what was said to him, and often it appears three or four minutes afterward. Although, according to Rimland, whose work is the classic on the subject, about half of all autistic children are mutes and remains so all their lives, we personally have been able to evoke considerable speech from some of them.[10] It is strange speech, full of exotic words at times, or unusual metaphors, sometimes interspersed with odd snatches of singing. But what strikes the observer especially is that the speech sounds dead, lifeless. There is no emotion or inflection in it. Here is a picture of one who spoke very little until treated:

> When we first saw Kipper, his parents' presenting complaints were that "he can't pay attention," has "no speech," shows "inconsistent hearing" and "other unusual behavior." In particular, his unusual behavior consisted of periods of "finger flicking" (strumming the index or small fingers of his left hand with the index finger or four fingers of his right hand), and periods of sitting very still and "staring off at something."
>
> He was essentially unresponsive and inactive during our initial evaluation. He sat where placed without moving. He showed no response to his name. When eye contact could be achieved, his face remained expressionless ("mask-like"), giving the impression of a "blank stare." He was heard to utter only a few random sounds. When tickled he made only a slight flinching movement. As far as could be determined, he showed no response to auditory stimuli or social reinforcers.[11]

The autistic child is a strange child, and he is sometimes very intelligent. It almost seems as though he is too hypersensitive to be able to bear the barrage of stimulation in which our children must live. Alexander Pope once wrote of the sensitive soul who "dies of a rose in aromatic pain." Autistic children are threatened by too much noise (and even a little noise is too much), too much color, too much movement, too many people— and sometimes even one parent is too much. They build walls around themselves, barriers to stimulation. Some of them do not seem to hear because they refuse to listen. Some of them sing the same little nameless tune over and over again to mask out the sounds and speech that can over-

---

[10] B. Rimland, *Infantile Autism* (New York: Appleton-Century-Crofts, 1964).

[11] R. Schell, E. J. Stark, and J. J. Giddon, "Development of Language Behavior in an Autistic Child," *Journal of Speech and Hearing Disorders*, XXXIII (1968), 42–47.

whelm them. Certain autistic youngsters concentrate on puzzles or mathematic manipulations to keep the world's fingers out of their lives. They may rock back and forth interminably to keep everything the same. Some of them do not talk at all or talk to themselves in a strange tongue. Other autistic children will talk a little, and even answer questions, but always in a detached and perfunctory fashion with a minimum of meaning and little feeling. They are strange children, not of this world. We have worked successfully with a few of them and have failed with more than a few. They require time and devotion which few of us can afford.

Negativism. Our culture demands much of its young. At the very time that the child is learning to talk, a hundred other demands are put upon him. He must learn how to eat at the table, how to control his bowels, how to be quiet, how to pick up his toys, how to behave himself. And this is the age at which we find out that we are *selves*, not objects, that we are important in our own right. This is the "bull-headed" obstinate age, when the child learns how to say that favorite word of his parents: "No!" There are children who fiercely resist the constant pressure to conform, who fight a gallant but losing battle against incredible odds. And there are a few children who actually win, by discovering the one way they can refuse and get away with it. They refuse to talk.

You can't make a horse drink. You can't make a child talk. The tenacity with which some children resist their parents' efforts to eliminate thumb-sucking is minor compared to that shown by some children who triumph by not speaking. It's a tough problem to handle, once it has existed for a few years. At times the negativism is widespread; often it seems to be focused on speech alone. First, we must convince the parents and associates of the child to stop making the usual demands that he say this and say that, and inhibit their complaining expressions of anxiety. We must remove the rewards which negativism brings. Here is one brief account of a child who had but one word in his vocabulary.

> The teacher said to the child in a rather peremptory tone, "Johnny, you go down to the drugstore this very minute and get yourself an ice-cream cone!" The child answered "No" and the teacher asked another child, who accepted and returned to eat the ice-cream cone under Johnny's regretful nose. Such a program soon brought a discriminatory answer to requests and commands, and when reward for positive response was added, together with humorous attitudes toward the negativism, the child's whole attitude changed, and his speech soon became normal.

Many of these children profit from a change in environment—placement in a nursery school—where they can learn from other children that speaking can be more pleasant than refusing to speak.

If we are to summarize these observations about the role of emotional disorders in the delay of language and speech, we would say first of all that most unpleasant emotionality involves human relationships. Communication also involves these relationships and it therefore is dependent upon them. If the very young child is immersed in negative emotion, he will have little inclination to learn language. If he is older when reality becomes unbearable to him, he will not use language enough to realize its fullest potentials.[12]

Experience Deprivation.   Some children are born into homes where conditions are unfavorable to speech development. There are silent homes where the parents rarely talk to each other. There are homes so confused with the noise and distraction of other children that the harried mother has no time to create the relationship out of which speech comes. Sick children are slow to talk, and there are sick homes too. Some children hear little but angry speech. One of our cases, who had lived with his grandmother, stopped talking when he was returned to his real parents, who were deaf-mutes. Often we have seen speech decay and disappear when an orphan child was shuffled from one foster home to another. When two languages are spoken in a home, one by the older children and the other by the parents, some children get too confused to talk.

If a child is to talk there must be some identification with the parent. We knew one little girl whose mother was a drunkard with whom no child could identify as she staggered around the house, dirty, cursing, and in half collapse. We have worked with children too hungry, too weak or tired to talk, and had to take care of these basic needs before they had a chance to learn. The county sheriff once brought us three almost-wild children from a hut in a swamp only a few miles from Kalamazoo. The father was a feeble-minded junk scavenger who fed them when he could. The mother had abandoned them. The tale is too incredible to put in a textbook, but those three nonspeaking children in the observation room were animal children. Yes, there are environmental conditions which prevent speech development.

Most of the research has clearly demonstrated that some children from the lower socioeconomic classes are delayed in language skills. As Bereiter and Engelmann show in their review, preschool-aged children from this sort of environment are deficient in vocabulary, sentence length, and complexity of grammatical structure.[13] In such life situations, there is often crowding, competing noise, and little time for a parent to give

[12] See G. L. Wyatt, *Language Learning and Communication Disorders in Children* (New York: Free Press, 1969).

[13] C. Bereiter, and S. Engelmann, *Teaching Disadvantaged Children in the Preschool* (Englewood Cliffs, N.J.: Prentice-Hall, Inc., 1966).

the sort of language stimulation that facilitates learning. Raph points up another obstacle:

> The culturally privileged child learns early that sentences are made up of words so that he imitates the noises that occur *within* words, but not the noises that occur *between* familiar words. Since he understands the single words he begins to use, he can then expand them into other combinations. The culturally deprived child, in contrast, tends to approximate the whole sequence of noises. Because of his lack of experience with verbally mature adults, his first words are likely to be composed of meaningless syllables which only vaguely resemble words and inflections he has heard, but does not understand. These sounds he uses lack distinctive parts he can use and recombine into new sentences. In part, the deprived child cannot understand a sentence that he is expected to imitate or repeat; and in part, since he cannot imitate or repeat it, this prevents him from learning to understand it.[14]

It should be made clear, however, that a gross injustice has been done to such ethnic groups as the black American, the Spanish-speaking American, and American Indian minorities by stating that they are linguistically delayed merely because they do not follow the grammatical standards of upper or middle-class American usage. These children usually possess a competence in their own variant of English which is quite as adequate as that of their other classmates, even though they may speak differently. For example, as Baratz has pointed out, the sentence spoken by a Negro child, "They don't have none" instead of "They don't have any" does not reflect linguistic incompetence but the standard usage of his community.[15] When such a child says, "He there" instead of "He is there," he is not violating the rules of the language spoken by his associates. Baratz's article is a healthy antidote for those who judge linguistic competence in terms of the upper-class white American standard.

TREATMENT OF DELAYED LANGUAGE AND SPEECH

As we have seen, these children with delayed language and speech present a wide range of problems. In helping them, we cannot prescribe a specific treatment plan which would be suitable for all of them. The

---

[14] J. B. Raph, "Language and Speech Deficits in Culturally Disadvantaged Children: Implications for the Speech Clinician," *Journal of Speech and Hearing Disorders,* XXXII (1967), 203–14.

[15] J. C. Baratz, "Language and Cognitive Assessments of Negro Children: Assumptions and Research Needs," *Asha,* XI (1969), 87–91.

medical model of disease is completely inappropriate here. If a child has diabetes, we can give him insulin and change his diet; if he has worms, a purgative will rid him of the parasites; but if a child has not managed to learn his language, we must try to determine the reasons for the delay, ascertain the particular deficits he shows, and then work out procedures that can help him to master this most difficult of all human achievements.

The Child Who Does Not Talk At All.   Among this population of children retarded in language development we find some who do not attempt to speak. They are essentially without language as we know it, although their gestures, grunts, jargon, and even screams may serve as a primitive means for expressing crude meanings. In this group we find mentally retarded, emotionally disturbed, autistic, deaf, and negative individuals; and our clinical problem is first to elicit some kind of consistent utterance. If this seems to be an insurmountable obstacle, let us say that we have not found it so; and a scrutiny of some of the case reports in our professional journals will bear us out. Rubin, Bar, and Dwyer, for example, provide this account:

> This boy produced nothing resembling our language and appeared disinterested in vocalizing until the clinician began to stimulate him with patterned babbling and repetitive sound-making. The child responded with similar activity and in a few months progressed to echoing behavior and subsequently to single words.[16]

Adams tells of a nonspeaking child who had spent eighteen of his first twenty-four months in a state school for the mentally retarded. Until he was seen by the clinician, there was no sign that he had developed any speech or gestures for communicating. Adams described her program and its results:

> This program consisted of two parts: (1) direct contact with him; and (2) counseling and demonstration for his grandparents, who lived in the area and visited him daily, and for the nurses caring for him. Therapy consisted of daily one or two hour sessions with him during which I emphasized names of common objects, demonstrated and labeled their uses, and gave him directions involving these objects. In addition, Gary was introduced to toys, books, noises, and other experiences available on a hospital ward. Nurses, patients, and visitors on the ward took an interest in him and attempted to follow through with similar activities for speech stimulation during the day.
>
> Within a week, Gary showed an increase in vocalization, and he seemed to recall previous activities and to become increasingly inter-

[16] "An Experimental Speech and Language Program," *op. cit.*, p. 246.

ested in new things. "Speech-like" movements of the tongue and lips, without sounds, were noted during the second week. By the end of the month he began imitating me in saying words with an initial bilabial consonant and vowel. His use of single words increased during the next two weeks, and at the time of his discharge from the hospital Gary consistently used approximation of at least seven words (hat, ball, book, and others). He sometimes accompanied his vocalizations with gestures and showed growth in recognition vocabulary and in his ability to follow verbal directions. His progress seemed to follow typical developmental patterns.[17]

The Operant Conditioning Approach.   Another approach has been to use operant conditioning procedures. The basic program consists of providing immediate reinforcement contingent upon vocalization and giving it consistently until the amount of vocalization shows an increase. Gestures are not reinforced. At times we must even return to a more primitive level of interaction, giving the reinforcement only when the child looks at us. Mild punishment or the withholding of reinforcement is applied when the child resorts to temper tantrums or other behaviors which make speech impossible. Once vocalization is achieved, the reinforcement is given only when some approximation to normal speech has been produced. The therapist may aid the child by providing prompts or aids by shaping his mouth with her fingers or other means, but these are gradually faded out as the vocalization comes more and more to resemble the utterance of single words. It is sometimes necessary to train the child to imitate before speech training is begun. Thus, contingent reinforcement may be given for any imitative behavior—for imitative bodily movements and postures to duplicative speech attempts.

Lovaas describes one such program consisting of a sequence of steps. In Step One the child was reinforced for all vocalization. Then when he was making more vocalization about every five seconds and watching the therapist's mouth more than half of the time, Step Two of the program was begun. In this step, the therapist (or parent) said a word once every ten seconds, and the child got his reinforcement only if he made some kind of vocalization shortly afterward. When this behavior increased to a substantial level, then Step Three was introduced. In this step, the child only got the reinforcement when he was able to match the adult's utterance. This was usually fairly simple and consisted of isolated sounds or syllables which were easily seen and could be facilitated by manipulating the child's mouth; or they were sounds the child had uttered before. When this was accomplished, Step Four was initiated, and this was followed by

[17] J. Adams, "Delayed Language Development," *Journal of Speech and Hearing Disorders*, XXXIV (1969), 170.

other steps which introduced new sounds and words and phrases according to the basic methods of reinforcement used in Step Three. This account illustrates the practices used by most of those who have attempted to get a nonspeaking child to talk through operant conditioning, though, of course, different children require different programs.[18]

They also require different reinforcers. Sloane, Johnson, and Harris describe some of these reinforcers as follows:

> A great variety of reinforcers were used, based upon what "worked." When a reinforcer no longer "worked," new ones were tried until something was found that seemed to exert control. Some children received one of their regular meals as a reinforcer; that is, the ordinary meal was delivered in small spoonfuls contingent upon appropriate responding. Other edible reinforcers used were candies (M & M's, Pez, Neccos), spoonfuls of sherbet or ice cream, small marshmallows, bits of graham cracker, milk, soda pop, water, pieces of dry cereal (especially sugar-coated cereals), and raisins.[19]

Some children respond to less tangible rewards—to social reinforcers such as praise or a smile of approval. Some will work hard to get tokens such as poker chips, which can be exchanged for opportunities to escape or to play or to use preferred toys for a time. It is usually wise to pair the clinician's approval with a primary reinforcer such as the candy so that the smile or "good boy" may later become effective controls. It is also important that the scheduling of these reinforcements be shifted from a consistent schedule—a marshmallow everytime he responds appropriately —to an intermittent or partial reinforcement schedule as soon as this can be done, if rapid extinction is to be prevented.

Hewett describes a rather drastic way of reinforcing an autistic child, although it is one which saddens us.

> Candy, however, would not control Peter's behavior. He was highly distractable, and his attention could only be engaged for brief periods with the promise of a candy reward. In an effort to reduce extraneous stimuli to a minimum and to introduce negative reinforcements as a lever for establishment of control, a special teaching booth was constructed for Peter. The booth was divided into two sections, joined by

[18] O. I. Lovaas, "A Program for the Establishment of Speech in Psychotic Children," Chapter 7 of H. N. Sloans and B. D. Macaulay, eds., *Operant Procedures in Remedial Speech and Language Training* (Boston: Houghton Mifflin Company, 1968).

[19] H. N. Sloane, M. K. Johnston, and F. H. Harris, "Remedial Procedures for Teaching Verbal Behavior to Speech Deficient or Defective Young Children," Chapter 5 of H. N. Sloane and B. D. Macaulay, eds., *Operant Procedures in Remedial Speech and Language Training* (Boston: Houghton Mifflin Company, 1968), p. 84.

a movable shutter ($2 \times 2\frac{1}{2}$ feet) which could be raised and lowered by the teacher. The teacher occupied one-half of the booth and Peter the other half. Each section of the booth was four feet wide, three and one-half feet in length, and seven feet high. The only source of light came from the teacher's side and was provided by two spotlights which were directed on the teacher's face. When the shutter was down, Peter's side of the booth was dark. When it was raised, light from the teacher's side flooded through the opening and illuminated a shelf in front of Peter. To the left of the shelf was a ball-drop device with a dim light directly above it. This device consisted of a box into which a small wooden ball could be dropped. The ball rang a bell as it dropped into the box and was held inside the box until released by the teacher. When released, the ball rolled out into a cup at the bottom of the box where it could be picked up. This ball-drop device was Peter's "key" for opening the shutter. When the ball was released into the cup, he picked it up and dropped it into the box. At the sound of the bell, the teacher raised the shutter and initiated contact between the two of them.

In this setting the teacher not only provided candy and light as positive reinforcers but also used music, a ride on a revolving chair, color cartoon movies, and a Bingo number-matching game which Peter liked. Isolation and darkness served as negative reinforcers and were administered when Peter failed to respond appropriately within a five-second period. Pilot trials with Peter and four other autistic children revealed the positive reinforcers to be effective in varying degrees and that all subjects would "work" to avoid isolation and darkness.[20] We personally do not use this kind of therapy.

Motivation Problems.   We have seen how the provision of contingent reinforcement is used to elicit vocalization that can then be shaped to produce the first imitation of words. Unless there is some need to talk, these children will not try to talk. They manage to get along without it, using gestures to supplement their grunts or garbled utterance. We might say that they have taught their parents or older siblings to understand their own primitive language. We have seen mothers aching and struggling to understand, trying desperately to translate the sounds and movements of such a child. Too often they succeed, thereby rewarding and reinforcing the garbled jargon or sign language.

Again, most of these parents have done much drilling, made many demands for display speech, asked for names, commanded utterance. "Say this and say that!" Their children, having a long history of failure in trying to please, give up. Attempting to speak has become unpleasant. There have

[20] F. M. Hewett, "Teaching Speech to an Autistic Child Through Operant Conditioning," *American Journal of Orthopsychiatry*, XXXV (1965), 929.

been too many such sessions ending in tears of reproach or frustration. Attempting to speak has become punishing.

Creating a Need to Communicate Verbally. Some of our delayed-speech children already have accomplished this aim. They cannot refrain from jabbering. But there are many others who have not realized how important and how satisfying a tool speech can be for manipulating their elders and satisfying their desires. They simply don't think that learning to talk is worth the trouble. They find it possible to get along without verbal communication. Pantomime and gesture are sufficient for a child in a home where everyone else tries to learn *his* language instead of the reverse. Parrots and myna birds have little incentive to talk, either, until their trainers pay some attention to motivation.

Another technique which creates a need to talk is to have the parent or therapist do a lot of self-talk, commenting on what they see or do. A sample of this running commentary is as follows:

> Mummy do dishes now. Wash cup . . . put cup here . . . Where glass? Oh, here glass . . . Glass dirty . . . Now glass soapy . . . Wash . . . Jerry wipe . . . Towel . . . Rub, rub . . . Glass clean . . . Glass on shelf . . .

If some of this simplified self-talk is done several times each day, the child who watches will begin to participate, first silently with inner speech and later aloud.

It is important in the speech therapy sessions that the therapist talk in this abbreviated way. Often in the first meetings it is wise to do as little talking as possible. Try to get down on the child's own level of nonverbal, gestural communication, then accompany gestures with single words, and then go to these brief phrases and sentences. The constant flow of adult speech is so fluent and complicated that most delayed-speech children feel it is too difficult to achieve. Once it is simplified it seems easier and within his reach. For the same purpose we should cut down on the amount of reading to the child that parents do. Its fluency provides an almost unobtainable goal. We have had several cases in which the elimination of oral reading by itself created the climate productive of spontaneous speech attempts.

In our own attempts to help these children who have no speech, we rarely begin with the operant approach, though we use contingent reinforcement later on when the child has shown a real desire to communicate and has started doing so. Instead, we try hard to establish the sort of relationship with a child that will make him desire to talk. We feel that most of them have already experienced altogether too many demands for utterance and for repeating what the parents have said. We are not interested in procuring parrot-like utterances that are not meaningful and then hoping later to attach some meaning to them. We have tried the operant approach, got our baselines, applied contingent reinforcements, and shaped the responses into something resembling words; but the results were far less satisfactory than when we created a real need for speech and provided simplified models in a hierarchy of developmental steps.

Here is a portion of a letter from a mother's report, which will illustrate some of the early procedures: [21]

> I did what you told us several times today, and even though it made me feel silly to be making animal noises and nonsense sounds, I could see that Timmy was enjoying it. I'd say "Bubba-bubba," give him a quick hug and then run off into the kitchen. Sure surprised him the first few times. Then I'd waggle my tongue up and down in the bathroom mirror while he was watching and say "lalalalalala." Also, when I heard him making sounds when he was playing on the floor, I'd go over there and make them too. Once when he was pounding with a spoon on the frying pan, I made some other sounds first and then said "Bang-bang" and he imitated me, I think. Finally we got to making faces at each other with sounds attached to the faces. There was a kind of back and forth talking in it, although he didn't say any real words. I've had to hold myself back to keep from asking him to say what I say, though.

However, we must do more than this. Speech must be made pleasant, it is true, but we must not forget that the child's jargon and gestural communication must be freed from its reinforcement. We knew one silly mother who had starved her boy for two days by insisting that he say the name of any food he wanted. And that he say it right! She came to us in tears, and we told her instead to pretend to misunderstand some of the boy's jargon when she really knew what he wanted, then aloud to try to guess what he was trying to say, and finally to say something like this: "Oh, you mean 'ball,' OK ball, here ball!" We asked her to put this delay and fumbling attempts at translation between his utterance and her fulfillment of his desire several times a day and gradually to increase the dosage. Children want what they want when they want it. The use of judicious delay, coupled with gradual translation into standard but simple English, will soon produce a real hunger to speak better.

Teaching the Child to Imitate. As in teaching the normal baby to talk, it is important that parents and therapists encourage all types of

[21] For an interesting account of how a clinician helped two children develop speech and language along these lines, see the article by J. N. Blake, "A Therapeutic Construct for Two Seven-Year-Old Nonverbal Boys," *Journal of Speech and Hearing Disorders,* XXXIV (1969), 363–69.

imitative behavior. We must identify with the child before he can identify with us. Accordingly, much of the early training of a child with delayed speech consists of sessions in which the parent or therapist shares the child's activities. If he scribbles, we scribble. If he explores the bottom drawer, we join him. If he hides under the table, under it we go. If he grunts, we grunt too.

Sooner or later he will engage in repetitive activities such as banging a pan on the floor, clapping hands, bouncing up and down. By interrupting these activities by our own performance of them, he will usually return to the same behavior with renewed zest. This means that he is actually duplicating our behavior as well as his own. It is the beginning of imitation. Soon we can be playing follow-the-leader in many ways, and he may occasionally enjoy being the follower. If such teaching of imitation in physical behavior is made very pleasant, it will soon generalize to speech behavior; and the child will enjoy imitating our speech. Most children respond to such play very swiftly.

Perhaps the following instructions that we gave to a student clinician who was about to begin working with a child with little speech will be illustrative:

> Most parents attempt to get a child to begin speaking by asking him questions. It has been our experience that this is not an effective procedure. Questions are demands. They immediately place the child in a subservient role, with the questioner in the position of power. Even when the child responds appropriately, the resulting relationship is one which immediately puts the questioner into the same category with other authority figures who have been controllers, a relationship which often regenerates the conflicts the child has previously experienced in threatening communication. If you ask what something is called and the child cooperates, he must either think that you must be stupid not to know its name or that you suspect he doesn't know it (which implies stupidity), or that you just want him to do a little verbal dance for your pleasure. If the therapist is to avoid these conflicts, he should seek other gambits for evoking communication.

> Moreover, eliciting speech by questions often yields very impoverished samples. At best, you'll just get a vocabulary item, not a good speech sample. Or, if you ask him a yes-no question, you'll get a yes or no answer, often the latter. Like a marriage, we do not feel that a therapeutic relationship should start with an invitation to say no. If the question is more elaborate ("What did you have for breakfast this morning?" "What did you do in school today?") the child has probably forgotten or finds it difficult to formulate, or feels that it's none of your business anyway. Especially with children for whom the acquisition of normal speech has been no easy accomplishment, any question

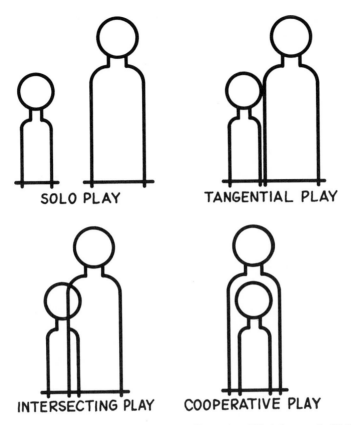

SOLO PLAY

TANGENTIAL PLAY

INTERSECTING PLAY

COOPERATIVE PLAY

FIGURE 12: *Diagram of Interaction Between Clinician and Child.*

tends to pose some threat. They have been bedeviled by too many questions from too many questioners, and when they have answered, their listeners have not always understood them or have rejected them. For these children the interrogative inflection is almost as potent a signal as the tone that makes the rat jump in expectation of shock.

How then should one begin? We suggest that you should simply greet the child, then do some simple *self-talk*, commenting on what you are doing, or perceiving, and with plenty of moments of comfortable silence interspersed, until you have him playing with his box of toys. And then, in the role of the adult playmate, you can play with those in your own box. Silently at first. No question. No demands. *Solo play!*

Once the child is comfortable in this activity, you should begin to put some self-talk into your own solo play; first noises (those of trucks, animals, etc.), then single words, then short phrases and simple sentences. All of these refer to what you are experiencing at the moment. Usually the child will begin to follow suit. His noises, his self-talk begin to flow. Next you should shift to contact play very gradually. Let your toy truck occasionally touch his fire-engine, or help him find a block, or put another one on his toppling pile, or straighten it up a bit so he can make it higher. When you feel the time is ripe in this *tangential contact play*, begin to accompany it with some noises or commentary, using *parallel talking*, telling him what he is doing, perceiving, or feeling, again making sure that you have more silence than speech.

From tangential play, you can often proceed rapidly to *intersecting play* in which your activity becomes a part of his. (Let your truck go over the bridge he has built or feed your doll or toy dog a piece of the play fruit he has put on the playhouse table.) Verbalize what you are doing. Next, seek to achieve *cooperative play*, assisting him to do the things he is doing. (Have your truck bring to him the blocks he needs to build his tower.) Usually by this time the child is speaking very easily and often copiously, your own verbalizations being primarily confined to reflecting what he has said. From this point onward, the communication can proceed fairly normally and naturally.

We hope we have not given the impression that this process is too time-consuming. Often we can accomplish all the progressive interaction in a single session and build a very warm communicative relationship in less than an hour. There are, of course, many children for whom so careful an approach may not be vitally necessary, children who have learned that big people always seem to have to ask stupid questions, children who are willing to dance when the interrogative strings are pulled, children who relate easily. Yet even with these children this approach seems to work very well. The relationship established is less superficial, more solid, more satisfying. We do not meet with as many moments of resistance or negativism later on in therapy.

Jargon.   Many children with delayed speech and language are not at all silent. Indeed, some of them jabber incessantly, using a completely incomprehensible jargon. Others may say many recognizable words, but only when echoing in a parrotlike way what has been said to them; and the words they emit have no more meaning than words uttered by the bird. Still others, as we have seen earlier, have developed a highly communicative system of gestures, most of which are accompanied by attention-getting grunts or meaningless sounds. Our task here is different from what it is with children who do not respond at all.

One of the basic reasons children remain fixed at the jargon level is that the models provided them by their parents and associates are far too complex to be matched. The child attempts to talk like the big people do. They jabber incessantly and so does he. We must therefore provide very simple models if we hope to have him change. With some cases we may speak only in single words for a long time. With others we can use simple phrases.

Self-talk and Parallel Talk. The speech models should have more than simplicity; they must also have utility. No child will ever learn to talk unless he sees that it is a useful tool. The way we teach him this lesson is through *self-talk* and parallel talk. By self-talk we mean that we talk aloud to ourselves, verbalizing what we are seeing, hearing, doing, or feeling. Here are some samples of a mother's self-talk and parallel talk.

> Where cup? Oh, I see cup. Cup on table. Here cup. . . . Milk in cup. . . . Mummy drink milk. . . . Johnny want cup? . . . OK . . . Johnny drink. . . . Milk all gone. . . . Give Mummy cup. . . . Mummy wash cup. . . . Here water. . . . Here soap. . . . Give cup bath. . . . All clean. . . . Where towel? . . . Here towel. . . . Wipe, wipe. . . . Give Johnny cup. . . . Put on table. . . . Johnny good boy.

This child was only making a few vowels, grunts, and gestures at the time but he was alert and interested. Note the mother's simple speech, within reach of the child's ability. Note the commentary accompanying what she did or saw. Note the recall and prediction. Here there is no demand for display speech. Here is self-talk used as verbalized thinking. It wasn't long before the boy was talking to himself too. Mothers and speech therapists must learn to talk this way for the time being, to build the bridge between where the child is and where he should be in language usage. He cannot jump the chasm. As he begins to talk, they can gradually increase the complexity of their models. With some children who are speaking only in grunts or gestures, we would begin therapy by doing our own self-talk in a similar fashion, then progress to single-word utterances, then to short phrases, and finally to sentences which gradually increase in complexity and completeness. We have to begin where the child is. We must join him before we can lead him.

A surprising bit of behavior comes when we get to the early sentence stage. If we occasionally fumble a bit, leave a self-talk sentence hanging uncompleted in mid-air, omit a key word, the child will often say it for us. When this occurs it is unwise to make much of an issue of the achievement. Just feel good and use the technique more often. If we put words in his ears he will find them in his mouth. This is especially effective when we are doing parallel talking.

In *parallel talking*, the mother verbalizes not her own thoughts but those of the child. She tells him what he is doing, what he is feeling. If he appears to be predicting that Jack will jump out of his box, she might say, "Jack pop out, pretty soon." If he is about to turn off the light, she says, "Light go away now." If he is remembering where she hid the cookie, she says, "Cookie in bag." As he bounces, she tells him what he is doing. When he tumbles from the chair, she says, "Johnny fall down. Ow, ow. Hurt foot. Ow!" Emotions can be expressed in self-talk and parallel talk too.

This parallel talking is fascinating stuff. Ideally, we should say the necessary word or phrase or sentence at the very instant that the child should be needing it. Practically, we seldom get the timing so precise. It is a skill which develops with use. We have known mothers to become wonderfully adept after a little practice. It requires careful study of the child and a lot of guessing, imagination, and the ability to identify with the youngster. Every speech therapist should learn the art, for it is very useful in treating the adult aphasic as well as the child who cannot talk. Training in empathy is vitally important in speech therapy.

We have spoken earlier of the importance of speech as a magical tool for controlling others. Nowhere do we see this so clearly as in delayed speech. As soon as we possibly can, we teach this function. We have used puppets, dolls, even ourself as our victims. We command these beings. We tell them to fall down, to cry, to clap hands, and they must obey! The child watches us and sees the power of speech. Soon he is commanding too. Our knees still creak from a session with a little boy who insisted that we get "Unduh taybo!" thirty-seven times by actual count. This spontaneously achieved command had been preceded by much self-talk on our part, commanding first a puppet and then ourself to follow orders.[22]

We also use self-talk to set models for egocentric speech, for the expression of the self. Yesterday, with the same little boy, we crouched on the floor and said, "I'm little. . . . I baby. . . ." Then we got up on all fours, and said, "I kitty . . . meow!" Then we stood up and said proudly, "I big man . . . big as a house." The boy liked the display and gestured that he wanted us to do it again. We looked puzzled, paused a bit, then said, "More? . . . You want more?" He grunted. So we did it again and again, and soon he was imitating first our postures and our animal noises, and finally a little of our speech. He climbed aboard the table, stuck out his chest and arms and crowed, "Man . . . bih MAN!" This was the beginning of speech as the display of the self.

We teach speech as communication a little later. Often it begins to come in by itself, once speech as thought and speech as social control are activated. Usually, we combine it with command at first. "Mummy blow bubble. . . . Big Bubble . . . Oh, oh . . . No more bubble. . . . All gone. . . . Go ask sister for soap. . . . Sssssssoap. . . ." If he's interested enough he might just possibly do it.

---

[22] A psychological rationale for commentary and command in self-talk in terms of "tacts" and "mands" may be found in the book *Verbal Behavior* by B. F. Skinner (New York: Appleton-Century-Crofts, 1957).

Echolalia and Jargon.   When we find a child fixated at the level of echolalia, we should understand that he has failed to perceive the usefulness of speech as a tool. He probably views speech as a display, as a verbal dance. He has been asked too often to say something after someone else. He obliges. The echoed words sound like speech, but they are not true speech any more than that of a parrakeet. His echoing has been too strongly reinforced. He plays a game of verbal ping-pong. Our task here is to stop rewarding this spurious verbalization and try to show the child how much more pleasurable it is to find that even a single word can command his elders and satisfy his desires. His first words should be "mand" words, commands, demands—words like "No!" "Want," "Gimme," "Go!" Since at first these words may be unrecognizable, we may have to shape them to more acceptable forms. Our own preferred way of doing this is to use a modification of the motokinesthetic method. As originated by Edna Hill Young, this method consists essentially of the manipulation, touching, stroking, or pressing the child's face and body by the clinician in such ways to provide tactual and kinesthetic cues for the sequence of sounds that compose the word. The clinician thus helps the child to locate the structures needed to produce the sound, indicates the direction of their movement, and gives some clues with respect to voicing, nasality, plosion, or continuousness. At the same time that the clinician is manipulating the child's oral structures, she is also clearly pronouncing the sounds of the word being produced.

We taught one nonspeaking child his first meaningful word "No!" by asking him if he wanted to stay on the table on which we had laid him, telling him that only if he said "No!" he could get down. We placed his fingers on our nose and lips as we slowly said the word. Then we took his forefinger, placed it alongside his own nose, and then shifted it and the thumb to round his lips. Next we showed him how we used these movements to form our own "No." Then, after asking him again if he wanted to stay on the table, we went through the same series of manipulations, he pronounced the word perfectly, and we let him get down and play for a time. To make sure, we asked him if he wanted to get back on the table, and it was interesting to watch him touch his nose and round his lips again as he said the word clearly. In that same session we also taught him "Yah" and invested it also with meaning. Throughout the half-hour period the boy would intermittently relapse into his usual jargon and gestures, but these we simply ignored. The boy's mother, who had watched the proceedings, then took over and successfully got both a meaningful "Yah" for a proffered bit of candy and a meaningful "No" when she asked him if he wanted to stay with us as she went home. For both words, the boy used his fingers on his face to help him say them, but the parent reported that within a week he was saying these words appropriately and without the motokinesthetic gestures. What was most important, the boy had learned that speech was a tool.

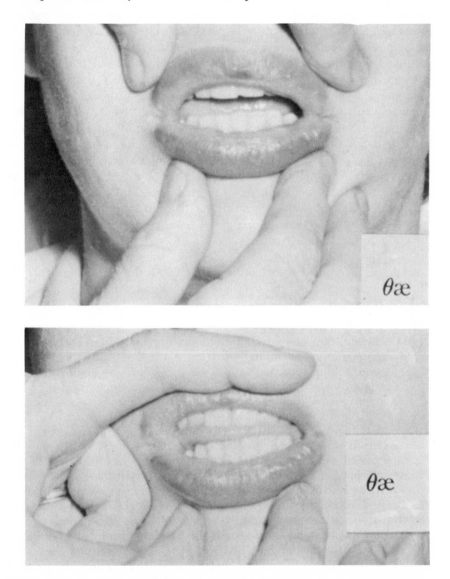

FIGURE 13: *The Motokinesthetic Method.* Reprinted from *Moto-Kinesthetic Speech Training* by Edna Hill Young and Sara Stinchfield Hawk with the permission of the publishers, Stanford University Press. Copyright © 1955 by the Board of Trustees of the Leland Stanford Junior University.

In addition to using these methods, the parent should occasionally talk gibberish herself, or use grunts and gestures, trying earnestly to get the child to understand. When he is thoroughly puzzled, she should catch herself and say, "Oh, I didn't say it right. What I mean is 'Bring me the shoe. Sh . . . oo. Shoe!" She does not ask the child to say it. She is merely creating a model for him to follow. She is showing him that even big people make mistakes and find it hard to make themselves understood if they don't talk right. She is showing him that it doesn't hurt to correct oneself. Later on, this can also be done on single words.

Gesture Language.   Some children, otherwise quite normal, learn a sign language rather than a verbal one, and some of them get surprisingly efficient in its use. They comprehend language very well, and we suspect that they just don't think that learning to talk is worth the trouble. They come from indulgent homes where the parents have learned the child's gesture language rather than the reverse.

Silent gestures must therefore remain unrewarded. The best policy to follow is to withdraw the parents' granting of the pantomimic requests in a gradual fashion. The first day, they pretend not to understand at least two gesture requests, guessing incorrectly until the child is pretty frustrated by their stupidity. The next day they do it four times, scattering the misunderstandings at random. Gradually most of the child's gesturing is being unrewarded. The guessing part of this technique should always be in single words:

Today I was carrying out your suggestions. Bobby wanted me to hand him down the ball from the shelf. He kept pointing and reaching and saying "a . . . a . . . a." I looked at him in a puzzled sort of fashion, saying, "Dish? Bobby want dish?" Then I tried "cap" and "cup" and "box," reaching up and taking down each, and pretending to be trying hard to understand. It certainly seemed cruel, but I did it. He finally got mad and began to suck his thumb. Is this what you want me to do?

It was, but it should not be used alone. All spontaneous utterance should be rewarded by providing attention, sharing through imitation, and a little extra loving. With a severe case, even grunts and babbling should receive rewards. If the child makes any attempt at all to say the right word, or indeed for some children who do not talk at all, if any utterance accompanies the gesture it should be reinforced by pleasantness.

Since one of the possible reasons for the child's use of gesture rather than speech is that the models of the speech he hears appear too complicated and difficult, we do everything we can to speak to him very simply. Let us therefore give another example of such simple self-talk by a mother:

Mummy do dishes now. Wash cup . . . put cup here . . . Where glass? Oh, here glass . . . Glass dirty . . . Now glass soapy . . . Wash . . . Jerry wipe . . . Towel . . . Rub, rub . . . Glass clean . . . Glass on shelf . . .

If some of this simplified self-talk is done several times each day, the child who watches will begin to participate, first silently with inner speech and later aloud.

For the delayed-speech case it is as necessary to teach a basic vocabulary of tool words as it is for the normal infant. Some of our delayed-speech cases already have a good many words when they come to us, but they are hidden and buried in the jargon. It is necessary to separate them out, get the child to use them meaningfully, and then reward them. Many of these children show great spurts of progress as soon as they come to realize that they can speak many words correctly. They also show surprise, since over-correction, rejection, or other penalties may have convinced them that they cannot talk correctly and they have accepted this judgment and made no further attempt to improve.

With the child who has little or no speech, it is necessary to teach the first words. The first project should not contain more than five or ten words, and they should begin with the easier sounds, *m, b, p,* or *w.* If possible, they should be monosyllabic or should consist of repeated syllables, such as *mamma.* They should be names of things or activities which the child enjoys. If the child has some distorted speech sounds which he habitually employs for naming favorite objects, it is wise to select new toys or new activities which he has not previously named. When this principle is followed, no unlearning is necessary.

In one case, the word *mop* was among the first five words to be taught. After the child had been given ear training in saying the *m* and *p* sounds by themselves, the therapist began the ear training necessary to the production of the whole word. She left the room in a very mysterious manner, returning with a bottle of colored water and a mop. As soon as she entered the room, she went solemnly to each corner and said "mop, mop, mop." Then she made another circuit of the room with the child, and in each corner she said the word *mop* into the ear of child. On her third circuit, she spilled a little water in each corner, uttering the same word three times, prolonging the *m* slightly and emphasizing the *p.* On the fourth circuit, she took the mop itself and wiped up the water with it, saying the word rhythmically as she worked. She motioned to the child to help her, and as he took hold of the handle he began to say the word in unison with her, somewhat to her surprise. In this case, the vivid stimulation and identification with an activity were sufficient to produce the spontaneous response.

Developing Language Mastery. If we have seemed unduly lengthy in our description of how to help the child acquire his first useful words, it is only because these words are crucial to all later speech and language development. However, we cannot be content to rest here. We must help him learn how to link words together. We must overcome the obstacles that prevent him from learning the rules of his language. Nevertheless, as clinicians, we always feel that once the child has acquired his first words, the greatest of these obstacles has been surmounted.

Many of the children with whom we work are not nonverbal. They come to us with a respectable vocabulary and even with primitive sentence structures, but they still are markedly handicapped in both receptive and expressive language. Our task with these, as with those who have just begun to speak, is to ascertain how far up the language ladder they have climbed and then help them climb higher. The Northwestern Syntax Screening Test (NSST) developed by Lee is a useful instrument in the general assessment of the child's competence and performance in language.[23] It consists of a set of pictures from which the child must make a selection by pointing when given a clue sentence (the receptive task) or to answer the question "What's this one?" when the examiner points to it (the expressive task.) Figure 14 illustrates the type of stimuli used.

The test, which can be administered in about fifteen minutes, provides percentile norms for "the comparison of receptive and expressive use of such grammatical features as prepositions, personal pronouns, negatives, plurals, reflexive pronouns, verb tenses, subject-object identification, possessives, *wh* questions, yes-no questions, passives, and indirect objects." The author states that the instrument should be considered strictly as a screening device for locating children with language deficiencies, but we have also found it useful in determining those deficiencies in an individual child. Other instruments for analyzing linguistic competence and performance are the Illinois Test of Psycholinguistic Abilities [24] and the Michigan Picture Language Inventory.[25]

Once we have located the basic deficiencies in language, we then help the child to recognize and to cope with them so that the proper linguistic models can be acquired. If the child, for example, seems to understand words but has difficulty recalling them when he needs them, we might use activities which involve associations.

---

[23] L. L. Lee, "A Screening Test for Syntax Development," *Journal of Speech and Hearing Disorders*, XXXV (1970), 103–112.

[24] S. Kirk, J. McCarthy, and W. Kirk, *The Illinois Test of Psycholinguistic Abilities*, rev. ed. (Urbana: University of Illinois Press, 1968).

[25] L. Lerea, "Assessing Language Development," *Journal of Speech and Hearing Research*, I (1958), 75–85.

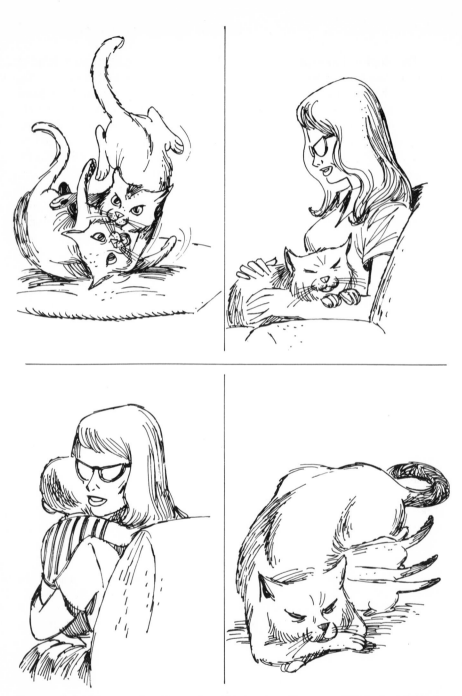

Figure 14: *Pictures for Receptive Distinction Between "This is Mother's cat" and "This is a mother cat."* From Laura L. Lee, "A Screening Test for Syntax Development," *The Journal of Speech and Hearing Disorders*, XXXV (1970), p. 107. Used by permission.

Billy knew the word "ball," could point it out, could say it after us, but always got frustrated whenever he wanted to talk about a ball, for he just didn't seem to be able to find the word. We had him repeat after us, as we played with all sorts of balls, such things as these: "A big ball; a little ball; a round ball; the ball is round; bounce the ball; hide the ball; ball in my pocket; throw the ball; yellow ball and red ball and the hard ball now. Balls are for bouncing. Balls are for throwing. Put the ball in the can. Take out the —— [Billy said it!] Going to put the [pause] under your shirt. [Billy said it again.] Kick the ——. [Billy said it and did it.]" Then we had him talk about what he was doing with the ball. We sat on the ball but didn't say anything. Billy sat on the ball and said, "Sit on ball." We threw the ball. So did he, and after this session he never had any trouble finding that word.

Some children have trouble with categories. When they do, we help them recognize that a shirt, or pants, or shoes, or stockings all belong together.

When I dress myself, I . . . [then we pantomime the activity and prompt the child to say], "put on my shirt, put on my pants, put on my socks and put on my. . . ." [He will usually say shoes.] We sort things according to function. "What things here in the playbox do we eat with?" We hunt for similarities and opposites. "Put all the big things in this box; put the small ones in this other box," and we have an assortment of pairs of big trucks and little trucks; big crayons and little ones; big pictures and little ones, and so on.[26]

Along with this attempt to overcome the child's basic deficiencies, we also begin our language teaching. Generally we begin where the child seems fixated in the developmental sequence of language acquisition. Thus, if a child has difficulties in verb tense, indirect objects, and prepositions but also shows impairment in relating subjects to predicates, we would work at the latter level first, since usually this stage of language mastery comes before the others. If the child is in the one-word sentence stage, we help him to develop noun and verb phrases. We start where the child is.

But what do we do? First of all, we stimulate him with the sort of material he should be mastering instead of talking to him in our usual complex fashion. If he is having trouble with such prepositions as *over* and *under*, we do a lot of crawling over and under the tables and verbalizing

---

[26] These few glimpses of how we try to help a child overcome some of his basic deficits only briefly illustrate the ways in which we work. For a more extended treatment of this subject, see D. J. Johnson and H. R. Mykelbust, *Learning Disabilities: Educational Principles and Practices*, Chapter 4 (New York: Grune & Stratton, Inc., 1967).

in simple phrases what we are doing as we do it. If his pronouns are all askew, we show him the differences between the correct and incorrect form by making errors and then correcting ourselves. We say, "Me go outdoors now . . . No . . . I go outdoors now," and the parent or clinician doesn't go outdoors until after she has corrected herself.

> Just last week we were working with a little boy who was thoroughly confused by plurals and possessives. So we emptied out his pockets and our own into one pile and said, "That's your . . . and that's *mines* . . . No, I mean that's *mine*. And that's yours, and that's mine. Yeah." Before the end of the session, the boy had recognized not only the difference between *yours* and *mine* but also that even while plural objects were designated, we did not add the *s* to *mine*. By demonstrating and self-correcting our own errors, we helped him recognize the correct usage as we took turns identifying the objects on the floor. And he also incidently learned some new words. In all of this interaction we never once corrected the child's usage; we merely corrected our own deliberate errors.

With an older child, we may work more directly, confronting him with his mistakes and providing the standard usage mold as soon as the error occurs. We play "Catch me!" games in which we deliberately make the mistakes, and they are his usual mistakes which he is to identify in order to get rewards. By "catching" these mistakes and having to show why they were mistakes and what the correct forms would be, most of these children learn the rules of the language very swiftly. They need help and they need careful teaching, but it is surprising how quickly they get the insights they need once the language task is simplified. Also, it has seemed to us that often the child seems to have already acquired the necessary linguistic competence, but has not been able to convert it into performance until we provide this focused sort of language stimulation:

> We were helping a four-year-old child who, among other problems, had shown great difficulty in getting his past tenses straightened out. After some prompting and error recognition activities which he enjoyed hugely, we were trying to get him to discriminate between "growed" and "grew." Suddenly, he grinned at us and said, "I growed-grew, knowed-knew that all the time. I knew it but now I got it." Unfortunately, the English language has many traps for the unwary, and we had to straighten out some tangles when he overgeneralized and told us how he "shew" his mother how well he could ride his tricycle. In Chaucer's time, he would have been correct.

In this introductory text we cannot possibly describe all the activities we use in helping these children to master their language. Each child presents his own particular pattern of difficulties, and the therapist must tailor the therapy to the needs. However, there is one problem that often presents itself—the problem of intelligibility. If we cannot understand the child when he really tries to talk to us, he will soon lose most of his motivation for learning language. The acquisition of the standard speech sounds is just as important in language development as any other linguistic feature.

The Alphabet of Sound. Many unintelligible children try to talk without enough sounds to talk with. They need more arrows in their quiver, more keys on their verbal typewriters. Any of us would have a hard time making sense if we had but seven or eight, or even fifteen sounds. They need to learn something about the characteristics of the individual speech sounds. They need to master the sound alphabet. This should be done in play sessions. Here is a picture of some of this therapy:

1. Blindfold the child. Make the sound from several different places in the room. Ask the child to point to where the sound came from or to find you.
2. Pretend that each of you is a certain animal or machine that makes the sound. Have him run around the room with you as you produce the sound.
3. Procure a calendar mailing tube or similar device. Hold one end to the child's ear as he winds a string upon a spool. The moment the teacher stops making the sound, he must stop winding.
4. Certain objects are set aside as demanding the hearing of the correct sound before they can be touched. Such rituals appeal to children and compel attention.
5. Prolong or repeat the sound rhythmically. Ask him to clap his hands or put his fingers in the ear whenever you make it very loudly.
6. Tell the child a story or rhyme and prolong the selected sound whenever it occurs in a word. The important thing is to accent the particular sound you are working on.
7. Tie a rope on the child and tell him to walk back and forth as you pronounce the sound. Whenever you cease making the sound, jerk the rope.

Indirect Methods for Combining Sounds and Movements. (Do these first in unison, making the sound a part of the activity.)

1. Snap off the light—say *ow.*
2. Shoot a toy gun—*bang, ba, boom,* or *pow.*
3. Turn an egg beater—any vowel on which you rhythmically change pitch.
4. Saw a board—*ee-ee,* or *ay-ay,* or *zzz-zzz.*

5. Hit piano or xylophone and sing any vowel.
6. Wind a toy—*mmmm-mmmmm.*
7. Pull the cork out of a bottle—*puh* or *buh.*
8. .Pull or push any toy animal and say its sound: Cow—*moo*, dog—*bow-wow*, and so on.
9. Move a zipper: *zzz* or *sss.*
10. Rock in a chair or bounce—any vowel or consonant.

Direct Methods for Combining Sounds and Movements.

1. For *m*: Have child flip or stroke your lips as you make the *m* sound. Then you stroke his lips as he makes it.
2. For *puh*: Have child hold his whole hand flat over your closed mouth with cheeks full of air. Ask him suddenly to pull it away as you explode the *puh* sound. Reverse the process.
3. For *buh*: Hold or have child hold a feather or strip of tissue over your mouth. Then explode the *buh* sound so that the feather or strip moves or falls. Reverse positions.
4. For *tik*: Cup hands around your mouth and ask the child to look inside and hear the clock. Say *tik-tik-tik*. Then have him be the clock.
5. For *dee*: By folding a cardboard provide yourself with a series of ten holes each large enough to insert a finger in. Have child hold it in front of himself, and as you insert your finger in each hole say *dee*. Then you hold it, refusing to let him hit the hole until he says *dee*.
6. For *nnnnnn*: Have child place finger on side of your nose as you open your mouth and say *nnnnnn*. Ask him if he feels the little noise. Then ask him to open his mouth so you can feel his little noise (and nose).
7. For *oo(w)*: Have child watch your rounded lips as you blow into a tube of paper or into a bag or horn. Then have him do it. Then blow the *oo* sound "out loud." Always call this the "blowing sound."
8. For *guh*: Call this the "squeezing sound" or the "choking or collar sound." Ask the child to choke you with both hands as you laugh and say *guh-guh-guh*. Reverse, but be gentle.
9. For *kuh*: Call it the "coughing sound," and play some sort of a coughing game. For example, put a feather into the mouth and cough it out with *kuh-kuh-kuh-kuh-kuh*.
10. For *f*: Call this the "blow on the finger" sound. Hold your finger laterally across the child's lower lip, pushing it inward. Then ask him to blow on your finger to cool it off. Then set his own finger in position and repeat.
11. For *v*: Ask him to watch you in the mirror as you "bite your mouth (or lip) and blow out loud." Then ask him to do it.

Vocal Phonics. Children during their third and fourth years are fascinated by rhymes and wordplay of every kind. They chant such sequences as these even when alone:

High chair, high tair, high bear, kigh kare,
  care care, bear tear, tear bear all up.
Sally, mally, silly sally, sabby, babby, sally babby.
I got a letter in the mail, in the pail, in the tail.
I like soup, sook, soos; do you like soot?

When their playmates seem puzzled by this punning, they laugh uproariously. If wordplay is the lowest form of wit, it may also be the earliest. But its major significance in the development of speech lies in its phonic training. Many children persist in their articulation errors because they never learn that words are composed of a series of consecutive sounds. They hear words as wholes—as chunks of sound. The word *fish* to these children is not a series of three sounds, *f*, ɪ, and ʃ, but a single sound. Thus the pronunciation of *fish* and *pish* if spoken quickly enough are much more alike than they are different, and the child fails to perceive any error. Very often, he may echo the word after his parent without error, and yet in the very next sentence he may use the *pish* again. Many parents consider these children obstinate because they do not use these words consistently with correct sounds. Yet, parrotlike repetition has little to do with mastery of true speech. The Mongolian idiot can often echo very long words and yet be speechless in the true sense of the word. The child must be able to perceive his own errors and to create his own standards of pronunciation before he can be expected to speak correctly.

The child must learn that words have beginnings and endings— heads, middles, and tails. He must learn that the word *fish* must start with the "lip-biting, breathy, finger-cooling sound" (or some similar identification) and with no other. He must learn that *cup* must end with a lip-popping puff of air. [kʌ] is not enough. There must be one more sound.

Most children learn these elementary facts of vocal phonics unconsciously through vocal play and listening. Many articulation cases never learn that words are made up parts, and that if one part is wrong, the whole word is incorrect. These observations may seem absurdly simple to the student of this text, but he will appreciate their truth once he starts to teach some lisper an *s* sound.

Say *sssssssssssss*.
S*ssssssssssssss*
Fine! Now say *soup*.
Thoup.
Oh, oh. You said *thoup*.
No, I didn't. I thaid it right: *ssssthoup*.

The best way of teaching vocal phonics to young children is through guessing games, rhyming, indexing, and rhythmic vocal play. Here are three typical vocal phonics games which we have used successfully with children of three to five years:

1. Make circles on the floor with chalk and give each circle a "sound name" (*ssss* or *mmmm*). The child must make that sound whenever he is in the circle. Thus, as he jumps from circle to circle, he could produce the word [s] [æ] [m] or *Sam*.

2. *Guessing game.* "Show me your *n-o-se* [noʊz]." Separate the sounds at first, but gradually shorten the intervals until the child realizes that [n-oʊz] is a slow way of saying *nose*. Then use other words such as [ʃ u], [f-eɪ s], [maʊɵ], and so on.

3. *Collection game.* Give the child some gaily covered boxes. Have him collect toys or objects whose names begin with an *s* sound and put them into the *m* box, and other objects whose names begin with an *m* sound and put them into the other box. Demonstrate first, and be sure to sound out the words so that he hears the *m* or *s* sound of the objects collected. Also demonstrate rejection thus: "Let's see. Here's a phone. Does this belong in the boxes? Let's see: *f-f-f-o ne*. No, that begins with a *fff* sound, not a *mmmm* or *ssss*. We don't say *mone* or *sone* do we? Let's just get things that begin with the *mmmm* or *ssss*. You bring them to me and I'll sound them out."

One reason why so many children develop a jargon or gibberish is that they fail to realize that a word is made up of a series of sounds blended together. They hear the word as a whole and pronounce some sound which bears a certain likeness to it. Some children can be taught some real words immediately by these sound-sequence games. The majority, however, need much practice in "vocal phonics," in combining and blending sounds without regard to meaning, before the true words are taught. Most successful teachers of delayed-speech cases first teach blending sounds as an interesting game and skill; then they teach sound combinations which they call nonsense names; then, finally, real and familiar words.

1. Let the teacher perform two of the previously practiced movement-sound combinations, then ask the child to imitate her. If this is too difficult, alternate before combining.

2. Let the child perform the activities while the teacher makes the sound, then reverse.

3. Trace a circle to form syllables. Have top arc of circle represent one sound, bottom part another. Trace slowly first, faster gradually for advancement, and divide circle into more parts and sides and sounds.

4. Have squares on floor for certain sounds. Say these sounds while stepping in squares. Form words or syllables.

5. Use different notes on the piano for different sounds.

6. Mount two or more cardboard bells on a piece of tag board so that they can be moved when strings are pulled. Color differently and let

each represent a sound. Have the child pull the strings as you make the sounds. Then exchange places.

7. Cut shapes of paper for various sounds. Arrange two or three in a row on the table for the child to sound out after he learns the sounds for them.
8. Roll a ball across the room, having the child say the sounds as the ball moves in the various spaces.

TERMINAL THERAPY: ITS PROBLEMS

Children differ in their response to treatment. Those whose delayed speech seems due to poor teaching methods and bad environmental conditions make the swiftest progress if these can be changed for the better. Those with emotional conflicts (with the exception of the autistic child) also progress very swiftly when the conflicts are resolved. They also speak very clearly. We have known many instances of children, whose voluntary mutism or infantile jargon made them nontalkers, who suddenly began to talk very well. The aphasic child and children with cerebral palsy, will make slow progress and need help for a longer time. So will the mentally retarded.

Among the problems which may be viewed as the residue or aftermath of delayed speech are severe articulation disorders: cluttering, stuttering, odd voices, and a pattern of behavior that has been termed "specific language disability." The latter is often designated by its initial letters SLD. Many of these unfortunate remnants of delayed speech can be prevented with proper understanding and treatment.

Dyslalia. This term, we wish to remind you, refers to the presence of errors of articulation due to functional causes. In the elementary grades of the public schools we often encounter children whose speech is barely intelligible. The use of language is adequate but there are so many errors of omission, distortion, and substitution that only the other children seem to understand them. In scrutinizing their histories we commonly find a history of delayed speech. Children who begin to speak at four or five years have a long way to go, a lot of sounds to master before they begin to read and write. They are usually children who have not had professional help. They come to us confused by too many targets in their mouths. Again, our task is to help them untangle the problem by helping them to recognize the different speech sounds, to analyze the sound sequences within words, and to build a basic nucleus of good speech.

Cluttering. When a child has discovered the pleasures of intelligible speech, he sometimes takes off like a skyrocket. He wants to talk all the time, to say everything at once. He grabs every ear in sight and fills it constantly. Communicatively, he has been starved and so he fills his mouth with too many words too fast. If, as often occurs in cluttering, there is a family predisposition and some evidence of minor brain damage, his speech will become almost incoherent the moment he speaks swiftly, although he can speak very well when he is careful. He falters, repeats, changes words, slurs his speech sounds, transposes syllables, and generally makes a hurried mess of his communication. This is cluttering. To some degree it may be prevented by removing the need for haste and by providing speech models which are themselves unhurried. The tempo of the home and the tempo of the mother's speech should be slowed. Parents should say that they do not understand the torrent of tangled syllables, show the child how he has spoken, and provide a willing ear which has plenty of time to listen.

Stuttering.   There are times when a child seems to travel a crooked path down which first delayed speech, then cluttering, then stuttering appear sequentially. In other children, the stuttering emerges directly from the delayed speech. Too much pressure for speech output by the happy parents who finally see their child beginning to talk may cause a need to talk without having anything to say. Such children will falter. We don't want them to learn a broken English, so we must counsel parents to wait rather than to urge. There are also many moments in learning to talk when words must be hunted, changed, revised in articulation, sorted out in sentences. This places a heavy burden upon fluency. Some children almost seem to face a choice between stuttering and defective articulation when they emerge from delayed speech. If there is such a choice, we would counsel parents to accept the defective sounds. Learning to talk takes time.

Voice Problems.   These are not common residues of delayed speech but they do occasionally occur. One of our six-year-olds who began to say his first sentences at five had two voices, his own and one that his mother called his "frog voice" because it was pitched so low and possessed a croaking sort of quality. David spoke an almost unintelligible jargon in his natural child's voice, but his frog voice spoke very good English. The problem was one of identification. He had been a very isolated child, living on a farm. Dave's mother worked in a drugstore during the day, and his father worked at night in a local factory but managed to care for him during part of the daylight hours. Dave had received help in the speech clinic and also at home under our guidance for several months, when suddenly he began to speak very clearly but in the deep bass croak of the frog voice. It became apparent that he was identifying intelligible speech with his father's speech and felt that he had to match it in pitch as well as in clarity and form. We got the child placed in a nursery school, and soon he was speaking well in his own voice. Other children finally learn to conform to adult speech standards but keep an infantile voice as a last defense against the pressures of a too-demanding environment. These are often the active ones. Autistic children who begin to talk also may show odd voices.

REFERENCES

Articles

1. Adams, J. "Delayed Language Development," *Journal of Speech and Hearing Disorders*, XXXIV (1969), 169–71.
   Describe the speech development of this mentally retarded boy.
2. Baratz, J. C. "Language in the Economically Disadvantaged Child: A Perspective." *ASHA*, X (1968), 143–45.
   What is the essential argument of this author concerning "language disability" of these children?
3. Blackman, R. S. and Battin, R. R. "Case Study of Delayed Language." *Journal of Speech and Hearing Disorders*, XXII (1957), 381–84.
   What were the emotional problems shown by this case?
4. De Hirsch, K. "Differential Diagnosis Between Aphasic and Schizophrenic Language in Children." *Journal of Speech and Hearing Disorders*, XXXII (1967), 3–10.
   What are the differences in the language characteristics of these two groups?
5. Dubner, H. W. "A Speech Pathologist Talks to the Parents of a Nonverbal Child." *Rehabilitation Literature*, XXX (1969), 360–62.
   What suggestions to the parents were given by the speech pathologist?
6. Furneaux, B. "The Autistic Child." *British Journal of Disorders of Communication*, I (1966), 85–90.
   How does this author describe the treatment of autistic children?
7. Gens, G. W. and Bibey, M. L. "Congenital Aphasia: A Case Report." *Journal of Speech and Hearing Disorders*, XVII (1952), 32–38.
   What, according to the authors, are the chief characteristics of congenital aphasia?
8. Greene, M. C. L. "Speechless and Backward at Three." *British Journal of Disorders of Communication*, II (1967), 134–45.
   How should the therapist examine these children? What should she investigate?
9. Hannigan, H. "*Rh* Child: Deaf or Aphasic? 3. Language and Behavioral Problems of the *Rh* Aphasic Child." *Journal of Speech and Hearing Disorders*, XXI (1956), 413–17.
   Describe the early speech development of these children and how they learn language?
10. Hegrenes, J. R., Marshall, N. R., and Armas, J. A. "Treatment as an Extension of Diagnostic Function: A Case Study." *Journal of Speech and Hearing Disorders*, XXXV (1970), 182–87.
    How did the speech therapists keep this child from being placed in a state institution for the mentally retarded?
11. Hewett, F. M. "Teaching Speech to an Autistic Child Through Operant Conditioning." *Journal of Orthopsychiatry*, XXXV (1965), 927–36.
    Describe the operant program in terms of schedules and reinforcements.
12. Johnson, W., Brown, S. F., Curtis, J. F., Edney, C. W., and Keaster, J. *Speech Handicapped School Children*. 3d ed., New York: Harper & Row, Publishers, 1967. Pp. 341–53.

Why were Bruce and Polly so retarded in learning to talk and how were they helped?

13. McGrady, H. J. "Language Pathology and Learning Disabilities." In Mykelbust, H., ed., *Progress in Learning Disabilities* (New York: Grune and Stratton, 1968), pp. 199–233.
Describe the deprivations which produce language pathology.

14. Palmer, M. "Educational Problems of the Aphasic Child." *Special Education,* LI (1962), 13–17.
What were the children like who attended this special school?

15. Picaizen, G., Verger, A. A., Baranofsky, D., Nichols, A. C., and Karen, R. "Applications of Operant Techniques to Speech Therapy with Nonverbal Children." *Journal of Communication Disorders,* II (1969), 203–11.
Describe how operant conditioning was used with these two cases.

16. Raph, J. B. "Language and Speech Deficits in Culturally Disadvantaged Children: Implications for the Speech Clinician." *Journal of Speech and Hearing Disorders,* XXXII (1967), 203–14.
What role should the speech therapist play in helping these children?

17. Stark, J. "Teaching the Aphasic Child." *Exceptional Child,* XXXV (1968), 149–54.
Describe some of the methods used in teaching these children to use language.

18. ———, Giddan, J. J., and Meisel, J. "Increasing Verbal Behavior in an Autistic Child." *Journal of Speech and Hearing Disorders,* XXXIII (1968), 42–47.
How did the speech therapist work with Kipper?

19. Werner, S. "Treatment of a Child with Delayed Speech." *Journal of Speech Disorders,* X (1945), 329–31.
Describe the child's behavior and how the therapist worked with her.

20. Wessell, M. H. "A Language Development Program for a Blind Language-Disordered Preschool Girl." *Journal of Speech and Hearing Disorders,* XXXIV (1969), 267–74.
Describe how this blind girl was helped to acquire language.

21. Wolf, E. G. and Ruttenberg, B. A. "Communication Therapy for the Autistic Child." *Journal of Speech and Hearing Disorders,* XXXII (1967), 331–36.
How can we motivate the autistic child to want to talk?

22. Wolf, M., Risley, T., and Mees, H. "Application of Operant Conditioning Procedures to the Behavior Problems of an Autistic Child." *Behavior Research and Therapy,* I (1964), 305–12.
What were these behavior problems and how were they solved?

Texts

23. Battin, R. R. and Haug, C. O. *Speech and Language Delay.* Springfield, Ill.: Charles C Thomas, Publishers, 1964.
A short book primarily intended for parents. Emphasizes good home practices, stimulation, and ear training.

24. Berry, M. I. *Language Disorders of Children.* New York: Meredith, 1969.
The third and fourth sections of this book provide some excellent case histories of language delay together with descriptions of treatment.

25. Johnson, D. and Mykelbust, H. *Learning Disabilities: Educational Principles and Practices.* New York: Grune and Stratton, 1967.
     Especially valuable is Chapter 4 in which the disorders of auditory language are presented together with some excellent suggestions for therapy.
26. Rimland, B. *Infantile Autism.* New York: Meredith, 1964.
     This is probably the clearest summary of the nature of autistic behavior that we possess.
27. Wood, N. *Delayed Speech and Language.* Englewood Cliffs, N.J.: Prentice-Hall, Inc., 1964.
     A survey of the basic information on speech and language delay. The material is slanted more toward diagnosis and nature than to treatment.
28. Wyatt, G. L. *Language Learning and Communication Disorders in Children.* New York: Free Press, 1969.
     This volume is noteworthy for its presentation of detailed case histories and accounts of diagnosis and therapy. The author's primary emphasis is upon the interaction of the child and an important adult. When this relationship is impaired, disturbances in speech and language ensue.

5

Voice Disorders

We worked once with a patient who had to spend most of his days and nights in an iron lung, although for a few hours each day he was able to use a chest respirator. We have never forgotten what he said to us about breathing: "Until I had polio I never knew what it meant to breathe. I didn't think about breathing. It was just there—naturally. Now I think about it all the time. It's the most important thing I do." Our task was to teach him how to speak while conserving his breath and how to produce voice with a minimum expenditure of energy. We have also had to do the same for many people who developed voice disorders because they had taken their voices too much for granted and had subjected them to incredible abuse. Perhaps only the professional speaker, singer, or actor really recognizes how vitally necessary voices really are; and many of these individuals, who of all people have so much to lose, fail to guard them appropriately, and so develop serious vocal problems.

But voice disorders may befall anyone. Most of us have experienced a temporary loss of voice after laryngitis, prolonged shouting, or having to speak continuously in the presence of loud noise. Few of us use our voices efficiently or pay any attention to them. When first hearing a self-recording, we are surprised and sometimes shocked to discover how our voices must sound to others. In part this is because we must use our ears primarily to hear our thoughts and those of others, and in part because we sense our vocal tones through bone and tissue conduction as well as from airborne sound. Also, the sound field is different, our ears being behind our mouths, but in front of the mouths of others. This peculiar distortion plus our inattention to how we sound doubtless may explain why some people are able to persist in using unpleasant voices that finally result in real disorders.

Chaliapin, the famous basso, once said that going to a party was like going to a symphony played by instruments all of which were out of tune. "All around me are voices blowing discords, squeaks, rasps, whines, grunts, and growls. I can hardly bear it." Fortunately for most of us, our ears are not so sensitive. His observation, however, is more accurate than our calloused ears would be likely to admit. All about us are voices which could be improved, made more pleasant and efficient. And there are some so markedly unpleasant or peculiar that they are referred to the speech therapist. The singing teacher gets some of these, the speech teacher gets another group, the physician sees the pathological ones, and the speech therapist is usually called upon last.

Since the human voice varies in pitch, loudness, and quality, the disorders of voice reflect these three features either separately or in combination. With respect to the latter, we remember very well a schoolteacher who lost his first job primarily because his voice was so unpleasant. His pitch level was not only too high; it possessed so little variability that his monotone put the students to sleep. The intensity was so weak that the students in the rear of the room could not hear half of what he said. What was most unpleasant of all, however, was the excessive nasal quality that permeated all of his speech. This weak little whiny high-pitched voice was unbearable, and the man was discharged after only two days of teaching. Like this man, other individuals show disorders of voice that are defective in more than one of the three features of pitch, intensity, and quality; but some of our cases show deviancy in only one of these aspects.

DISORDERS OF INTENSITY

We begin our presentation of vocal disorders with *aphonia*—the lack of voice—not only because it is probably the most serious of all the voice disorders but also because it reveals how important phonation is to normal living. The person with aphonia is greatly handicapped as this man's written comments demonstrate. He had to write these thoughts, for he could not speak, his entire larynx having been removed because cancer had developed on his vocal folds.

They told me I had cancer of the throat and that they would have to take out my voice box immediately. First I thought, "No, let me die!" I was scared to the marrow of my bones. How could I make a living? I could never talk again to my wife and children or to anyone. I thought of shooting myself and getting it over quick. That biopsy suddenly turned my whole existence upside down. What was I to do? My confusion and depression were so great that I just went along with the doctors. And so I found myself there in the hospital bed with my wife holding my hand; and I tried to tell her not to cry, but nothing came out of my mouth—just a rush of air out of the hole in my throat under the bandage. I could move my lips, but there was no sound. Then I cried—but silently. I was mute. I was not me.

It was unfortunate that this man had not been able to talk to a speech therapist prior to his surgery or to another laryngectomee who had learned to speak again with the vicarious esophageal voice. Most surgeons try to arrange for this before the operation, since it is possible to develop a different but usable kind of phonation by learning to trap air within the upper part of the esophagus, and to "burp" it out in a controlled fashion sufficient to provide enough sound for speech. All of us have been able to produce sound in this way. As infants, we were burped after every bottle and some of us, as adults, have found ourselves making similar sounds after drinking too much of a different liquid or partaking too heavily of a hearty meal. The possibility therefore exists for the acquisition of a substitute voice even when no vocal folds are present, and the upper end of the airway from the lungs ends in a hole in the neck. This new voice is called the *alaryngeal* or *esophageal voice*. For those who have lost a larynx and have complete aphonia, the esophageal voice may be the way back to a normal life; but it must be learned, and usually it must be taught, although a few laryngectomees manage to discover it by themselves.

The Artificial Larynx.   Another method for producing vicarious voice involves the use of an artificial larynx, one of which is illustrated in Figure 15. The first such device we ever saw was a most cumbersome instrument consisting of a bellows held under the arm, and a mouth-tube probe which contained a reed similar to that used in the ordinary harmonica. By inserting the tube into the corner of his mouth and pumping the bellows with his upper arm, the patient who owned it was able to talk intelligibly, though somewhat weakly. We now have much better artificial larynges, most of which use an electrically activated diaphragm or reed as the sound source.[1] In the instrument illustrated below, one of those most commonly used, the battery is contained in the case; and the buzzing diaphragm at its end is held against the neck. By articulating carefully, the sound thus produced can be turned into usable speech. Other electrolarynges have the vibrating mechanism built into the bowl of a tobacco pipe, with the stem transmitting the sound into the mouth, or even into the upper plate

---

[1] The electrolarynx was evidently discovered by Gilbert Wright, who noted while shaving that when he pressed his buzzing electric razor against his throat and pantomimed talking while holding his breath, he could produce intelligible speech.

of a denture. Some devices are held in the hand while a small plastic tube carries the sound into the corner of the mouth.

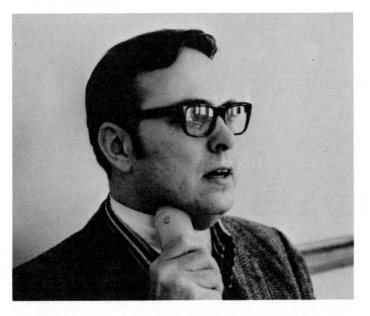

FIGURE 15: *Artificial Larynx; How the Electrolarynx Is Used.* Reproduced by permission of the Western Electric Company.

Comparison of Methods for Producing Vicarious Voice. Neither esophageal speech nor that produced by an external vibrator are ever as good as the voice which was lost. The esophageal voice, at its very best, is often low pitched and hoarse. It is often difficult to master, and many laryngectomees give up before they achieve any real competence. Martin writes:

> Many esophageal voices, even though loud enough, are neither of such quality as to be adequate for practical needs, nor acceptable from the social standpoint. Other laryngectomees simply cannot achieve any usable esophageal speech, no matter how long or how hard they try. These unfortunates obviously should be urged to give up further public attempts at this form of artificial speech and rely entirely on the electrolarynx for all but family and other intimate contacts.[2]

[2] H. Martin, "Rehabilitation of the Laryngectomee," *Cancer*, XVI (1963), 323–41.

Some of the features of esophageal speech which often appear during the learning process and which are regarded as objectionable by the laryngectomee are these: the gulping sound as air is taken into the esophagus; the weakness of the sound produced; the very low pitch (often about an octave lower than the normal male voice); the hoarse quality; the contortions such as lip-squeezing or extending the neck with the head thrown back; the whoosh of air through the opening in the neck that accompanies the speech attempt and causes the little gauze apron covering the hole to flap; the feeling of abdominal distension when air is swallowed and collected in the stomach; the effort and carefulness required; and finally the flatulence or borborygmus that may occur. The latter refers to the abdominal noises which all of us experience at times when we have fed too well. The old limerick says it best:

I sat by the Duchess at tea
She was haughty and proud as could be
But her noises abdominal
Were simply phenomenal
And everyone thought it was me.

Nevertheless, despite these hurdles, some laryngectomees manage to acquire an esophageal speech so fluent and good that their listeners do not realize that they are speaking in a different way. They sound as though they have laryngitis, but they talk very well. One of our cases could make himself heard and understood in a large auditorium and could say Gilbert and Sullivan's classical definition of a falsehood on one air intake: "Merely corroborative detail intended to give verisimilitude to a bald and unconvincing narrative." William White, one of the instructors in our department of speech pathology and audiology for a time, was a laryngectomee whose esophageal speech was so fluent and clear and free from mannerisms that all of us, students and colleagues alike, found it hard to realize that he was speaking differently than we were. The best esophageal speakers are very, very good, and they possess a sense of triumph over adversity which is very impressive. Some of them have better lives after the operation than they had before. We have met many of them who have dedicated their lives to helping speech therapists teach other laryngectomees how to use the substitute voice. Some of them have organized Lost Cord or New Voice Clubs, where those who have just had surgery can find understanding and help. We once took a recording of sample communications from a local Lost Cord Club to a similar group in Melbourne, Australia, and we have never forgotten the way those Aussies closed their meeting with the same esophageal utterance of the Twenty-third Psalm ("Yea though I walk through the Valley of the Shadow of Death, Thou shalt comfort me . . .") that was used in our own group so far away. If any student can attend a meeting of some local chapter of the International Association of Laryngectomees (IAL), he will find it inspiring—and he will certainly quit smoking cigarettes.

Nevertheless, most of the evidence indicates that far too many laryngectomees fail to achieve good esophageal speech. Putney reported that 140 out of 440 laryngectomees failed to acquire any esophageal voice at all;[3] Gardner and Harris found that 40 percent of their patients failed to get intelligible esophageal speech.[4] We worked very hard with several who never got a decent esophageal tone. One was a refined elderly lady to whom a burp was an utter disgrace; another was too depressed to try; another was so tense the sphincter muscles of the cricopharyngeus at the upper end of the esophagus would clamp shut so hard no vibration was possible. Still another, a successful business executive, was so impatient that when he found that he could not immediately transform his first brief burst of esophageal sounds into long sentences, he left the clinic. More than half of our own patients have acquired fair to good esophageal voices and are able to speak in phrases and sentences loudly and clearly enough for ordinary communication. The others have had to learn to use the electrolarynx either as a supplemental aid when telephoning or trying to talk in a noisy environment, or they use it as their sole means of communicating. What is most important is that they are not aphonic and that they can speak. To be mute is to be touched by death.

The kind of voice and speech produced by the various electrolarynges is felt by most speech therapists to be less satisfactory, and generally we recommend that the patient use the electrolarynx only when it becomes clear that he cannot learn esophageal speech.[5] Some workers recommend that the electrolarynx be used immediately by the laryngectomee while he tries to master esophageal speech; but others protest that if this is done, he will tend to rely upon the easier mechanical aid and will never learn it. Our own practice has been to postpone its use until we are pretty certain that no adequate esophageal speech will be acquired. In its present form the artificial larynx has many shortcomings. It is conspicuous and immedi-

[3] F. J. Putney, "Rehabilitation of the Postlaryngectomized Patient; Specific Discussion of Failures, Advanced and Difficult Technical Problems," *Annals of Otology, Rhinology and Laryngology,* LXVII (1958), 544–49.

[4] M. H. Gardner, and H. E. Harris, "Aids and Devices for Laryngectomees," *Archives of Otolaryngology,* LXXIII (1961), 145–52.

[5] R. L. McCroskey, and M. Mulligan, in their article, "The Relative Intelligibility of Esophageal Speech and Artificial Larynx," *Journal of Speech and Hearing Disorders,* XXVIII(1963), 37–41, showed that naïve listeners felt that speech produced by the electrolarynx was more intelligibile than esophageal speech, while students and speech thearpists made just the opposite judgments. Earlier M. Hyman, "An Experimental Study of Artificial Larynx and Esophageal Speech," *Journal of Speech and Hearing Disorders,* XX (1955), 291–99, found the same results.

ately makes clear that the person is disabled. The buzzing noise that accompanies all speech detracts from communication. The sound produced seems very different in quality from normal speech, and although some speakers become highly proficient in varying the pitch of the buzz, the inflections leave much to be desired. It tends to be monotonous. As Greene writes:

> The voice artificially produced by means of the various types of electric vibrators available is a poor substitute for esophageal voice and will never be mistaken for the normal voice which is hoarse from laryngitis. The voice generated artificially is always bizarre.[6]

Nevertheless, for many persons the electrolarynx has helped them return from alaryngeal muteness to a place in a communicating world.

Learning to Use Esophageal Speech. The clinician who seeks to help the laryngectomee acquire esophageal speech need not himself be able to produce it, though we have found our own ability to do so has contributed much to the patient's early progress. What is necessary is the provision of an adequate model such as that by some other skilled esophageal speaker or at the very least some tapes or films of such speakers. Also, the clinician must understand the basic principles for the intake of air into the upper esophagus and have some systematic sequence of subgoals such as the four basic skills listed by Berlin: (1) ability to phonate reliably on demand; (2) ability to demonstrate short latency between inflation of the esophagus and vocalization; (3) ability to maintain an adequate duration of phonation on the vowel [a]; (4) ability to sustain phonation during articulation of syllables, words, and phrases.[7] Other clinicians prefer other sequences, but all of them start with the goal of being able to take air into the esophagus and to expel it in the production of tone.

In an introductory text such as this one, it would be unwise to go into too much detail; but there are at least three alleged methods for trapping enough air into the esophagus to permit vocalization. In the first, the inhalation method, the sphincters of the esophagus must be relaxed, and then, as the diaphragm descends, air is naturally gulped into the esophagus. Then the sphincters of the cricopharyngeus are tightened and vibrate as the diaphragm returns upward. The second procedure is termed the "injection procedure" or the "glossopharyngeal press." [8] In this method, the lips and soft palate are closed, and the cheeks are contracted simul-

---

[6] M. C. L. Greene, *The Voice and Its Disorders* (Philadelphia: J. B. Lippincott, Co., 1964), p. 311.

[7] C. I. Berlin, "Clinical Measurement During the Acquisition of Esophageal Speech: I. Methodology and Curves of Skill Acquisition," *Journal of Speech and Hearing Disorders*, XXIII (1963), 42–51.

[8] P. H. Damste, *Oesophageal Speech* (Gronigen, Holland: Hoitsema, 1958).

taneously with an upward and backward bunching of the tongue. This forces or injects the air that was trapped within the mouth cavity down into the esophagus. Good esophageal speakers can use the concomitant constriction of their plosive sounds to pump small amounts of air down into the esophagus, thus continually replenishing the supply, and so speak continuously. A third but less advisable method is based upon swallowing.

We have found our work with laryngectomees to be challenging and rewarding. It is challenging because there are many problems which must be solved: the need to provide motivation in the face of repeated failure, the need to relieve these patients of their emotional storms, the need for repeated restructuring of tasks and goals. With one of our cases, we discerned a deep resentment in him whenever we used a normal voice, but found that when we spoke esophageally or wrote out what we had to say, thereby sharing his problem, he could make real achievements. We kept some of these written records, and they run as follows:

> *Therapist*: I'm getting tired of using my esophageal voice. Let's write for a while. You got a pretty good tone on both the *ah* and the *ee* just then, but I felt you waited too long after the air intake. Try to let it come out as soon as it comes in. Don't hold it. In and out, like this . . . (*demonstrates*).
>
> *Patient*: (writing): I get tired too, but that was better, wasn't it? Although I got tensed up too much.
>
> *Therapist*: Yes, much better. Try letting your arms and shoulders go limp even if you press your lips and tongue to charge the esophagus with air. Like this . . . (*demonstrates*). It's like the old trick of patting your head and rubbing your stomach at the same time. We've got to squeeze the cheeks and mouth to inject the air, but we've also got to keep the esophagus from squeezing shut at the same time. Try it again.
>
> *Patient*: It's so hard. I get discouraged.
>
> *Therapist*: It *is* hard at first, but it'll get easier. Remember how impossible is seemed at first to get any sound at all. Now you can always get it but we have to find ways of lengthening it, letting it leak out, and not wasting it. I'll bet you can say "pie" (*patient does and is surprised and delighted*).
>
> *Patient*: Look: I'll say "I" and "pie" with a pause in between, and you put in the word "want" so it makes "I want pie."

An understanding therapist can make the difference between success and failure and it is very good to know the joy of helping a fellow man to speak again.

Learning to Use the Artificial Larynx. It is much easier to learn to produce speech by the use of this instrument than to master intelligible esophageal phonation. One needs only to press the button on an electro-larynx and hold the diaphragm end of the device flush with the surface of the neck while articulating to be able to achieve some communicative ability. Many users have had no more training than that provided by the instruction booklet which comes with the instrument. The speech therapist however can make the difference between inferior speech and highly in-telligible speech by helping the patient to find the best areas of contact. He can show the patient how to turn on the apparatus intermittently rather than continuously and thereby prevent some of the droning buzz which often interferes with communication. The patient also needs training in mastering the pitch variations that enable him to produce the inflections required by questioning and other prosodic features of normal utterance. Phrasing can also be taught, but perhaps the major contribution a clinician can make is improving the intelligibility of the artificial speech. By helping the patient to articulate the consonants precisely and carefully, the therapist can improve the speech greatly. It is difficult for the user of an electrolarynx to achieve the full potential of this instrument by himself. He needs a therapist.

Hysterical Aphonia.   This disorder, the loss of voice due to emotional stress, usually begins suddenly. The person may begin to talk, then sud-denly find himself unable to finish a sentence with any phonation. One of our cases went to bed, quite happily he told us later, and arose to find him-self unable to speak aloud. A schoolteacher lost her voice in the middle of an explanation of a geometry problem. A preacher who had just conducted the opening exercises and participated in the singing was unable to produce even a squeak of sound when he started his sermon. A housewife about to give her mate a good calling down for coming in late at night found herself unable to say anything except in a whisper. A lieutenant in the jungle of Vietnam started to give the order to his men to enter a par-ticularly dangerous thicket and found that he was not even able to whisper the command, that his mouth moved but no sound came out. Many hy-sterical aphonias arise from laryngitis or colds, the illness creating the necessary explanation for voice failure, though the real reasons lie deep in basic emotional conflicts. We also meet cases where the aphonia comes and goes intermittently. Here is one:

> Wilma's parents and grandparents had been schoolteachers, and they desired her to follow their profession. Her college education had been financed on that understanding. But Wilma didn't want to be a schoolma'am. As soon as she entered college she became engaged to a young man and thought she might escape the horrible prospect of teaching by becoming a housewife. However, in her senior year, he suddenly decided to enter medical school, a decision which meant that

she would have to support him by teaching for several years. She fought the decision but finally acquiesced. It was in her first week of practice teaching that her voice began to go. She would begin her sentences all right, but after saying a few words, she could only whisper. At times longer words would be uttered with the first syllable voiced and the other syllables produced in pantomime. No organic cause was evident. She dropped out of school, and he dropped her; we don't know what happened thereafter.

The medical reports on these cases usually state that no laryngeal pathology is present or that in attempted phonation the vocal folds are bowed. Occasionally the laryngologist will say that though the vocal folds are easily abducted (moved apart), they do not meet in the midline when the patient attempts to produce voice for speech, although they do so in coughing or clearing the throat. Indeed many of the more naïve hysterical aphonics can hum or sing without difficulty. These features indicate that the disorder is not of organic origin, and so also does the use of pantomime speech when it is present. We do not find persons with a true laryngeal paralysis who cannot produce at least a whisper or airflow during attempted phonation.

Treatment of Hysterical Aphonia.   Since this type of aphonia must be viewed symptomatically as a protective device to cope with real or imagined difficulties that have become intolerable, some psychotherapy is often necessary; and the speech clinician may need to refer the patient to a psychiatrist or clinical psychologist and work closely with them. However, there are some cases whose loss of voice persists even after the conflict situation has been resolved; and these provide some of the most sudden and dramatic cures known to speech pathology. At times even in a single session we have been able to help them "find" their voices again and to leave us talking as well as they ever had. When recurrences and relapses occur (and they do not always take place), we can be pretty sure that deeper psychotherapy or environmental change will be required. The largest number of our own clients with hysterical aphonia have been schoolteachers who just needed a rest from their duties for a time. They often come to us in March when summer vacation seems too far away, and they cannot bear to cope with "the little savages" in their schoolrooms another moment. The speech therapy gains time, and the speech therapist provides understanding and hope; often this is all which is required. Greene recommends the use of breathing and relaxation exercises and some counseling interviews. She says, "Relaxation should be followed by breathing exercises while still lying on the couch, and then an attempt at vocalization made, breathing deeply and sighing, then strengthening the sigh till it becomes an audible sound. The therapist may gently manipulate the lower thorax with the hands or massage the throat to reinforce the suggestion of what is wanted. The confident and convincing manner in which she introduces the exercises is of course far more conducive to results than the exercises themselves." [9]

Suggestion is frequently used with hysterical aphonias. Physicians often use a faradic current or ammonia inhalation or massage as the culminating procedures in a period of treatment marked by complete cessation of speech attempt and strong cumulative suggestion. In many instances, coughing is used to demonstrate to the patient that voice exists. Persons who have once had such aphonia are likely to have it again unless the cause is removed. In some instances, when the cause cannot be discovered, a relapse is prevented by having the individual perform some simple vocal ritual each day, such as prolonging each of the vowels for ten seconds.

Some quotations from an article by Sokolowsky and Junkermann will illustrate some of the methods for treating hysterical aphonia:

> First, we administered breathing exercises in connection with a systematic speech and voice retraining . . . (using a humming, or breathy, speech attempt while "pressing together the hands of a nurse standing behind him";) . . . By means of this phonetic reeducation we succeeded in restoring the voice to about 60 percent of our aphonics, a rather meager result considering the relatively tiresome treatment which sometimes lasted several weeks.

> Induced by the publications of Muck and his extraordinary results, we then tried his method—the introduction of a pellet or small ball into the larynx between the vocal cords in order to bring about a sensation of being suffocated which superinduced a cry of fright. We have to confess that our own results with Muck's ball were not very encouraging.

> As soon as the anamnesis pointed to a psychogenic aphonia and the laryngoscopic mirror confirmed this assumption, a short remark such as, "You will be all right quite soon," or, "You will be getting your voice back quite soon," was made. After that the patient was not permitted, so to speak, to "collect his wits." All manipulations such as setting the head in proper position and pulling out the tongue were carried out as quickly as possible, and accompanied by short, crisp and somewhat commanding words. Then followed the deep introduction of the mirror and the attempt to obtain a vocal retching reaction. After this was accomplished, it was brought into the consciousness of the patient with short, crisp remarks, such as "Here we are," "Now your voice is back," or "Do you hear your voice?" After that it required but relatively little effort (the mirror, of course, remaining

---

[9] M. C. L. Greene, *The Voice and Its Disorders* (Philadelphia: J. B. Lippincott, Co., 1964), p. 154.

continually in the throat) to elicit from the patient the unpleasant gag-reminding but nevertheless audible "ah." [10]

In our own practice, we have not needed to resort to such procedures. If the patient has had his unconscious profit from the aphonic symptom and is ready to get rid of it because it is a nuisance, we usually can find some way to restore phonation either through sighing, singing, or humming; the prolonged clearing of the throat; or especially through the use of the *vocal fry*. This term refers to the clicking, tickerlike phonation many of us have used while playing lazily with our voices when relaxed. We have found it very useful in modifying many kinds of voice disorders. All students of speech pathology should learn to produce it. For our patients it is wise to set up some home practice in voice-finding, some routines and exercises for voice-strengthening, and to arrange for several appointments in advance so that further opportunity for counseling can be provided and any relapses taken care of. One of the favorable prognostic signs when the voice does come back is the ability to produce it without tension. If the voice is strained or forced, our experience is that relapse is inevitable.

Spastic Dysphonia.   In this disorder, we have a mixture of aphonia and a strained, tense, vocalized whisper. The person labors hard to squeeze out some voice. It sounds like the strained speech of someone performing tremendous strenuous muscular effort and trying to speak at the same time. The mountain labors and produces a mouse of sound. At times there are facial contortions almost as in the severe stutterer. Fear of speaking is present, but usually not fear of words. This is also to be found in the cerebral palsied or some other type of central nervous system disease.

Unlike hysterical or alaryngeal aphonia, the person with spastic dysphonia often can produce voice at times. Indeed, he may often begin a sentence with easy and normal phonation, then begin squeezing out his speech with progressively greater tension until finally no sound at all is produced. Thus the term *dysphonia* rather than aphonia. The disorder has been called "vocal stuttering," and there are several resemblances between it and stuttering. Often the person may be able to sing easily or say non-meaningful asides with good phonation, only to strain and struggle greatly on meaningful utterances. Although many authors have felt that spastic dysphonia has an emotional origin, recent studies seem to indicate that it may reflect neurologic lesions probably in the pyramidal tract of the brain and that it may be related to the essential tremor syndrome.[11]

[10] R. R. Sokolowsky, and E. R. Junkermann, "War Aphonia," *Journal of Speech Disorders,* IX (1944), 192–208.

[11] E. Robe, P. Moore, and J. Brumlik, "A Study of Spastic Dysphonia," *Laryngoscope,* LXX (1960), 218–23, R. Luchsinger, and G. E. Arnold, *Voice–Speech–Language* (Belmont, Calif.: Wadsworth, 1965), pp. 328–33.

Aronson, Brown, Litin, and Pearson found no significant differences between persons with spastic dysphonia and normals on the Minnesota Multiphasic Personality Test.[12] Fortunately the disorder is rare, for the prognosis is very poor and speech or voice therapy has had little success. We have worked hard with eleven of these persons and completely in vain. Our reason for describing the disorder here is to help other therapists recognize its distinctive features so they might be spared some of our own heartache at being so ineffective.

Phonasthenia. This term refers to the voice that is too little and too weak to carry the normal burdens of communication. Voices which are not loud enough for efficient communication are fairly common, but they seldom are referred to the speech therapist. Imitation, overcompensation for hearing loss, and feelings of inadequacy leading to retreat reactions account for most of them. Many pathological reasons for such disorders are common, but they are frequently accompanied by breathiness, huskiness, or hoarseness, or other symptoms sufficiently evident to necessitate the services of the physician, who should rightfully take care of them.

> One individual with a history of prolonged laryngitis, but with a clean bill of health from the physician, claimed that she was afraid to talk loudly because of the pain she had experienced in the past. Something seemed to stop her whenever she decided to talk a little louder. She constantly fingered her throat. She declared that she was losing all her self-respect by worrying about her inability to speak as loudly as she could. Use of a masking noise during one of her conferences demonstrated to her that she could speak loudly without discomfort. Under strong clinical pressure, she did make the attempt, but the inhibition was automatic.

When we speak we expose ourselves, and the louder we do it, the greater that exposure is. The insecure, withdrawn person finds even ordinary levels of intensity almost unbearably revealing. His very nature resists the display of self. Usually he has good reasons for his inhibited utterance, although they may remain hidden until counseling makes them bearable and manageable. An emotionally healthy person enjoys a certain amount of display speech. One who is not finds it traumatic. And once again, we find that even when psychotherapy is successful, often there is need for voice therapy to enable the person to use an adequate vocal intensity.

Where there is no organic pathology such as vocal modules, paralysis, or contact ulcers, we can assume that the person does possess an adequate

---

[12] A. E. Aronson, J. R. Brown, and J. S. Pearson, "Spastic Dysphonia: I. Voice, Neurological and Psychiatric Aspects," *Journal of Speech and Hearing Disorders,* XXXIII (1968), 203–18.

voice. Our task is to help him find it. Often we discover that emotional insecurity lies at the bottom of the problem, and we must provide opportunities for exploration and release of these feelings. These people often are fearful of establishing close relationships, and their barely audible voices reflect this fear. A warm, permissive therapist can make the vocal therapy itself a means of creating at least one nonthreatening relationship. Often the speech therapy is less important than the case's testing of the therapist's acceptance, but we use the vocal exercises as the pathway to reassurance. By extending the therapy to other communicative situations, the person comes to find that the world may not be as threatening as he had supposed.

But there are often habits involved too. Whatever the original cause of the weak voice, these people often show inefficient forms of breathing when speaking. They may habitually exhale much of the inhaled air prior to vocalization (air wastage), or make a series of small inhalations rather than one large one (staircase breathing), or speak on the very end of the exhaled breath, or speak while the chest is expanding (opposition breathing). A certain amount of air pressure is needed for adequate phonation, and these methods of speech breathing make it difficult to speak loudly enough for communication. We seldom need to teach the person how to breathe; but there are times when we have to teach him to stop breathing in an abnormal way. Once he knows what he is doing wrongly and recognizes the moments of normal breathing which he always shows occasionally, the normal patterns will return.

Often, the problem may consist of the use of improper pitch levels. The person who speaks at the very bottom, or very top, of his pitch range, for any reason, cannot have normal vocal intensity. We may therefore have to change the habitual pitch. We have had cases referred to us as having weak voices who merely were fearful that if they spoke in their usual way, they would have pitch breaks upward into the falsetto. With these, it was necessary to work on pitch control and to ignore the intensity. Generally, intensity becomes louder as the pitch rises. By prolonging tones and then introducing rhythmic pulses of pitch rises which go higher and higher, the intensity of the pulses becomes louder and louder.

Certain voice quality changes can also increase the intensity. By making the voice less breathy or aspirate through the use of very sudden bursts of sound, the voice becomes louder. Increasing the nasality a bit also helps. We once solved the problem of a foreman in a steel mill who was constantly losing his voice and could barely speak above a whisper due to the constant strain to make himself heard. We trained him to speak with a nasal twang while he was on the job.

Also the duration aspects of voice should be explored. By prolonging the vowels a bit, the carrying quality of the voice can be improved. Most public speakers have learned this technique. Also, a slowing down of the rate and the use of longer pauses seem to aid intelligibility.

Some of these cases are difficult to hear merely because they speak with their mouths almost shut—because they do not articulate with any energy. Putting a stopper in any horn diminishes the loudness of its tones. We teach these people to uncork their mouth openings. Also, by making the plosives distinctly or by stressing the fricative consonants, we can compensate for the lack of vocal intensity. Many of the bad habits of utterance are due to excessive tension in the mouth, tongue, or throat; and by relaxing these focal points of tension, the voice becomes freer and louder. One of the common areas of excessive muscular contraction is the region just above the larynx and below the chin. The larynx is often raised almost into the position for swallowing. When a person habitually assumes this abnormal posture prior to vocalization, it is difficult to produce normal voice no matter what effort is expended. Again, we must identify this abnormal behavior and bring it up to consciousness so that it can be brought under voluntary control and eliminated. Voice should not be squeezed out. It needs an open, relaxed, natural channel. At times we have these persons talk while chewing to discover the normal function. Some of our voice cases have forgotten how to produce voice normally. We must show them.

A few of our voice cases, especially those who have some paralysis of the vocal folds, need more energy rather than less, and they need it in the right places. Certain pushing exercises with the arms or legs, or sudden contractions of the fists may aid if they are accompanied by phonation. Also we have found that certain large body postures facilitate louder and freer voices. One of our cases first found his natural voice while on hands and knees with arms extended forward and his head backward. Once he had found it, he gradually became able to produce it in any position.

Finally, we use masking noise to prevent self-hearing when we feel that the person can really produce normal voice but inhibitions prevent it. We ask such a case to continue reading aloud while we gradually introduce a masking noise from an audiometer or tape recorder into both ears. Usually, the person's voice grows much louder as the noise level increases. When we feel that sufficient change has occurred we suddenly shut off the noise, and he hears himself speaking with a normal voice. One of the author's cases was "cured" when he suddenly emerged from a noisy factory and found himself shouting.

Pitch Disorders

There are four fairly common types of pitch disorders: (1) the habitual pitch level which is too high, (2) the monotonal or monopitched voice, (3) pitch breaks, and (4) the falsetto which is usually a disorder of both pitch and quality. There are also several less common ones: (5) the tremulous voice, (6) peculiar and stereotyped inflections, and (7) too low a pitch level in children or females.

Habitual Pitch Levels. The concept of a habitual pitch level must be clearly understood. Except in the case of monotones, it does not refer to a certain fixed pitch upon which all speech is phonated. It represents an average or median pitch about which the other pitches used in speech tend to cluster. For example, in the utterance of the sentence, "Alice was sitting on the back of the white swan," the fundamental pitch of each vowel in any of the words may differ somewhat from that of the others. Moreover, certain vowels are inflected—that is, they are phonated with a continuous pitch change which may either rise, fall, or do both. Of course, each inflection has an average pitch by which it may be measured, if the extent of the variation is also considered. If all the pitches and pitch variations are measured and their durations are taken into account in the speaking of the preceding illustration, we shall find that they cluster about a certain average pitch, which may be termed the "key" at which the speaker phonated that sentence. It should be understood, of course, that different pitch levels will be used under different communicative conditions. Nevertheless, each voice can be said to have a habitual pitch and a habitual pitch range in which most of the communication is phonated.

The pitch of the normal human voice presents many mysteries, and much research needs to be done before we can hope to understand its abnormalities. We know that the voice of a young child is high-pitched when compared with that of the adult, and that in old age it tends to creep back again to higher levels. We know that the major pitch changes occur at puberty, the bottom of the girl's pitch range descending from one to three tones with an equivalent gain at the upper limit. Boys' voices usually drop a full octave, and there is a less marked but noticeable loss at the upper end of the pitch range. Usually, but depending upon the onset of sexual changes, the voice changes occur in boys between the ages of thirteen and fifteen with the girls showing the same basic changes a year earlier. Occasionally, the change of voice has been known to occur very suddenly (usually when puberty comes late), but most frequently it takes from three to six months on the average.

Why do some people fail to make the normal pitch change? There are several reasons besides delayed sexual development. Some cases have voices which are high-pitched primarily because of infantile personalities, because they cannot or prefer not to grow up. This case study may help to make the point:

Charles J. was first referred to the public-school speech therapist for his articulation difficulty at the age of twelve. He substituted *w* for *r* and *l*, *t* for *k*, and *d* for *g*. He had a marked interdental lisp. He sucked his thumb and cried easily. He preferred the company of very young children and still played with dolls at home. He was rejected and despised by boys of his own age and bore the nickname of "Sister." He was an only child, pampered and babied and overprotected by an anxious mother. Although intelligent, he had failed the third grade twice. He was absent from school a good share of the time for chronic headaches and stomach upsets. The articulation defects were very resistant to therapy, and the child was not cooperative. Consequently, he was dismissed from speech therapy classes and referred to the school psychologist, who was unable to solve the home problem because of the mother's attitudes.

At seventeen he was again referred to speech therapy, this time at a college clinic. No articulation defects were present, but the voice was very high-pitched, rather nasally whiny, and weak in intensity. The secondary sex characteristics were present, and he was quite fat. The personality was still infantile.

In such cases psychotherapy is the indicated treatment, although vocal training may be used along with it, either to make the psychotherapy more palatable or to help the person to make changes in the habitual pitch as he comes to accept and solve his psychological problem.

Another common cause of the high-pitched voice is tension. The tighter the vocal cords are held, the higher is the pitch of the tone produced. Tension in any area of the body tends to flow toward and focus in the larynx. Many individuals who, in their occupations, are compelled to speak very loudly will raise their voices to make themselves heard, and this raising also lifts the habitual pitch. Speech therapy will be of little avail unless the underlying cause of the tension can be eliminated or reduced. Some case presentations may help us understand the problem.

Joan P., a high-school senior, referred herself to the speech clinic after hearing a recording of her voice. "Why, I sound like a little first grader," she complained. "After hearing that voice I'll never dare talk to a boy again over the telephone. Please do something!" Analysis of the average pitch levels used by the girl showed that she phonated about the pitch of middle C, a level which is well within the normal range for females of that age. When the test recording was played back, she said, "That's funny. That's a little bit higher than I thought I talked but not so high as the other recording." We then made another recording, in front of a class, and this time the average pitch level did reach F above middle C. We explained to Joan that most females hear their recorded voices as seemingly higher in pitch just as most males hear themselves as possessing a deeper voice than they expect. We also explained the effect of tension and fear on the pitch level and the need for learning to adapt to the pressures of confronting a group. A series of experiences in making recorded talks to a group while trying to use the middle-C habitual pitch of her conversational voice proved successful, and no further difficulty was experienced.

Most of us tend to raise the pitch of our voices when communicating under fear or stress, or when trying to speak loudly. In examining a voice case, we must always be alert lest the case's uneasiness give us a false picture.

A boy of seventeen was referred to us as a monotone, and most of his speech was pitched at D above middle C. He tended to use loudness instead of pitch variations to give the meaningful inflections necessary in asking questions, making demands, and so on. For example, he would say this sentence with each syllable pitched at the one note, but saying the last word quite loudly. "Are you planning to GO?" The effect was often one of hostility, which he did not mean to convey at all. The voice quality was rather harsh. Most strange, he was able to sing in a very high tenor voice and sing very well. A series of counseling interviews and examinations resulted in our refusal to accept him as a case for therapy at that time. A year later, he was reexamined and his voice was entirely normal, being pitched at B below middle C, with a range of an octave and a half, and normal inflections and quality. He had meanwhile started to shave.

As the foregoing case implies, pitch levels are dependent upon many factors. The case mentioned was slow in acquiring the secondary sex characteristics. His larynx, at the time of our first examination, was childlike and underdeveloped. Highly conscious of this, he had endeavored to compensate for the natural high pitch by speaking at the very bottom of his range.

Monopitch. We have never seen a case whose voice could be viewed as strictly monopitched, although we have known many whose voices were highly monotonous. All of them were capable of some pitch change, and all of them had some inflection. The key characteristic was the narrow range of inflection and pitch change, often no more than one or two semitones. Also, these individuals often substitute a change in intensity for the pitch change, and this creates the impression of deviancy. Many persons whose voices strike us as entirely lacking in inflection are merely those with stereotyped inflections. These are the ones whose voices fall after every pause, comma, or period. There is deadly monotony, to be sure, but not monopitch. Nevertheless these restricted, lifeless voices are miserable to listen to, and they interfere with communication by sheer lack of variety.

The causes of monopitch are (1) emotional conflicts, (2) lack of physical vitality, (3) hearing loss, and (4) the use of habitual pitch levels too near the top or bottom of the pitch range. The role of emotional causation in producing the monotonous voice has been described by various authors and researchers. Diehl's review of the literature indicates that individuals who are in states of depression and schizophrenics tend to show this type of voice.[13] We have also found it in paranoid or suspicious individuals or those who are barely able to keep their emotions under control, as a defensive mechanism to prevent others from knowing how they feel.

Undernourished, sick, or fatigued persons also tend to show little range of pitch or inflection. They seem to have insufficient energy available for the normal melody of speech. Those who are very hard of hearing also present the picture of monotonous voice, although careful scrutiny often reveals certain stereotyped inflections, most of which are alike and yet unlike those of the normally hearing person. Finally, when the habitual pitch for any reason is either too near the ceiling or floor of the pitch range, we find a tendency toward monopitch. We need voice room to maneuver. If we cannot go downward, we do not go upward. Falsetto voices often show this feature.

Pitch Breaks.   Most of us tend to think of the change of voice as occurring abruptly when it does occur, and the "pitch breaks" have been the subject for a good deal of humor in our culture. However, recent unpublished research has shown that most children, boys and girls alike, do have these sudden shifts of pitch as characteristic of the period of voice change; and also, some children as young as seven and eight can show similar sudden shifts of pitch. We also are prone to think of the pitch changes as always shifting toward the higher notes, but when this does occur consistently, it does so only toward the end of the puberal period. Voice breaks can be downward as well.

The majority of the pitch breaks that do occur are generally an octave in extent in most children. They occur involuntarily, very suddenly, and the child seems to have little control over them, reacting at first with great surprise. The upward pitch breaks of boys, according to Curry, start when the word spoken is pitched below the habitual pitch of the moment. It often seems as though, in the attempt to return to the level they feel most natural, they overshoot their mark. In a few children the experience is so traumatic that they resort to a guarded monotone, and develop a very restricted range.

The cause of the puberal pitch changes is not entirely understood, though we do know that profound alterations in the organs of voice occur at this time. The male larynx grows much larger, and the vocal cords longer

[13] C. F. Diehl, "Voice and Personality," in D. Barbara, ed., *Psychological and Psychiatric Aspects of Speech and Hearing* (Springfield, Ill.: Charles C. Thomas, Publisher, 1960), Chapter 9.

and more suddenly; the female larynx increases more in height than in width, and the vocal cords seem to thicken. The male vocal cords lengthen about one centimeter, the females only a third as much. At the same time, the child is growing swiftly in skeletal development. The neck becomes longer, and the larynx takes up a lower location relative to the opening into the mouth. The chest expands greatly, and perhaps one of the causes of voice breaks is the greater air pressure that suddenly becomes available. The following case may be illustrative:

> One of our cases was a boy who had been delayed markedly in physical growth until his sixteenth birthday, at which time a great spurt of development occurred. He grew six inches in three months and his voice seemed uncontrollable as far as pitch was concerned, so much so that he developed a marked fear of speaking and a profound emotional disturbance. Speech therapy was ineffective until he was taught by the speech therapist to fixate the chest and to use abdominal breathing as exclusively as possible. Immediately the pitch breaks disappeared, and the technique tided him over the next six months, at which time he returned to his normal thoracic breathing pattern without difficulty.

The above case illustrated another of the characteristics of the truly abnormal voice. Not only did he have many more pitch breaks than does the average boy, but also he showed shifts of pitch which were not of the usual type. Sometimes the break in pitch was of fourteen semitones. The speech therapist can often distinguish a pathological case who will not "outgrow" his adolescent pitch breaks by listening to the type of pitch shift which occurs. Curry cites the following similar case from the German literature:

> Case four is that of a 23-year-old girl with a mutation disorder; since age eight her voice had been continuously hoarse and accompanied by many involuntary breaks. These breaks from a higher to a lower pitch took place so rapidly that the voice was originally diagnosed as diplophonic (two-toned). In this instance, however, the apparent diplophonia is due to a rapid succession of different fundamentals rather than to different rates of vibration of the two individual cords. This case is of especial note because the difference between the two frequencies is not necessarily an octave.[14]

Public-school speech therapists who have to make surveys of large populations of school children should recognize the fact that the control

[14] T. Curry, "Voice Breaks and Pathological Larynx Conditions," *Journal of Speech and Hearing Disorders*, XIV (1948), 356–58.

of pitch during puberal development can vary widely from day to day. Very often there is less control early in the morning than later in the day. We have also found that anger, excitement, fear, and other emotions may give a false picture of the severity of the problem. Laughter, especially if uncontrolled, will also produce an unusual number of breaks.

Too high a pitch in some individuals, either male or female, may be the result of failure to make the necessary transition to the adult voice. The social penalties upon the male with a voice pitched too high are severe in our culture. Indeed, an old name for this voice problem was the "eunuchoid voice." The penalties upon the female are less severe. An occasional male may even find a "baby voice" as attractive as a "baby face." Nevertheless, the high-pitched voice is rarely much of an asset. We have seen some marked tragedies resulting from the disorder. Personalities have been warped by social rejection; vocational progress has been blocked; self-doubts have destroyed the person's ability to cope with the demands of existence. There is nothing humorous about a high-pitched voice.

The Falsetto.   This voice is one which is available to all of us. We may not be able to yodel, but we can at least use the falsetto at will, both in speech and song. Authorities are not agreed as to the manner of its production, but it is most easily produced when the throat and laryngeal muscles are fairly relaxed. Some individuals use only this particular adjustment of the larynx habitually in the production of voice, and its oddness in speech can provoke much distress. It usually begins in puberty and is more frequently encountered in the male.

The causes of the habitual falsetto voice appear to consist of (1) emotional factors as a protest against sexual or social maturity, (2) use as a defense against pitch breaks, and (3) use as a method for preventing the hoarse or husky voice. The first of these presents a problem in counseling and psychotherapy in some cases and professional help may be needed.

> R. James S., III, came to us with a very high-pitched falsetto whose only inflection was at the end of his phrases and sentences. He was a fat boy at eighteen, and he was a boy rather than a youth. His divorced mother had spoiled and babied him for years, and he was almost totally unable to cope with his freshman year in the university. She phoned him every evening and wrote to him every day. He refused to eat in the dormitory, to have a roommate, and often to go to class. In our examination, he wept easily and frequently and also in a falsetto. We recorded his voice, played it back to him, and then referred him to a psychiatrist. He dropped out of school and we lost track of him for a year. When he returned, he told us that he had continued his psycho-therapy, had cut his ties with his mother, and was working as a janitor. His psychiatrist reported that he was now ready for voice

therapy. Within a single week he found his deep bass voice. It was one of the easiest bits of therapy we have ever had. Had we attempted to work with Bob, as he had finally come to call himself, earlier, we are sure we would have been unsuccessful.

This case points up another significant bit of information. Abnormal voices can persist of their own momentum and habituation long after the original cause has ceased to exist. They perpetuate themselves by the reinforcement they get from successful consummation of communication.

In some of our cases, the falsetto appears to be the result of a defensive reaction against the traumatic experience of pitch breaks. It is not pleasant to have one's voice flop around, especially when this behavior provokes mockery and social penalty. By using the falsetto, one can prevent these breaks; and some beginning adolescents use it for this purpose, only to find that they have lost the ability to find the normal adult voice. They fear to use the low-pitched voices we can teach them fairly easily, and our problem is to help them realize that the pitch breaks can be controlled and prevented. We use a lot of negative practice in working with these individuals, deliberately practicing the pitch breaks and desensitizing them. Chanting and singing on the lower pitches is useful. These same basic principles are employed when working with a person whose falsetto is a defense against hoarse or husky voice qualities.

Other Pitch Disorders. The tremulous voice may be due to paralysis, muscular dystrophy, or other similar neurological disorders. It may also be due to cerebral palsy on the one hand, or to fearfulness on the other. Referral to medical or psychological services is indicated. Females or children with very low-pitched voices should be referred to a physician before undertaking speech therapy; often glandular and hormonal problems are present. Stereotyped inflections may be due to foreign-language influence, to psychological conflicts, or to hearing loss.

Treatment of Pitch Disorders.[15] When the problem consists of an habitual pitch which is abnormally high in the male or abnormally low in the woman, the clinician's basic task is to discover ways of helping his case produce a more optimal pitch level. First, there must be some confrontation through tape recording, an experience that often shocks the case terrifically, for he has not really recognized before how his voice sounds to others. We have also found the use of the delayed auditory feedback apparatus very effective in this regard, especially when longer

---

[15] For an excellent discussion of the causes and treatment of pitch disorders due to failure in voice mutation, see the following references: D. A. Weiss, "The Pubertal Change of the Human Voice (Mutation)," *Folia Phoniatrica,* II (1950), 126–59, M. C. L. Greene, *The Voice and Its Disorders* (Philadelphia: J. B. Lippincott, Co., 1964), Chapter 11.

delay times (at least one second) were used. When appropriate, we have even recorded the voice and then played it back with strong amplification. This confrontation in other persons must be done less drastically; but unless the individual really recognizes his pitch deviation at the time it is occurring, he will rarely have the motivation to change.

Our next task is to help the person vary his pitch levels, to explore the range of pitches of which he is capable but has not discovered. The pitch of the voice usually varies with the intensity. By increasing the loudness, the tone will usually be made to rise in pitch. Even high-pitched falsettos will shift downward if a tone is first initiated very loudly, then gradually softened as it is prolonged. Pitch rises when the laryngeal musculature is tensed, and we can use this feature in therapy. Tension in almost any part of the body seems to be reflected and finds some focus in the larynx. By asking the person to pull upward on the seat of his chair, or to push down on the table, we can increase the tension of the vocal folds and raise the pitch of a sustained tone. This works best if the effort is applied in pulses. Conversely, if we wish to lower a pitch, we can begin by using strong muscular contractions and let go jerkily in a series of relaxations.

The self-perception of pitch is still mysterious. We still do not know why some individuals with excellent hearing seem to be unable to match a given pitch or to locate their own voices on a scale. They sing off key and do not know it. However, there seems to be some evidence that pitch perception is tied in somehow with body postures and kinesthesia. Even little children who have never seen a musical scale lift their heads and rise on tiptoe when they reach for a high note. When we try to sing very low, we tuck our chins in, lowering our heads. At any rate, we have found that by having the case follow our head or arm or body movements as we show him how his pitches are rising or falling or being sustained, we can improve his faulty pitch placement. Here is a brief transcript of part of a session with such a person whose pitch breaks were driving him crazy.

> *Therapist:* Now lower your head way down like this, then bring it up in three steps as we sing together do-me-sol.
> *Case:* doh-fa-la.
> *Therapist:* OK. You went up—but you took too big steps. Raise your head in smaller steps. Here, I'll hold your head and move it. . . .
> *Case:* doh-fa-sol.
> *Therapist:* That's better. The first and last were all right. You sang do-fa-sol. It should be do-*me*-sol. Let's make the second movement smaller. . . .

We stopped the transcript just in time. The case sang, "doh-la-tee." This is patient work, this voice-retraining—but we have succeeded often when our first attempts seemed to reveal a hopeless prognosis. With real motivation, surprising results may be had. In this regard, we find that a prime motivation is the opportunity provided by a permissive therapist for the case's singing. These sour-toned people love to sing, and they've been penalized and frustrated most of their lives because their "pear-shaped tones" turn out to be lemons. So we let them sing a lot and do some voice therapy when we can. Another similar method consists of pitch-writing. We take the case's hand as he holds the pencil or chalk and tell him to go up and down or hum or sing his own invented tunes. Then we trace the variations and provide a graphic record.

Although the above method for teaching a new pitch level is most effective, there are several others. One frequently employed uses the vocalized sigh or yawn to produce the desired pitch. These sighs and yawns must be accompanied by decreasing intensity and relaxation in order to be most effective. Another method employs exclamations of disgust or contempt in order to provide a lower pitch. Still another makes use of the grunts and noises symbolic of relief or feeding. Clearing the throat may also be used to provide a lower pitch. These methods are often effective with true monotones when the former stimulation or matching method fails. Many of the techniques included in the stimulation method are combined with the biological-activity methods in order to provide the necessary stability of performance.

An example of some actual therapy which produced a change from a high falsetto into normal male phonation within a single hour may now be given, though it should be understood that further work was necessary to stabilize the new voice thereby obtained.

T. J. was a nineteen-year-old boy with a high-pitched monotonal falsetto which was inconsistent in that occasionally nonfalsetto tones were heard, although they, too, were spoken at the same high level. After the usual ear-training in identifying the problem, we had a session in which we demonstrated the following kinds of phonation and asked him to join us and to duplicate what we heard: (1) We asked him to do some vocalized donkey-breathing, alternately on inhalation and on exhalation, and very rhythmically. As we produced the model, we occasionally changed the pitch of the exhaled sound, using first the falsetto ourselves and then lower normal tones. Several of his tones were very good. (2) We asked him to retract his head as far as he could, then to bring it forward until it dropped down on his chest, producing a long sigh as he did so. We showed him and first did what he did so far as sound was concerned, then gradually let our own pitch fall as the sigh ended. He followed us and ended with a weak, breathy, but very low tone. (3) We showed him some stretching and yawning and asked him to join us, saying "Awwwww" in the middle of the yawn. (4) We placed some tissue paper over a comb and asked him to buzz it, using a prolonged *z* sound with his lips against the paper. The tone we used was of low pitch, and so was his. We then asked him to say *zzzeeezzz* and *zzzooozzz* and then *zzzzoooooo* as he buzzed the comb. This failed, for he used a falsetto buzz. (5) We asked him to duplicate a vocalized clearing of the throat as he held his fingers in his ears. It was very low-pitched and without any falsetto. (6) We then taught him the clicking vocal fry until he could sustain it for several seconds, then had him open and shut his jaws and lips during the fry phonation. In this activity we heard normal phonation along with the vocal fry. (7) We demonstrated head- and jaw-shaking from side to side while we produced various vowels of different pitches. (8) As he duplicated our model by head- and jaw-shaking in unison with us, we slowly said, "I am using my real voice," and he echoed it in the new low pitch. (9) We played back the recording of his voice to him, called it quits for that session, asked him not to speak very much until we saw him again, and made an appointment to do so.

DISORDERS OF VOICE QUALITY

There are five major disorders of voice quality: hypernasality; denasality; the breathy, husky voice; the harsh or strident voice; and the hoarse voice. In addition, there is a peculiar throaty or guttural voice which is actually a low-pitched falsetto, and it is treated accordingly in another section.

Hypernasality. This problem is not an uncommon one. It occurs primarily because the back door to the nose fails to close sufficiently. The contraction of the soft palate and pharyngeal muscles which elevate, spread, and squeeze the rear opening to the nasal passages may be said to constitute that door. Research has shown that the closure need not be complete on all sounds to prevent hypernasality, but there are definite limits to the amount of opening permitted. Certain organic conditions reflect themselves in excessive nasality because they make it difficult to close this valve-like mechanism sufficiently. The person with an unrepaired cleft palate shows hypernasality; so does the person whose soft palate has been paralyzed or made sluggish by poliomyelitis or other disease. Investigations have also revealed that hypernasality tends to occur after the adenoids have been removed, a process which leaves a relatively larger channel than had previously existed, due to the adenoid mass.

Hypernasality, when excessive, creates a voice quality which most listeners find unpleasant, although the vocal yokel who loves hillbilly ballads may deny this. It has some virtue in enabling the speaker to get his message across in the presence of masking noise, for it carries piercingly. Auctioneers and barkers at carnival side shows find it useful, if not ornamental.

Assimilation Nasality. Hypernasality may be general and exist on most of the vowels and voiced consonant sounds, or it may be restricted only to the sounds which precede or follow the nasal consonants *m, n,* and *ng.* This latter type is termed assimilation nasality. Many speakers of general American English show some assimilation nasality in such a sentence as "Any man can make money." This is because of the need for alternate openings and closing of the velopharyngeal opening. In the word *man,* the passageway to the nose must be open on the *m,* closed on the *a,* and opened again on the *n.* It's easier just to leave the space open. Also, even on a word such as *and,* we tend to prepare for the *n* opening while we're still saying the *a,* and this may cause a premature lowering of the soft palate, thereby producing the sound nasally. The assimilation may thus be either forward or backward. Hypernasality of either type seems to be more likely to occur on certain sounds than on others. High back vowels such as *oo* [u] and *o,* show less hypernasality than do the lower front vowels such as A [e] or *an* [æ] as in *cat.* The consonants *z* and *v* tend to show more hypernasality on them than do the other consonants. It is possible to have much hypernasality without ever having any airflow coming out of the nose because it is the resonation of the sound, not the air flow, which creates the unpleasant voice quality. The louder the voice, the more prominent the hypernasality appears.

There are other causes besides the organic for hypernasality. Through imitation and identification, children can learn the excessively nasal voices of their parents or associates. Low vitality and fatigue also tend to produce more of the problem, for it takes energy to make the swift adjustments needed. Finally, whining children and adults have whining voices; complaint prefers the trombone of the nose. Certain stereotyped rising-falling inflections along with the hypernasality tend to identify this causation. It is different from that shown by the organic cases.

Denasality. This is the voice of the head cold, of the hay fever, victim, of the child with enlarged adenoids. The nasal passages are occluded, perhaps by growths within the nostrils, by congestion in the nasal cavities above the roof of the mouth, or by adenoids in the rear passageways. Often some of the nasal consonants are affected, the person saying "Mby syduhzziz are killig mbe." The voice sounds are dulled and congested. Listeners desire to clear their own throats or to flee. Again, as we have found before, denasal voices may be maintained long after the cause has ceased to exist.

The Breathy, Husky Voice. This disorder often coexists with other problems. It may show itself in intermittent aphonia, in cases of weak intensity, in conjunction with the hoarse voice. Its major characteristic, as the name implies, is an excessive output of air flow along with the phonation. Breathy voices are not whispered, but they are aspirate in quality.

Phonation is present, but the rush of air is obvious. At times, the huskiness accompanies the tone; at other times the constricted hissing of the air precedes or follows the tone. There is air wastage. In some cases, a sort of gasping series of short inhalations throughout the person's speech produces the impression of huskiness. When this occurs, the phrases are short and choppy, and the rhythm of utterance is disturbed. From this description it is obvious that there are different types of breathy voices.

The causes of the breathy voice may be either organic or functional. A paralyzed vocal cord may fail to join its twin at the midline for part of its length, thus leaving a gap through which the airflow may leak. A vocal nodule—a tiny corn-like growth on the edge of a vocal cord—may prevent complete closure. Certain diseases may inflame or swell the membranes of the vocal cords so that they vibrate inefficiently. Excessive strain may make them weak—as it does any muscle when overloaded too long. Whenever you meet such a disorder, you should first make sure that the person hasn't just been yelling too long at a football game or has a bad cold, and then, if the condition has persisted or is getting worse, the case should be immediately referred to a physician.[16]

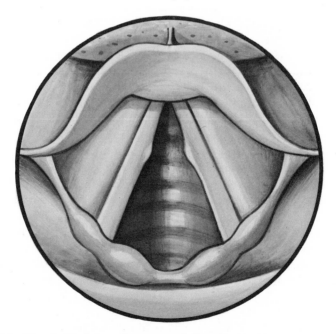

FIGURE 16: *Vocal Nodules.* Courtesy of Dr. P. N. Damste, University of Utrecht.

[16] For a more thorough explanation of the organic causes of defective voice quality, see the following references: R. Luchsinger and G. E. Arnold, V*oice–Speech–Language* (Belmont, Calif.: Wadsworth, 1965), pp. 176–86, 218–47; and P. Moore, *Organic Voice Disorders* (Englewood Cliffs, N.J.: Prentice-Hall, Inc., 1964), Chapter 6.

There are also other causes. We have known individuals whose breathy voices were being produced and maintained solely by improper habits of vocal attack. They always began voicing with a preliminary exhalation of air. We had to teach them to start speaking without this preparatory windup. Some persons use a breathy voice because of the fear of being heard or exposed. And a few of them employ it deliberately. The following case illustrates the latter point.

> Ruth, a rather plain high-school girl, was referred to us by the English teacher, who reported that her voice was so husky she was unable to make herself heard in class. We examined the girl and discovered not only the huskiness but also a low, habitual pitch level with certain inflections which were unmistakable. She could sing well and without any breathiness. A bit of sympathetic interviewing explained the situation. "The boys like this kind of voice," she said grinning. "I'm not too attractive, but a moose is a moose and they come when I call." We found out later that the boys called her "Hot-breath Harriett." We kept her secret.

The male has also been known to mistake asthma for passion.

The Harsh or Strident Voice.   There are voices which are so rasping and piercing that they repel listeners. The basic characteristic of these voices is the presence of what is called the "vocal fry," because, perhaps, it sounds like the sizzling of bacon in the frying pan. It is hard to describe but fairly easy to produce. By opening your mouth and making a ticker-like, crackling sort of sound, you can produce it and even slow it down until the separate clicks can be distinguished. When this vocal fry is fast, however, and accompanied by great tension, we have the basic quality of the strident or harsh voice. It is often accompanied by strain localized about the larynx, and often this structure is pulled up almost into the position used in swallowing. If you will place the tip of a finger against your Adam's or Eve's apple and produce a very harsh voice, you will know what we mean.

Along with these features we also find the presence of what is called the "hard attack." Normally, the vocal folds should be brought together almost simultaneously with the pulse of air pressure. In the aspirate or soft attack, as we have already seen, the vocal folds close *after* the air has begun to flow. In the hard attack, the folds are closed and held tightly prior to the breath pulse. To break them open and start them vibrating from this tight position requires extra effort. If you will squeeze and hold your vocal folds tightly closed and suddenly utter a vowel, you will hear the little strained click that indicates the hard attack. It is not a good way to produce voice; vocal nodules or contact ulcers may result from the strain.

The usual causes of the harsh voice are imitation, personality problems involving hostility and aggression, the need to make oneself heard in the presence of masking noise, and the use of improper pitch levels. We need not belabor the obviousness of the first two of these causes, but some comment on the others is necessary. Strident voices seem to be able to make themselves heard more easily than normal voices, even though the effect is often unpleasant. In this regard they are somewhat like hyper-nasality. They're harsh but you can hear them. Those of us whose profes-sions demand constant speaking in noisy situations often develop them, and sound more aggressive than we are. One of the nicest persons we have ever known was a lady who was in charge of the woman's swimming classes at our university, and she sounded like a witch until she developed vocal nodules and had to have voice therapy as well as a change of jobs. The only way she had found to pierce the echoing noise of the splashing, squealing girls was to scream at them harshly. One of our cases was a foreman in a noisy factory whose harsh straining voice finally gave out due to the formation of contact ulcers near the back ends of his vocal folds. Those of us who become teachers or speech therapists must remember to take care of our own professional tool, the human voice. It cannot be abused with impunity.

Finally, let us say something of pitch levels. Some persons, for one good reason or another, may lower their habitual pitch level nearly to its floor. If you will attempt to speak loudly at your own lowest note, you will find harshness and the vocal fry coming into your voice. You will find strain. Most of us, however, tend to raise our pitch level when we speak loudly. This too can lead to screaming stridency. It is possible to speak very loudly at your own natural pitch level, but some of us never discover this skill.

The Hoarse Voice. Acoustically, the hoarse voice may be said to be a combination of the breathy and the harsh voice quality disorders. In it you can hear the air wastage and also the straining vocal fry of the strident voice. When voices suddenly become hoarse, we look for evi-dence of overuse or abuse. Most of us have become hoarse from too much yelling at one time or another but not from praying. Usually with rest the hoarseness disappears. You've got to stop calling the pigs from the back forty, Ma. The same situation occurs as the result of a severe cold or laryngitis. Many boys develop a hoarse or husky voice just before puberty in an effort to assume the deep, low tones of the adult male or to demon-strate their toughness. This too shall pass. But we wish to sound a strong note of warning about hoarseness. When it persists long after the abuse or laryngitis has disappeared, and there seems to be no apparent reason for its continuance, referral to a laryngologist should be made. Cancer of the larynx often shows its ugly head first in this form.

A hoarse voice may also be produced through ventricular phonation. By this term we refer to the vibration of the false vocal folds which lie above the true ones. It is uncommon but we have found it in some few bedeviled children who suffered many penalties. The following account by Voelker may illustrate the problem.

> One patient complained of dropping his voice at the end of sentences, and it was found that he did not lower his vocal cord pitch, but actually stopped using his vocal cords at the end of the sentence and substituted for them a ventricular vibration. An actor, with an excellent stage voice, complained of hoarseness only in conversation. It was found that in intimate and quiet conversation he used a ventricular voice to "save for his art" his stage voice. A youth was criticized by his parents for having a high and squeaky voice and acquired ventricular phonia in order to lower his voice to a normal pitch. Thus, instead of lowering his voice to a normal pitch of perhaps 150 cycles, he lowered it to one of between 48 and 57 cycles. A similar case was found in which a man thirty-one years old, who had a deaf wife, became self-conscious about his yelling, and outside his home developed phonation with the ventricular bands to subdue his voice. A college student raised the pitch of his voice to read aloud or to recite but used a ventricular tone in conversation. Sometimes it is found in careless conversation only. A five-year-old boy was kidded by his playmates for having a high voice, and he lowered it by acquiring a ventricular voice. An eighteen-year-old youth, with a eunuchoid quality, substituted ventricular phonation for his weak and strident vocal cord voice and thought his new hoarse voice gave the impression of virility.[17]

Treatment of Voice Quality Disorders

Speech therapists who have watched professional singers working hour upon hour to perfect their tone, practicing scales, spending long hours with their voice teacher sometimes envy that teacher. To find the same devotion in a person with a voice disorder is unusual. Even when the person has a falsetto or a husky voice due to severe vocal nodules, it is difficult to get him to work hard enough to hope for a favorable result. The reason for this state of affairs seems to lie in the relative lack of attention we pay to our voices. We listen to our thoughts rather than to the carrier waves on which they ride. In the expression of emotion, we are more concerned with the cargo of anger rather than the voice vehicle which carries it. In most communicative interchanges, the basic message is carried by the articulation rather than the tones; and unless the voice is so weak it cannot be heard, the fulfillment of communication generally rewards unpleasant voices as well as good ones. It is only in display speech

[17] C. H. Voelker, "Phoniatry in Dysphonia Ventricularis," *Annals of Otology, Rhinology, and Laryngology,* XLIV (1935), 471–72.

such as that of the teacher or actor that a poor voice is a major handicap. Our society seems to be more tolerant of deviant voice than of deviant articulation or timing or language. For these reasons, then, it is always wise to explore the amount of motivation we can expect before undertaking therapy with our voice cases.

Identification of the Problem.   One of the best ways we have found to motivate these cases is to have them hear their own voices on tape recordings, not once but over and over again. Once we put a schoolteacher with a very hypernasal voice into a booth, locked the door, and piped in her own recorded voice a bit amplified for fifteen minutes. From then on she worked very hard. We also have a delayed-speech apparatus which echoes what the person says about four seconds later. But best of all is a therapist who can imitate almost exactly the voice he hears. We train our own student therapists in this skill so that they can be the echo machine. Amplification, by means of one of the new binaural auditory training units, can be very effective, especially if the therapist joins the person and first uses the abnormal voice, then shifts to a better one. The same effect can be had by having the person cup his hands to make a channel from his mouth to one ear, then the therapist alternately puts his echo and his normal voice into the other ear as they read in unison. At other times we feed a masking noise into the person's ears from an audiometer as he is speaking, and then suddenly turn it off so the person hears his voice more vividly. Since much of the inability to hear one's voice comes from the adaptation to the usual conditions of phonation, almost anything which alters the usual conditions helps one to hear it as it is. Radio announcers long ago found that they could hear their own voices better by cupping one ear to alter the sound field. We use this device and occasionally employ a hearing aid to help the case identify his problem. It has been said that voice is monitored by bone conduction rather than by air-conducted sound, although the research on this is not definitive. However, we have often found that having the person plug his ears with his fingers makes it possible for him to hear his defective voice more clearly and to modify it.

Analyzing the Deviancy.   We find that often the person is unable to recognize the deviancy in voice until he is trained in its analysis. One has to know what to listen for. One needs training. The therapist must train the case to do this analyzing, patiently providing examples of what is wrong, checking their occurrence in the person's voice. Let us give a description of this analyzing process as it would be done in hypernasality.

Recognition of Defective Quality.   In order that the student may learn to recognize the unpleasant voice quality whenever it occurs in his speech, the vowels that are least defective should be used. The therapist should imitate these vowels as the student produces them, and then repeat them, using excess nasality. The student will readily recognize the difference. He should be required to produce these vowels first normally and then with excess nasality, carefully noting the difference. Lightly placed thumb and forefinger on each side of the septum, or the use of the cold mirror placed under the nostrils, will provide an accessory check of the presence of the hypernasality. The student should then listen to the therapist's production of his worst vowel, with and without nasality. If difficulty is experienced in recognizing this, the student can correlate his auditory judgments with the visual and tactual sensations received from the use of the mirror and finger-septum contact. Requiring him to close and open his eyes during alternate productions of the vowels as the therapist uses the mirror under his nostrils will soon provide adequate discrimination.

After some of this training has been successfully completed, the therapist should read a passage in which certain vowels are underlined and are purposely nasalized. The student should listen carefully, checking on a copy of the passage all vowels in which he hears the unpleasant quality. Many of the games and exercises used in the ear training of articulatory cases can be modified to teach the student better discrimination and identification of the good and bad voice qualities. Although at first the therapist will need to exaggerate the hypernasality, she should endeavor to decrease it gradually until the student is skilled in detecting even a slight amount of it. After this has been done, the student should read and re-read a certain paragraph, making judgments after each word as to whether or not excess nasality occurred. These judgments may be checked by the teacher, and the percentage of correct judgments ascertained. This procedure will serve as a motivating device. The student may also be required to repeat series of words or isolated vowels, using the mirror under his nostrils and making his judgment of normal or nasal voice quality before opening his eyes to observe the clouding or nonclouding of the mirror. Much home practice of this sort can be used.

The same sort of self-scanning should be used with other voice disorders. Unless the person comes to hear what is wrong, he will not correct it. There is one caution we wish to leave with you. Occasionally, a person may feel that he is becoming much worse as the result of the recognition training. All that has happened is that he has become more conscious of what has always been there before; but it is wise, early in treatment, to warn him that this may occur and that it is a good sign of improvement. Similarly, some of our voice cases may become rather emotional and rejecting of themselves as the defective voice becomes more apparent to them. However, if the therapist is able to share the problem, using the abnormal voice calmly and without anxiety, the person usually soon becomes desensitized to it. We have found it wise from the beginning examination to present the task as a joint endeavor. We explore its causes together, and together we work to modify the voice.

Discovering the New Voice.   Each of us is the potential possessor of many voices. We can all vary our pitch, intensity, and quality pretty much at will, although few of us have ever felt that it was possible or necessary to learn a new habitual voice. When this necessity becomes apparent, as a result of the training in awareness, we might think that little further difficulty in procuring cooperation would be necessary. However, a storm of resistance usually arises at this point. This is what one of our cases said to us:

> Yesterday, when we made that tape recording of my new voice and I heard it, I felt all mixed up inside. I told you it sounded much better, and it does. Compared to my old voice, it's a great improvement. But it isn't ME! It just isn't. I sound like a phony or like an actor playing a part. I know it's better, but I don't want to talk so strangely. I just couldn't keep my appointment with you today because I'm so upset about it. I'm even thinking of quitting. I know you said I'd get used to it, but right now I don't think I ever could.

She got used to it, and now it is the old voice which seems unbelievable to her. But this is a problem to be faced. The voice is closely integrated with the personality. Its inflections, volume, and quality have been used since childhood to express emotion. The old voice has a long history of being associated with basic feelings. It does not yield easily to modification, but it does yield. The important thing is that both the therapist and the person with the voice problem must anticipate this resistance and be prepared to cope with it.

Variation.   One of the ways to overcome this built-in rigidity and resistance is to begin by exploring all the possible ways of producing phonation. We must share together in free variation, almost in tonal play, trying one vocal variation after another. Van Riper and Irwin describe this process as follows:

> First we can get the case to run through his entire repertoire of possible phonation, locating within it the desired target tones. Few individuals are entirely consistent in their abnormal voice. Some vowels, for example, may be less nasalized than others; in certain activities, such as sighing, no hard attacks or tension may make the tone strident; in shouting, no breathiness may occur; in humming, a higher pitch level may be used. By varying the postural, breathing, pitch, intensity, or quality factors we may be able to locate within the individual's own phonation the voice we need to use as a standard, as a goal.[18]

[18] Charles Van Riper, and John V. Irwin, *Voice and Articulation* (Englewood Cliffs, N.J.: Prentice–Hall, Inc., 1958), p. 285.

Let us view some of the specific ways by which we might help our voice case vary his phonation in his search for a better voice.

Nowhere will we find resistance to change as tenacious as in voice quality. A habitual voice quality seems as much a part of the person as his nose, and unconsciously the case seems to say, "Keep your therapeutic fingers off my proboscis!" It has been so closely associated with egocentric speech, with emotional expression, with communication, that it is almost a basic feature of the self. Even when the case hates her voice, a better voice sounds so strange and artificial that she tends to sabotage any attempts to change it. We have found it essential to verbalize this, to predict the resistance, and to help the case understand it. It is unwise to ask the person to use new voices in communication, in social gesture, in emotional expression until this phase of resistance has passed.

Accordingly, our first experimentation with change in voice quality should be confined to play, to fantasy, to imitation of animal noises, or imitation of other people. The therapist must set the appropriate models, and he must be in command of almost as many voices as a professional actor. We have trained our majors in speech therapy in these skills so that they can provide these variations in voice quality. Too many beginning therapists try too soon to get a better voice quality from their clients. First their clients must discover how many voices they own; first they must vary and play with their own voices.

This variation should first of all involve changes in pitch and intensity, which are easier to accomplish. Then perhaps a falsetto or a hypernasal voice can be attempted. Then a denasal or throaty (low-pitched falsetto) or harsh or hoarse voice can be assumed.

After these gross variations, we have found it useful to go with the client into stores and to study and later to imitate the voices of various clerks. We help the person to learn the technique of silent echo-speaking, pantomime in subvocal form the speech of the person being heard. Then we use playlets or dialogues, taking various parts and adopting the voices most appropriate. Again the therapist must share the variation and set the models.

Out of all this variation training comes the firm understanding that voice change is possible. The experiences have been pleasant. The person realizes for the first time that he has not one voice but many—and that he has a choice!

Fixation. Once the person has come to identify his abnormal voice and has learned to vary it, our next task is to get him to locate and fix solidly his new voice. The process is at first a bit like target shooting. He may miss the bull's-eye of the new voice quality more than he hits it. His voice gun tends to wobble. New patterns of muscular contractions and of laryngeal or pharyngeal postures must be learned. It is the therapist's role to help him know how far off the mark his vocal attempts have been. Patiently the therapist makes suggestions, points out the extent of the difference between the voice produced and that desired.

In this process it is helpful if the therapist is able to imitate with some fidelity the case's various voice productions and also to present a model of the voice to be attained. We use a tape recorder more often with voice cases than with any other of the speech disorders. Usually it is possible, even very early in treatment, to get a sample or two of the desired voice. This we isolate from the rest, make a loop of tape bearing the good sample, and use this as our target.

At this phase of treatment every session begins with a playing of this model loop, and we use it often to provide the bull's-eye. We also often make a tape recording which has on it, first a vivid sample of the abnormal voice at its worst, then a series of graduated and numbered voice samples that progressively come closer and closer to the voice desired, which forms the terminal example. After the case becomes familiar with this "measuring tape," he is able, with fair consistency, to evaluate any vocal attempts in terms of its proximity to the desired new voice. Strong motivation is thereby procured.

Progressive Approximation. Let us say here again, that speech therapy is not a matter of exchange of one type of speech for another, but a process of progressive approximation. Therapists who have only *good* and *bad* or *yes* and *no* in their professional vocabularies should exchange them for *closer* and *farther* or *hotter* and *colder* as in the old nursery game. In voice therapy, we work with little shifts, and we reinforce with our approval those vocal attempts that come closer to the desired goal. This holds for disorders of pitch, intensity, and quality and for all types of variant human behavior seeking to modify itself.

To aid in getting this concept across (for the case, too, tends to make judgments in terms of black and white) it is well for the therapist to present models of these miniature modifications that change in the direction of the goal. It is the client's task to judge whether they approach or retreat from the goal. By using large changes first, and then smaller ones, the case's perceptions and discriminations are sharpened, and he can then evaluate his own attempts with objectivity.

One of our favorite ways for using progressive approximation in voice therapy is to use a binaural auditory trainer. We then feed in the case's voice into one ear and our own voice into his other ear, thereby permitting simultaneous comparison. We usually begin by joining the case as he reads or phonates a tone, imitating him closely so both voices harmonize in unison, then gradually we change our own voice in small steps in the direction of the desired voice. Perceiving the difference, the case often shifts unconsciously to bring both voices together again, and so a progressive approximation has occurred. Often it is necessary for the therapist to rejoin the case and use the latter's voice again before attempting another shift. But careful training in this way, along with commentary, breaks for relaxation, and suggested corrections, can be very effective. There is also in this procedure a basic psychotherapeutic healing. The case is not alone. Someone is sharing his problem, someone is identifying with him who knows the path out of his troubles.

If no auditory trainer is available, the case may use his cupped hands to bring his voice to one ear while the therapist puts his mouth to the other.

Stabilization.   New voices are weak and unstable. They need careful tending at first. We have found it wise to insist that the case use it at first only in the therapy sessions where we can concentrate on its motor and acoustic aspects and make it stronger therein.

Once we feel the case has the new voice fairly solidly and can use it consistently in therapy when he's listening to himself, we introduce masking noise into his ears so he can monitor it by proprioception alone, by feeling the vocal postures and muscle tensions. Often at first, this masking tends to create a regression to the old voice, so we introduce the masking noise gradually and intermittently. No one can ever come to use a new voice habitually if he must constantly listen to it. We have to use our ears to hear what others are saying and, indeed, to discover what thoughts we are verbalizing! Let's not burden the ears too much. It is also necessary to be sure that the case can use the new voice at his natural tempo or speed of utterance. It must not be labored or too careful. It cannot be confined to a monotone or chant. All these motor and acoustic variations need some attention.

Next we attempt to stabilize the new voice in display speech, and we like to make recordings of the new voice so the person can listen to them and feel good. Role-playing, orating, readings, all can be used for this purpose. Often at this point we ask the person to give us a verbal autobiography, and to use the new voice while doing so. This should run for several sessions. We do this so as to help to identify the new voice with the self. The perpendicular pronoun "I" especially should become colored with the new role. This provides an opportunity for some mild psychotherapy at the same time. However, as we shall see, we prefer at this stage to keep emotional expression fairly innocuous.

Next we like to stabilize the new voice in the thinking aspect of speech. We show slide films, provide problems, and ask the case to keep a running commentary going in the new voice. At times we even have him do a lot of free or controlled association, saying whatever thoughts that come. It is interesting to watch a case whispering and pantomiming, in the new voice. We cannot hear it, but he insists that it is *there*; and when we suddenly signal for him to vocalize, it appears. Pantomimic speech is close to thought.

When we feel definite progress has been made in the foregoing aspects of speech, we stabilize it in communication. We ask the case now to use the new voice outside the therapy sessions—but at first only when he talks to strangers. We do this to avoid the listener's shocked surprise that often greets a voice case when he confronts them with a new voice. The father of a young man who had never known anything but a high falsetto voice stormed into the bathroom one morning to find out what strange man was in the house at seven in the morning. The boy had only said something to the family dog.

Once the new voice has been used easily with strangers, it can be brought out in the circle of acquaintances and friends or family. It is wise to suggest that the person speak of his voice therapy casually or use it as a conversation piece. Most people are very interested. About this time (and perhaps we have protracted the process unduly in describing it, for at times we have changed voices in a single hour), the new voice becomes stabilized and is felt as natural as the old one had been. There will be a few momentary relapses, usually in emotional expression, but the task has been accomplished.

REFERENCES

Articles

1. Adler, S. "Some Techniques for Treating the Hypernasal Voice." *Journal of Speech and Hearing Disorders*, XXV (1960), 300–302.
   What are these techniques?
2. Arnold, G. E. "Vocal Nodules and Polyps: Laryngeal Tissue Reaction at Habitual Hyperkinetic Dysphonia." *Journal of Speech and Hearing Disorders*, XXVII (1962), 205–17.
   What are the causes of vocal nodules and polyps, and how should they be treated?
3. Aronson, A. E. "Speech Pathology and Symptom Therapy in the Interdisciplinary Treatment of Psychogenic Aphonia." *Journal of Speech and Hearing Disorders*, XXXIV (1969), 320–41.
   Summarize the kinds of emotional problems presented by these cases, and describe the kind of treatment offered them.
4. ———, Brown, J. R., Litin, E. M., and Pearson, J. S. "Spastic Dysphonia." *Journal of Speech and Hearing Disorders*, XXXIII (1968), 203–31.
   Is spastic dysphonia primarily a neurotic disorder?
5. ———, Peterson, H. W., and Litin, E. M. "Voice Symptomatology in Functional Dysphonia and Aphonia." *Journal of Speech and Hearing Disorders*, XXIX (1964), 367–80.
   What are the varieties of symptoms shown by these cases?
6. ———. "A Case of Hysterical Dysphonia in an Adult." *Journal of Speech and Hearing Disorders*, XV (1950), 316–23.
   Why was this case diagnosed as a functional aphonia, and what type of treatment was required?
7. Bangs, J. L., and Friedinger, A. A. "Diagnosis and Treatment of a Case of Hysterical Aphonia in a Thirteen-Year-Old Girl." *Journal of Speech and Hearing Disorders*, XIV (1949), 312–17.
   Describe this case and what was done to help her.
8. Brodnitz, F. "Functional Voice Disorders." Chapter 13 in N. Levine, ed., *Voice and Speech Disorders: Medical Aspects* (Springfield, Ill.: Charles C Thomas, Publisher, 1962).
   What information is presented in this chapter which has not been given in our own text?
9. ———. "The Holistic Study of Voice." *Quarterly Journal of Speech*, XLVIII (1962), 280–84.
   What does the author mean by "holistic," and how does this concept apply to treatment?
10. ———. "Vocal Rehabilitation in Benign Lesions of the Vocal Cords." *Journal of Speech and Hearing Disorders*, XXIII (1958), 112–17.
    Describe the voice training for these cases. When should it begin, and what should be done for those who, like professional singers, must be especially careful of their voices?
11. Burkowsky, M. R. "Vocal Ulcers in a Seventy-One-Year-Old Male."

Journal of Speech and Hearing Disorders, XXXIII (1968), 268–69.
What produced these ulcers, and how were they treated by the voice therapist?

12.   Canfield, W. "Dysphonia Associated with Unilateral Vocal Cords Paralysis: A Case Study." *Journal of Speech and Hearing Disorders,* XXVII (1962), 280–82.
How did the therapist work with this woman?

13.   Curry, T. "Voice Breaks and Pathological Larynx Conditions." *Journal of Speech Disorders,* XIV (1948), 356–58.
Are pitch breaks confined to the pubescent male only? How can they reflect laryngeal pathology?

14.   Dowie, L. N. "Functional Dysphonia." *Speech Pathology and Therapy,* VIII (1965), 18–22.
Describe the three cases presented.

15.   Engelberg, M. "Correction of Falsetto Voice in a Deaf Adult." *Journal of Speech and Hearing Disorders,* XXVII (1962), 162–64.
How did the therapist work with this difficult problem?

16.   Fox, D. R. "Spastic Dysphonia: A Case Presentation." *Journal of Speech and Hearing Disorders,* XXXIV (1969), 275–79.
In the case mentioned, what was the evidence that organic or emotional factors were involved?

17.   Freud, E. D. "Functions and Dysfunctions of the Ventricular Folds." *Journal of Speech and Hearing Disorders,* XXVII (1962), 334–40.
Describe the voice problem of the thirty-seven-year-old woman.

18.   Gardner, W. H. "Voice and Articulatory Defects from Paralysis by Glomus Jugulare Tumor." *Journal of Speech and Hearing Disorders,* XXXIV (1969), 172–76.
How did the speech therapist work with this unusual case?

19.   Goldstein, L. P. "A Case Report of an Edentulous Aphasic Laryngectomee." *Journal of Speech and Hearing Disorders,* XXIX (1964), 86–89.
Faced by two speech disorders, how did the therapist begin, and what was the final result?

20.   Hauley, C. N. and Manning, C. C. "Voice Quality After Adenectomy." *Journal of Speech and Hearing Disorders,* XXIII (1958), 257–62.
Summarize their research findings.

21.   Morris, H. L. "The Oral Manometer as a Diagnostic Tool in Clinical Speech Pathology." *Journal of Speech and Hearing Disorders,* XXXI (1966), 362–69.
How valuable is this instrument in diagnosis and treatment?

22.   Moser, H. M. "Symposium on Unique Cases of Speech Disorders: Presentation of a Case." *Journal of Speech Disorders,* VII (1942), 173–74.
What is the vocal fry, and how is it used?

23.   Perkins, W. H. "The Challenge of Functional Disorders of Voice." Chapter 26 in L. E. Travis, ed., *Handbook of Speech Pathology* (New York: Appleton-Century-Crofts, 1957).
What new information not contained in this text did you find in this chapter?

24.   Rees, M. "Harshness and Glottal Attack." *Journal of Speech and Hearing Research,* I (1958), 344–49.
Summarize this research.

25.   Rubin, H. J. and Lehrhoff, I. "Pathogenesis and Treatment of Vocal

Nodules." *Journal of Speech and Hearing Disorders*, XXVII (1962), 150–61.
What kind of treatment do the authors recommend for vocal nodules?

26. Shryock, R. H. "Speech Without a Larynx." *Hygeia*, XXV (1947), 725.
Recount this man's experiences after his larynx was removed.

27. Van Riper, C. *Speech Therapy—A Book of Readings*. Englewood Cliffs, N.J.: Prentice-Hall, Inc., 1953.
Read Chapter 4 and write up your discovery of new information.

28. Wilson, D. K. "Children with Vocal Nodules." *Journal of Speech and Hearing Disorders*, XXVI (1961), 19–26.
Summarize the information given in this article.

Texts

29. Brodnitz, F. S. *Vocal Rehabilitation*. Rochester, Minn.: Whiting Press, 1960.
Although this book was written primarily for the physician, it gives the speech clinician much of the basic information he needs about the vocally disordered patients he may have referred to him by the medical profession.

30. Greene, M. C. L. *The Voice and Its Disorders*. 2d ed. Philadelphia: J. B. Lippincott Co., 1964.
The first part of this book gives a good review of normal voice production, and the second part presents the disorders of voice, and their causes and treatment. Medical aspects are stressed. A valuable book.

31. Luchsinger, R. and Arnold, G. E. *Voice–Speak–Language*. Belmont, Calif.: Wadsworth, 1965.
Probably the classic book on voice and voice disorders, one which should be in the library of all speech pathologists. Information is presented in the first section which is unavailable elsewhere. It summarizes both the "European and American" contributions.

32. Moore, P. *Organic Speech Disorders*. Englewood Cliffs, N.J.: Prentice-Hall, Inc., 1971.
A comprehensive survey of all the organic voice disorders and the determinants of normal phonation.

33. Moses, P. J. *The Voice of Neurosis*. New York: Grune and Stratton, 1954.
A curious and intriguing book that seeks to show how emotional disturbances are reflected in voice.

34. Murphy, A. T. *Functional Voice Disorders*. Englewood Cliffs, N.J.: Prentice-Hall, Inc., 1964.
A broad survey of the nonorganic voice disorders. Reports of actual casework and diagnosis are given. Emphasizes therapy.

35. Sokoloff, M. "Phonatory and Resonatory Problems." In Chapter 14 of R. W. Rieber and R. S. Brubaker, eds., *Speech Pathology*. Amsterdam: North Holland, 1966.
A summary of the research on functional voice disorders.

36. Van Riper, C. and Irwin, J. V. *Voice and Articulation*. Englewood Cliffs, N.J.: Prentice-Hall, Inc., 1958.
Chapters 8 and 9 of this book present the various disorders of voice and detailed suggestions for their treatment.

Laryngectomy References

37.   Gardner, W. H. "The Whistle Technique in Esophageal Speech." *Journal of Speech and Hearing Disorders,* XXVII (1962), 187–88.
      How was the whistle used and for what reasons?
38.   Gardner, W. A., Hill, S. D., and Carano, H. N. "Esophageal Speech for a Ten-Year-Old Boy." *Journal of Speech and Hearing Disorders,* XXVII (1962), 227–31.
      How did the clinician help this boy to talk again?
39.   Hauser, P. "The Talking Frog of Marion County." *Journal of Speech Disorders,* XII (1947), 8–10.
      Is this incredible tale true? Could a person really talk by putting a frog in his mouth?
40.   Hyman, M. "An Experimental Study of Artificial Larynx and Esophageal Speech." *Journal of Speech and Hearing Disorders,* XX (1955), 291–99.
      Which of the two types of speech seemed most easily understood, and which was most acceptable to the patient and why?
41.   Lauder, E. "The Laryngectomee and the Artificial Larynx." *Journal of Speech and Hearing Disorders,* XXXV (1968), 147–57.
      What are the arguments for and against the use of the artificial larynx?
42.   Palmer, J. M. "Clinical Expectations in Esophageal Speech." *Journal of Speech and Hearing Disorders,* XXXV (1970), 160–69.
      Describes how this person without a larynx learned to speak again.
43.   Shames, G. H., Font, J., and Matthews, J. "Factors Related to Speech Proficiency of the Laryngectomized." *Journal of Speech and Hearing Disorders,* XXVIII (1963), 273–87.
      What factors contribute to better esophageal speech?

Texts for Speech after Laryngectomy

44.   Diedrich, W. M. and Youngstran, K. A. *Alaryngeal Speech.* Springfield, Ill.: Charles C Thomas, Publisher, 1966.
      Chapter 7 of this book, most of which is devoted to research, contains an excellent discussion of esophageal speech and speech with the electrolarynx. Failures are analyzed.
45.   Levin, N. ed., *Voice and Speech Disorders: Medical Aspects.* Springfield, Ill.: Charles C Thomas, Publisher, 1962.
      Among the many topics treated in this book are the effects of paralysis, surgery, stenosis, and endocrine disturbances on the voice. Chapter 10 by Levin, "Esophageal Speech," and Chapter 13 by Brodnitz, "Functional Voice Disorders," are noteworthy.
46.   Snidecor, J. C. *Speech Rehabilitation of the Laryngectomized.* Springfield, Ill.: Charles C Thomas, Publisher, 1962.
      Chapters 7 through 10 of this book describe the methods for learning and using esophageal speech and the electrolarynx.

6

Disorders of Articulation

Of all the speech disorders, the articulatory disorders are by far the most frequently encountered. They comprise the great bulk of all the cases treated by the speech clinician in the public schools, for over 75 percent of all the speech problems are articulatory in nature. Although generally these persons respond readily to systematic treatment, some of the hardest cases we have ever worked with have possessed persistent articulation errors.

One of them, a man thirty-one years old, had only two defective sounds, the s and the z; but both of them were emitted laterally around both sides of an upthrust tongue, and they were characterized by a very abnormal slushy, mushy sound with an accompaniment of bubbles of saliva. No hearing loss or organic abnormalities were present. The man was highly intelligent and strongly motivated. He wanted to be a teacher rather than a truck driver so badly that he had worked his way through college by driving at night. He was married and had two children. All in all, a very well-adjusted, fine man. We worked personally with him for two years, three hours a week, before we were able to help him acquire adequate sibilants. This man finally responded to a program of operant conditioning based initially on modified whistling. Everything else we tried had failed, and we marveled at his persistence in the light of our evident incompetence.

Most clinicians feel that their articulatory cases are the easiest ones they have to treat, but some of them are really tough.

With some exceptions, most of us when we are learning to talk go through a period of some years during which our speech shows deviant articulation. Only a few children speak clearly from the first. They omit sounds; they substitute easy sounds for difficult ones; they distort other sounds. But gradually they overcome these errors and become able to produce the standard sounds of our language easily and automatically. In many ways the whole process of speech sound mastery is a mysterious one and cannot readily be explained solely in terms of conscious learning or parental correction. For one thing, the coordinations involved are tremendously intricate, and the discriminations required are often very difficult. You will realize that this is true if you ask another person to say a random series of paired syllables such as *van-than, thee-vee*, or the prolonged isolated sounds of *vvv* and *th*, then try to identify them. Unless you look at the speaker, the *v* and the voiced *th* will sound very much alike. Most children must learn to make such discriminations as these from samples hidden in the ceaseless, fast-flowing speech of others, which is almost like trying to identify swiftly flying birds from a momentary glimpse of them as they pass through shrubbery. To cite another example, we would wager that though you have uttered the various *r* sounds a million times, you are still completely unable to tell anyone else how you actually produce these sounds. Trying to help another person to correct his defective sounds is not as easy as one might think.

How important is it to be able to articulate the speech sounds correctly? In early childhood, society's toleration for errors of articulation is much greater than it is with increasing age. We expect very young children to make these mistakes, but we also expect that they should be able to overcome them at least by the time they enter school or soon after. After this time, the child becomes subjected to strong penalties from his parents and peers.

Defective articulation can be profoundly handicapping. In order to communicate, a common verbal code is necessary. We have worked with adults who were almost completely unintelligible. One of them is shown in our Ciba film "Introduction to Speech Problems: Physical Diagnosis," and we hope you can see it sometime. The man shown in the film was almost completely unintelligible, seemingly speaking a language only remotely similar to standard English, yet his wife and children had learned his language. They could understand him and translate to others what he was saying. He had been reared on an isolated farm with his major contact being a congenitally deaf mother, and evidently he had learned his language from her. His unintelligible jargon was very fluent, and so long as he remained there on the farm or did his day labor at a winery where he did not need to communicate, he managed to get along. But one day he had to hitchhike to town, and then his garbled utterance suddenly created conditions in which he was placed in the jail where we found him. The officers thought he was crazy.

It should be understood, of course, that most of our clients with articulation disorders are not so severe. We can usually understand the person who lisps, even though all his sibilants are defective. However, we will have real trouble comprehending a person whose incoordinations due to cerebral palsy distort most of his speech sounds. Generally, the more defective sounds shown by a person, the less intelligible he becomes and the more penalties and rejection he experiences. As anyone knows who has tried to understand a young child whose speech is still filled with errors of omission, substitution, and distortion, an articulatory problem can be extremely frustrating to both the speaker and the listener. In the adult even the smallest articulatory error is viewed as an unnecessary blemish. We expect the person with whom we converse to use the same sounds we do, unless he speaks a foreign language or has some other good reason for not doing so. We view articulation errors as unnecessary and even perhaps as signs of gross immaturity, mental retardation, or general incompetence. People who have them need help.

Dysarthria and Dyslalia

As in the case of voice disorders, the terminology which has grown up about the disorders of articulation lacks precision. Although we continue to use the terms "lisping" to indicate sibilant errors and occasionally "lalling" to describe sounds that are defective primarily because the tongue tip fails to execute its necessary lifting, we rarely use a term such as "baby-talk," for it tells us little about the actual errors employed. Two terms, however, are in common use: *dysarthria*, which refers to disordered articulation due to brain or nerve damage, and *dyslalia* for articulatory problems that have no organic origin. The dyslalias are by far the most frequently encountered. They arise primarily from failure to learn the standard speech sounds; they represent those failures in the acquisition of speech sounds which cannot be accounted for in terms of neurological impairment. In contrast, a child with a partially paralyzed tongue or with cerebral palsy is said to show dysarthric errors. In adults who formerly spoke perfectly before they contracted multiple sclerosis or muscular dystrophy, we find dysarthria rather than dyslalia. It should be understand that these are etiological (causal) terms and that they do not describe different types of defective sounds. The defective *r* and *l* sounds in a person with dyslalia may sound no different from those of a person with dysarthria. In many ways these terms seem rather superfluous and imprecise. There are many so-called dyslalics who show a certain clumsiness in coordinating their tongues, which probably contributed to their failure to learn the more complicated speech sounds, and yet who manifest no other abnormal neurological signs.[1] In this text we shall use these terms sparingly.

The Causes of Defective Articulation

It is very difficult to pin down the actual cause or causes in a specific case of articulatory disability. Who can really know what happened long ago in the child's development that caused him to fail to learn the standard phonemes of his language? The many researches dealing with causation have compared groups of persons with normal speech with those with misarticulation; but the cases have been examined long after the errors have become habituated, and all sorts of articulatory problems have been lumped together in the defective groups. Winitz has reviewed all of this research very carefully, and he has shown clearly that there seems to be no single cause for disorders of articulation.[2] Winitz also concluded that significant differences between groups of misarticulating and normal subjects have not been consistently found for any of the following: general motor skills; oral and facial motor skills; laterality; intelligence; kinesthetic sensibility; dental abnormalities; oral and facial structures; tongue-thrusting; developmental progress; illnesses; auditory memory span; personality; and language adequacy. Certain studies have found such differences; others have not, but generally no real support for any of these presumed etiological factors has been conclusively demonstrated. The one major factor that appeared to be reasonably significant was auditory and pitch discrimination, but as Winitz points out, this may be due to the articulatory errors themselves. If you cannot articulate a certain sound correctly, you will tend to have trouble distinguishing it from others that closely resemble it.

The clinician should not conclude that these research findings make it entirely unnecessary for him to investigate these etiological factors in his clients. The design of these researches leaves much to be desired. Moreover, the lack of group differences does not always reflect the impact of any certain factor or a group of factors in an individual case. For example, although persons with articulation disorders generally cannot be distinguished from normal speakers in terms of intelligence, when we find a person so low in intelligence that he has little interest in communication, we would not expect him to master the standard speech sounds. Although only a few of our cases have shown poor auditory memory span, some of

[1] Muriel Morley, the British writer, in her book *Development and Disorders of Speech in Childhood* (London: Livingstone, 1957), has described some of these cases under the headings of *developmental dysarthria* or *developmental dyspraxia*.

[2] H. Winitz, *Articulatory Acquisition and Behavior* (New York: Appleton-Century-Crofts, 1969).

them were so deficient in this ability that they could not possibly retain the auditory image of a sound long enough to use it as a model, until we trained them to do so. Most of our cases of misarticulation show no signs of organicity; but there are some with grossly abnormal oral structures or neurological involvements, and these must be considered in any therapeutic program. These are not the ordinary run of clients but often are those who cause us the most therapeutic difficulty.

Investigating for Causal Factors. The clinician, when confronted by a person with a severe problem in misarticulation, does not begin immediately to work on the speech itself. Instead he tries to discover *why* this particular individual failed to master his speech sounds. He investigates the past history of his client and administers tests as well. To illustrate some of the contributions of the case history of this investigation we provide the following survey.

Parental and Family Influences

Names. If the names of the parents are foreign, the child's consonant errors might possibly be due to imitation of parental brogue, or to the learning of similar consonants belonging to another language. Thus, in one of our cases, the child who substituted *t* for *th* [ə], did so because he imitated his father's pronunciation of *th* words. The father's name (which gave us the first clue) was Molo Zymolaga.

Age. When the age of the parents seems somewhat unusual in terms of the child's age, certain emotional factors may be influencing the latter's speech development. Thus, Peter, age, seven, had parents aged twenty-two and twenty-four, and (as we found out by following the clue) was an unwanted child, neglected, unstimulated, and untrained. His articulatory errors were easily understood against this background. Or, consider Jane, who astonished her forty-nine-year-old father and forty-five-year-old mother by being born. Their excessive attention and demand for adult speech standards drove the child too early into a negativism which made her reject their constant corrections and persist in her errors.

Speech Defect. Imitation is often a causal factor in articulation, but we must be sure that the symptoms are similar. All five children of a family living on an isolated farm had nasal lisps. Organically, they were perfect specimens, but their mother had a cleft palate. It is often wise to explore to ascertain whether or not the parents had possessed a speech defect in their own childhood, since such an event would affect their attitudes toward the child's difficulty.

Physical Defects. If the mother is deaf, we can easily understand how a child's articulatory errors would receive little attention from her. Here are two other items from our case history files which had significance in our understanding of the child's speech problem: a father whose tongue tip had been shot off in a hunting accident; a "nervous" hyperthyroid mother so unstable that she screamed whenever the children made noise or mispronounced a word.

Emotional Conflicts. Conflicts between one parent and the other, or between parent and child, can arise in each of the other areas mentioned in the case history: handedness, religion, education, occupation, and so on. Other people living in the home or closely associated with the child may have significant harmful influences on the child's speech development.

DEVELOPMENTAL HISTORY

Birth History. Severe birth injuries may have malformed the mouth cavity and wrecked the alignment of the jaws or teeth. They sometimes produce, through their injury to the brain, not only feeble-mindedness but the unsure, trembling, or spastic coordinations of cerebral palsy.

Physical Development. When we learn that a child was delayed in sitting alone, in feeding himself, in walking, we usually probe to discover whether the speech development was similarly retarded. Almost any factor that retards physical development also retards speech. Many articulation cases with sluggish tongues and palates have histories of slow physical development.

Illnesses. These have importance according to their severity and sequelae. Certain illnesses such as scarlet fever may impair hearing. Others may so lower the child's vitality that he does not have the energy to learn the difficult skills of talking correctly. Prolonged illness may result in parental attitudes of overconcern or of overprotection. The parents may anticipate the child's needs so that he learns to talk relatively late. They find it difficult to "correct" the speech of a sick child. If illness occurred during the first years of life, the child may not have had the necessary babbling practice. Injuries to the tongue may make certain sounds defective. One child who had burned his tongue started immediately to lall and continued in this articulatory disorder long after the tongue had healed. Many children lose their speech after a prolonged illness with high fever and find it difficult to master it again.

Mental and Educational Factors. It is often the unpleasant chore of the speech correctionist to help parents face the fact that their child is feeble-minded, and that his general retardation is not solely the consequence of his delayed speech. When we find such children, we usually postpone speech therapy until they have a mental age (on a nonverbal test) of from five to six years.

Failures in school subjects, especially in reading, may be a direct consequence of defective articulation, and remedial reading can frequently be combined with remedial speech. Children who fail in school are likely to be resistant at first to speech correction. If they have been penalized for their school failure, they may become so emotional over their speech handicap that their tension prevents new muscular adjustments of the articulatory organs. One of our cases made no progress in his speech until he was transferred to another grade. The hatred he felt toward his teacher constantly reflected itself in our work with him.

Play. Children adopt the consonant errors of their playmates as well as their grammatical errors. In one instance, children from three different families in the neighborhood acquired a lisp by identification and imitation of a dominant older boy. It is said that *s* and *z* are pronounced as *th* [θ, ð] in Castilian Spanish because a certain king of Spain lisped, and his courtiers adopted his pronunciation of the sibilant sounds. Little tyrants in every child kingdom similarly impose their speech peculiarities upon their subjects.

Home Conditions and Emotional Problems. A knowledge of the home conditions, the tempo of life lived therein, and the attitudes of its inmates is often vital to the understanding of the articulatory problem. Parents may bedevil a child for his social blemishes merely because they are sensitive about their own. An unhappy home can make our speech correction difficult. The list of emotional problems given in the case history can give us some indication of the child's reaction to his speech defect. The child who is always fighting, hurting pets, setting fires, or performing similar aggressive acts must be handled very differently from one who withdraws from the challenges of existence. Articulatory disorders, as well as stuttering, can be primary or secondary, according to the manner in which the child regards his difficulty. We have known lispers to substitute easier words for those which included sibilant sounds. One boy's speech was so halting that he was referred to us as a stutterer. Extremely maladjusted and antagonistic, he avoided speech whenever he could. Asked to recite in school, he would growl, "I don't know and I don't care." Investigation showed that he had been penalized severely by his classmates for his lisp. His breaks in fluency and his behavior problem disappeared simultaneously with his lisp.

Language Development. In exploring this area, we sometimes find not only that the child was delayed in the onset of the first words but also that he was a very quiet child showing little babbling or vocal play. Or we may discover that the normally developing speech was suddenly interrupted, that he regressed to gesture or jargon or even became mute. There may be in the history certain periods or episodes in which he seemed to fail to understand or be interested in the speech of others. The parents may tell of speech reversals and confusions in sentence structure. They may describe the picture of idioglossia in which the child invented his own names for things. One of our cases, for example, insisted that bed was *tubboo* and refused to call it anything else. Or perhaps, other children in the family may have done all the talking for the child or competed so successfully for attention and communication that he had no opportunity to learn normal speech. This may be one of the lonely children, the isolates. Or he may be a twin and prefer twinlingua to English. Or he may have been the teacher rather than the pupil, his parents learning to understand his mutilated speech. Indeed all the factors which we have described as being important in creating delayed speech may be said to be productive of sound errors. What we are saying is that these matters should be explored rather than ignored. It is not enough to examine the child's present picture; we must also know something of his past if we are to treat him intelligently.

Organic Abnormalities

The role of organic deviations in the production of defective articulation has always been a favorite belief of parents and teachers. All children who do not talk clearly are suspected of having a tongue-tie or shortened frenum, that little cord beneath the tongue which most of us visibly possess. Tonsils have been removed, teeth straightened, and tongues trained gymnastically because of this belief, even when these structures were within the normal range. Yet there are many persons possessing such organic abnormalities or deficiencies who speak well. Speech therapists are usually conservative in attributing the defective sounds to organic factors. They know that the matter is not so simple. It is possible to produce the speech sounds in many ways—as the ventriloquists can show us. It is possible to compensate. A perfectly good *l* sound may be produced with the tongue tip down or even outside the mouth. An adequate *f* or *v* can be made upside down. We have known adults without a tooth in their heads who could produce every speech sound correctly. In our clinic cupboards we have tapes of men and women without tongues or with only half of their tongues who speak with intelligibility.

Do these observations mean that organic abnormalities play no part in causing or maintaining articulation errors? The answer is no. Only extra effort, only extra learning can overcome these obstacles. Many of our cases have not put forth this effort, and no one has helped them learn the necessary compensatory movements required. It is important therefore that we examine our cases to ascertain the organic deviations which are present.

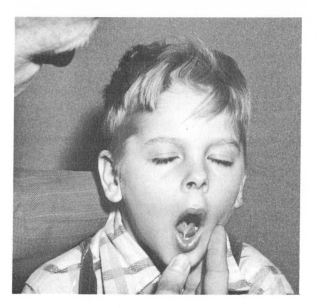

FIGURE 17: *Tongue-tie: Laller*

Orthodontia and Surgery, Physical Therapy. In recent years, orthodontia has made great strides, and almost unbelievable changes in dental,
palatal, and jaw structures have been accomplished. The speech-therapist
should refer all children with marked mouth deformities to these specialists
and should begin her work after the reconstruction has been carried out.
Unfortunately, such reconstruction is expensive, and many cases cannot be
taken care of in this way. Nevertheless, the speech therapist should acquaint herself with the resources in the orthodontic field so that she will
not waste months of effort in teaching compensatory movements to a
child whose speech problem can be taken care of through surgery or the
displacement of structures. Similarly, she should realize that palatal abnormalities are frequently associated with those of the jaws, and that orthodontic projection or retraction of the jaw can facilitate tongue contact with
the roof of the mouth. Modern surgery also offers a wide variety of repair
and reconstruction techniques. Scar tissue can be excised, and grafts can
be made that will provide the necessary mobility. High palatal arches can
be lowered, and the velum can be modified to almost any desired degree.
Much of this work should be done early in childhood, and the speech therapist is often responsible for seeing that it is done. Frequently, parents postpone such remedial work until too late, but they may often be convinced
of its necessity by the teacher who points out the social maladjustment
which such defects may produce.

Paralyzed structures occasionally can be helped by exercises, and a professional physiotherapist should be consulted in planning a remedial program if the physician's report indicates a possibility of success. Such remedial work usually consists of recourse to the more biological functions and the tying up of the specialized movement with gross muscular action. Spaced practice, well motivated by graphs of successes, is advisable.

Teaching Compensatory Movements. As we have said, many cases showing severe organic defects cannot be helped by the orthodontist or plastic surgeon because of age or financial reasons. The picture is by no means hopeless, however, since all of the speech sounds may be made in various ways. The art of the ventriloquist demonstrates compensatory activity of the tongue for that of the lips and jaws. Many normal speakers have profound anatomical abnormalities, occasionally so marked as to excite wonder in the speech correctionist familiar with the ordinary production of the speech sounds. Perfect *t* and *d* sounds, for example, have been made by individuals so tongue-tied that they were unable to lift the tongue tip to contact the upper teeth. Inmates of prisons frequently learn to talk out of the side of the mouth—the one farthest away from the guard—with just minor jaw movements.

In order to teach compensatory or nonstandard ways of making any speech sound, it is first necessary to make a phonetic analysis in terms of the type of sound to be produced. For example, the production of an *s* sound requires the propulsion of a narrow stream of air past a cutting edge. The cutting edge should be placed at about right angles to the air stream in order to produce a clear *s*. The average person produces this narrow stream of air by placing the sides of the tongue along the side teeth, thereby cutting off all lateral escape of air, and by grooving the center of the tongue so that the air stream is projected directly past the cutting edge of the front incisors. Lacking these front teeth, or having them widely spaced, the person can get an equally good *s* by directing the air stream past the cuspids or bicuspids on the side of the mouth having the better teeth. This new procedure, however, is not quite so simple as the preceding sentence might imply. The tongue must adjust itself so that on one side it makes a larger occlusion and the groove is diagonal. The lips must plug the former opening and part at the appropriate side. Frequently the mandible must be moved sidewise so that the best upper teeth and lower teeth will be brought together. Thus the therapist must plan the type of compensatory mechanics necessitated by the particular mouth deformities involved. In this plan, the teacher should take into account or seek to minimize as far as possible the following factors: complexity of performance (the fewer adjustments, the better), ease of transition from other sounds, amount of facial contortion, distinctness of kinesthetic and tactual sensations, and the motivation and cooperation of the subject.

In teaching compensatory mechanics, then, the therapist should follow this general outline. (1) Note how the student articulates the defective sound. (2) Make a phonetic analysis to determine what the essential mechanics of the sound must be. (3) Discover what structures the student might possibly use to satisfy these requirements. (4) Give the student a thorough course in ear training, stimulation, and discrimination along the lines of the program sketched on pp. 210–215. (5) Through manipulation, phonetic diagrams, mirror work, imitation, and random activity, try to get the student to produce a sound similar to that made by the instructor. (6) Once achieved, do not let the student move a muscle of face or body until he prolongs, repeats, and uses it in nonsense syllables many times. (7) Build up its strength through techniques suggested in the next section. (8) Do not worry about exaggerated movements used by the student in making the sound. At first, most students will use facilitating movements of other structures as a baby uses gross movements prior to specialization. We frequently encourage head and jaw movements or modifications of smiling, chewing, biting, and swallowing as accessory tools. These extraneous movements drop out as the new performance pattern becomes habitual. (9) Increase the speed with which the new performance pattern can be initiated. No compensatory movements will become habitual if they cannot be used quickly and easily.

Motor Deficiencies. Articulation cases are occasionally seen who could truly be called the "slow of tongue." They can scarcely protrude the tongue even in the expression of impudence without having it lall around and droop over. Sometimes these poorly coordinated movements seem to be localized about the mouth. The tongue, jaw, soft palate—all are sluggish. But in most of these "clumsy-mouthed" individuals the other coordinations are similarly affected.

Not all articulation cases are thus poorly coordinated, but those who are so handicapped must be given therapy devoted to their needs. In earlier speech correction, tongue exercises had the status of a religious ritual. All speech defectives were given rigorous training in this routine. In modern speech therapy, the emphasis on tongue exercises has almost disappeared. Yet for certain of the "clumsy-tongued" individuals with whom we work, modern forms of these exercises are very valuable.

A good many diseases and defective neuromuscular conditions reflect themselves not only in muscular incoordination but also in distorted speech. The speech therapist is often able to refer them to the physician they need. The student should therefore be able to recognize the general symptoms of paralysis, both flaccid and spastic, and pronounced neuromuscular incoordinations. Simple activities that demonstrate poor coordination are: walking a straight line; extending arms above head and dropping them suddenly; beginning with hands resting on knees as one sits in a chair, alternately touching nose with forefinger of each hand; standing first on one leg and then on the other, with eyes closed; skipping; standing on tip-toe for five seconds.

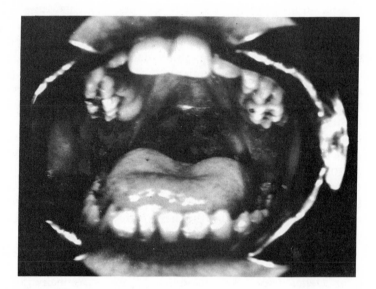

FIGURE 18: *Mouth of a Child Who Suffered a Severe Lye-Burn*

We find persons who articulate fairly well when speaking slowly but whose errors increase terrifically with each increase in speed. Some are just slow-moving children, whose tempo of living should be unhurried. Most of us make slips of the tongue when we try to talk at a rate far beyond that of our usual speech, and so do they. Geared up by competition for speech, by impatient listeners, by parents who themselves talk very swiftly, these children race their speech motors beyond their normal capacities, and so they fail to articulate. By measuring the diadochokinesis (the speed of repetitive movement) of the tongue, lips, and jaw, and by observing the general rate of other motor behaviors, we can determine the importance of this factor.

Accuracy. We have spoken of the clumsy tongue. By this we mean that the coordinations of that member lack precision and accuracy. We see this very clearly in the speech of cerebral palsy or other forms of dysarthria. The child finds it difficult to curl up the tip of the tongue, to swing it from side to side, even to hold it fixed in an out-thrust position without trembling. He may find the location of contact points within the mouth to be very difficult, even when he watches himself in the mirror or attempts to touch the spot stroked by the examiner's tongue depressor. He overshoots or undershoots. He cannot maintain a necessary posture. It wobbles. These phenomena are not found in all articulatory cases, but when they are present, they must be considered in therapy.

Lack of Differentiation.   When the baby first lifts his tongue, he probably lifts his legs and curls his toes. When he cries, he cries with his whole body. Later, we find less gross bodily movement involved. What has happened? Essentially the child has learned to differentiate the finer movement from those larger ones out of which it emerged. We find this process of differentiation in all motor skills, in handwriting, in playing badminton, in speaking. In our consideration of all the aspects of speech we must not forget that one of the most fundamental is the motor aspect. Accordingly, we should scrutinize our cases to determine whether there has been a failure in differentiation. When the child lifts his tongue, does he also lift his jaw? When he lifts his jaw, does he also round his lips? Does he still show an infantile swallow in which the tongue is protruded? We have worked with college students who could not produce an *r* or *l* sound without lifting the jaw and pursing the lips as in sucking. This is a disability almost as important as the inability to move the forefinger without moving the arm. What happens usually in these cases is that they do not lift the tongue and the speech becomes lalled and slurred. It is important for good articulation that the tongue be able to move independently of the lips and jaws.

Training in Motor Coordination.   Since we frequently find in persons with motor disabilities that other motor activities are also slow, imprecise, or undifferentiated, it is often necessary that we begin our training first with the larger motor skills. It might seem odd to the observer to discover the speech therapist teaching children to dance, to swing, to balance, to do rhythmic calisthenics. But the clumsy body often carries a clumsy tongue. Fortunately, as general bodily coordinations improve, so too do those of speech.

It is often necessary however to work directly on the coordinations of tongue and lips. Tongue exercises have in the past been much abused. Only a relatively few of our cases need them. But there are some. They are the ones whose tongues do not move with the speed and precision demanded by good speech. They can assume only the simplest tongue positions. Therefore, they raise the front or middle of the tongue instead of the back, and protrude it rather than lift it. It is difficult for them to curl the tip or groove the tongue. Tongue exercises are useful and necessary for these cases.

The exercises that follow are given in a form suitable for adults where we may be direct in our therapy. For children, it will be necessary to cast the same activities in the form of games. The principles governing the use of tongue exercises are as follows:

1. Learn to recognize the movement as part of some familiar biological movement such as chewing, swallowing, coughing, or others to be mentioned later. Practice these basic activities.
2. The finer movements should be taught first in conjunction with larger movements, then alone.
3. The movement should be used with increasing speed, strength, and accuracy.
4. The movement should be combined with other movements (breathing, phonation, and so on) used in speech.
5. The emphasis in this training should be on the activities (lifting, thrusting, drawing, tip-curling, and grooving), the contacts (upper gum ridge, lower teeth, interdental, palatal), and the positions actually used in speech, rather than random and generalized tongue movements.
6. Not only the tongue tip, but the blade, middle, and back of tongue should be exercised.
7. In any drill period, use a few from each of the lists of exercises under each major activity heading rather than complete one section at a time.
8. Avoid fatigue and hurry. Identify movement by imitation or mirror observation rather than by oral description. Identify contacts by stroking or pressure. Identify new positions in terms of their variation from other well-known positions.
9. After movement is well learned, combine it with production of other speech sounds.
10. Compare, contrast, and combine the various movements.

ACOUSTIC AND PERCEPTUAL DEFICIENCIES

Hearing Loss.   In our discussion of developmental factors we pointed out the necessity for exploring the histories of our articulation cases to determine whether or not temporary hearing losses might have occurred during the speech learning period. It is equally important, in examining our person with sound errors, that we ascertain if such losses are still present. Certainly if a child cannot hear a sound with fidelity it will be difficult for him to produce it correctly. While we shall discuss this topic in more detail later, we should make clear at this point that some children have a loss of acuity that affects all the sounds of speech, while others may hear certain sounds very well, yet be unable to identify the characteristic features of others. In high-frequency hearing loss, for example, the vowels and voiced sounds may be heard very clearly, while the unvoiced sibilants such as *s* or *sh* may be so faintly heard as to be nonexistent. Shouting at such a person will only amplify sounds which he can already hear and perhaps mask out those he hears weakly.

Auditory Memory Span.   There are some few children who find it very difficult to remember sounds even when they can hear them. Sounds disappear very swiftly once they are spoken. In the swift rush of conversation the life of a given consonant is very brief—much shorter than a fruit fly's. Most of us find it easy to hold a familiar sound in memory, but have great difficulty in hanging onto one that is strange. It seems to fade so fast. We even find it difficult to repeat a snatch of our own free babbling or jargon after a short period of silence. Most children with articulation errors do not have defective auditory memory spans. They can hold a sound as well as we can. But there are others who have much difficulty. They may remember the meaning but not the characteristics of the sounds which have been spoken. Indeed, often they cannot even recall how they have uttered their own sounds. We can readily see how such a disability would make it difficult to correct articulatory errors. Fortunately, it is possible to improve this deficiency through training.

Difficulties in Phonetic Discrimination.   It is not enough merely to be able to recall a given sound. We must also learn to distinguish it from others. Each sound, like each Chinaman, has its own distinctive features. To some of us, all Chinese look alike, and we probably look alike to them. As we become acquainted and familiar with specific individuals, we discover that there are great differences, and we wonder why it took us so long to see them. Some of the people with whom we work find a similar difficulty in recognizing the differences between sounds. They have not learned to look or listen to the distinctive differences. Some of them can tell these differences when the sounds are paired and compared in isolation, yet show a remarkably poor performance when defective sounds are incorporated within the sentence. The distinctive characteristics seem to get lost in the flow of speech just as individual faces in the photograph of a crowd seem much alike. At any rate, we find such difficulties in phonetic discrimination and when we do, we must take steps to provide the necessary training. Many of the ear-training techniques to be described later in this chapter are devoted to the improvement of phonetic discrimination.

Difficulties in Phonetic Analysis.   In our discussion of how children learn to talk we stressed the importance of vocal phonics, of learning to recognize that words have heads and tails and middles. Lumps of sound are difficult to analyze for errors. Words are little melodies of successive phonemic notes. If one of those notes is sour, it should be corrected; but all of us have heard singers who cannot carry a tune, who blithely flat or sharp a pitch and never know it. They sing "Home on the Range" with gusto, but not with precision. Only through the reactions of others do they come to realize that they do not sing well. When queried, they cannot analyze their tunes to locate the mis-sung notes. A similar difficulty exists in the articulation problem of some of our cases. They find it very difficult to analyze words into their component sounds, and so they have trouble in correcting their errors. In helping these individuals, specialized training in vocal phonics is essential.

Articulation Testing.   One of the vitally necessary tasks in dealing with persons with misarticulations is to determine what the errors are, how many there are, and the type and consistency. In diagnosing an articulatory disorder we attempt to assess its features in terms of its conspicuousness, its effect upon intelligible communication, and the amount of emotional maladjustment. We need to know how others react to it and how they view the problem. We try to ascertain the degree to which it would interfere with social and scholastic success. Will it or has it affected the ability to read, to participate in group activities, to earn a living? How aware is this person of his errors? Does he have a distorted self-image as well as distorted speech sounds? Does the severity change with different condition of communication? Is this the sort of speech that would evoke penalties or produce frustration? Is there evidence of anxiety, guilt, or hostility? What is the big picture?

Number of Defective Sounds.   We do not remain content with this overall scrutiny; we must also do a careful analysis of the speech itself. Our first item in such an analysis is the determination of how many speech sounds are defective. A crude measure of severity consists of this very counting. The more defective sounds the person has, the more severe a problem he possesses. Each additionally defective sound adds to the conspicuousness, to the unintelligibility, to the probability that the case has experienced penalty and frustration. One of the crude devices we have to predict the successful maturation of articulation or to prognosticate the success of therapy is to determine how many different speech sounds are defective. The fewer, the better. When a child comes to the speech therapist with eight or nine sounds misarticulated, we know that we have a real job before us.

Type of Error.   Although the above principles are generally true, we must also consider the type of error, since certain errors are more difficult to eradicate than others. Distorted sibilants as in lateral lisping or the distorted *r* and *l* sounds as in lalling may be very resistant to therapy even when they are the only errors present. Some of the sounds used by our cases as replacements for the standard sounds are much more difficult to change than others. An interdental lisp, for example, is usually easier to work with than is a nasal or lateral lisp. The child who substitutes a *t* for the *k* should have less trouble in conquering that error than if he substituted the little cough-like glottal catch. It is necessary, therefore, to scrutinize the error sounds.

Phonemic Approximations.   It is very important that we analyze the actual sounds used by our cases as replacements. Unless we are careful, we may fail to detect that the error is a distorted approximation of the standard sound. Few children ever say *wabbit* for *rabbit*. The initial sound they make is usually a bilabial *r* with rounded lips. Often as a child makes progress in mastering a new sound, he proceeds through a whole series of gradual approximations, one different distortion after another, all of which progress in the direction of the standard sound. They seldom jump from the error to the correct sound; they make progressive approximations. If the therapist is not alert, these little shifts may be unnoticed and unrewarded. A child can make progress even if his standard sounds are not being produced perfectly by modifying his errors in the direction of the correct sound. When a new case comes to us, we can use this analysis of approximation distortions to tell us how far he has to go.

Phonetic Analysis. Speech therapists tend to make their phonetic (phonemic) diagnoses more accurately than a mere listing of defective sounds would permit. They also want to know the type of phonetic error. If the *k* is defective, is it distorted or omitted? Is some other sound used in its place? Is the utterance defective because other unnecessary sounds have been added or inserted?

These are some of the questions the speech therapist must ask himself in sizing up an articulation problem. He must analyze the phonetic errors in terms of substitutions, omissions, insertions, and distortions. The child who says, "Tally taw me tee-tawing," is substituting the *t* for the *s*. We record this: t/s. The child who says, "Oh ook at the itto doggy," is omitting the initial *l* sound but substituting an *o* for the final *l*. We would record this as: — l(I) and o/l(F). The letters in the parentheses indicate the location of the error. We use *I* (for "initial") if the error is found at the beginning of words, *M* if in the middle, and *F* if in the final position. The minus sign(—) indicates that the sound has been *omitted*; the plus sign (+) represents an *insertion* such as the pronunciation of "blue" as "brrlue" (+ r); the diagonal represents a *substitution*; th/s equals a frontal lisp; *distortions* are substitutions of sounds foreign to our language, and we use adjectives or symbols to describe them.

A lingual-frontal lisp is a substitution: (th/s). Let us now analyze a lateral lisp which has distortions. We have no unvoiced *l* in our language. Welshmen do, and much of their speech seems lisped to us. One common variety of our lateral lisping is the use of a whispered *l* for the *s*. If you will attempt to say "LLLLLLLee the LLLLun" and whisper the L sounds, you will be saying "See the sun" with a lateral lisp. These are distortions, and so we write them: S (I, lateral-emission), or more simply: — s — (I). If the *s* were laterally emitted in every position of the word, it would be recorded: — s — (I,M,F). If the student has mastered the International Phonetic Alphabet with its modifying marks, he can record many of the distortions as substitutions. For example, it is difficult to record on paper the *l* produced by holding the tongue tip down and using the middle of the tongue for making the contact against the palate. It seems to be a distortion. The best we could do is to call it "a dark *l*" or a "retracted *l*."

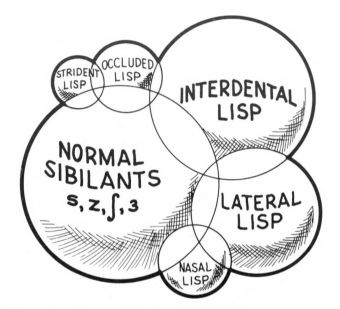

FIGURE 19: *Types of Sibilant Errors.* Where circles intersect, blends and distorted approximations or combinations of errors are found.

An alternative method for recording distortions is by the use of intersecting circles representing the sounds nearest to the error. Many distortions are actually homogenous blends of two standard sounds. The diagram in Figure 19 illustrates the various distortions by the intersecting arcs. For example in the intersected area of the circle [θ], for *th*, and the large circle for *s* represents a very common error, much more common than the substitution of a pure *th* for the *s*. Few children really say *thoup* for *soup*; instead they use a replacement sound which is this combination of *th* and *s*. You can duplicate it by protuding your tongue slightly and still trying to prolong a *ssss* sound. It has the characteristics of both. It is a distortion.

To summarize, we cannot understand or diagnose an articulation case without making a *phonetic* analysis of his speech in terms of (1) the sounds which are defective; (2) the type of error in terms of substitution, omission, insertion, or distortion; and (3) the location of the error within the word (initial, medial, or final). This sort of analysis is not academic.

It has vital importance for therapy. It helps us answer such questions as: "With what sound or sounds should we begin? Does the case ever make the sound correctly? How much ear training will be required?"

> One of our student speech therapists gave an articulation test to a boy of seven and came out with the astounding summary that although he had thirty-two defective sounds, his speech was perfectly intelligible. When we checked her findings we found that the child actually was doing only one thing incorrectly: He was *forming* the final sounds of every word, but he was not pronouncing them audibly. The student therapist had been right in finding that thirty-two sounds were defective, but this actually had no significance or importance. Our therapeutic task was clearly to teach the child to strengthen his terminal sounds.

To show you what a brief report of a typical phonetic analysis would be like, we submit this one of an eighteen-year-old college student whose tongue had been badly cut during the first grade of his schooling:

Name of case: K. J.   *Examiner:* Leith   *Date:* 1/4/63   *Rapport:* OK

Summary of errors: y/l(I,M); o/l(F)
w/r(I,M); — r(F)
t/ch(I,M,F)
— s — (Lateral, I,M,F)
— z — (Lateral, I,M,F)

Why are these sounds defective? Besides a phonetic analysis such as we have described, we also need a *kinetic* analysis. It is important to know which sounds are being misuttered, but we need also to know how they are being produced. The label "lisp" is a *phonetic* term; the modifying adjectives "lateral," "occluded," "interdental," or "nasal" are *kinetic* terms. They describe how the error is being made. They refer to the *manner of production.* The term "lalling" is such a kinetic or kinesiologic term. It refers to the type of speech produced when the individual characteristically makes most of his speech sounds without raising the tip of the tongue from the floor of the mouth. It tells us only that his tongue position is at fault. If you were told that a child was a *laller,* all you could guess about his actual speech would be that certain of the consonants which normally are made with an elevated tongue tip would be defective. You could be sure that the *r* would be defective; the *l* probably would be poor, and perhaps the *ch* and *j* or even the *t, d,* and the sibilants. Those would be the probabilities, but you could not be certain. Only by analyzing the manner of error production could you know what the person is doing incorrectly.

Each of the speech sounds can be incorrectly produced in several ways. The most frequent error of such *stop-plosives* as *k* and *g* seems to be due to (1) the wrong location of the tongue contact. Other errors include (2) the wrong speed in forming the contacts; (3) the wrong structures used in contacts; (4) the wrong force or tension of the contacts; (5) too short a duration of the contacts; (6) too slow a release from contacts; (7) the wrong mode or direction of release; (8) the wrong direction of the air stream; and finally (9) sonancy errors in which voiced and unvoiced consonants are interchanged. Examples of these errors are now given for illustration:

1. The child who says "tandy" for "candy" is using a tongue-palatal contact, but it is too far forward.
2. A breathy *k* sound [*xki*] for [*ki*], results when the contact is formed so slowly that fricative noises are produced prior to the air puff.
3. A glottal catch or throat click [¿æt] for [kæt] is often found in cleft-palate cases. They make a contact, but with the wrong structures.
4. Insufficient tension of the lips can result in the substitution of a sound similar to the Spanish *v* [ø] for the standard English *b* sound.
5. When the duration of the contact is too short, it often seems to be omitted entirely. Thus the final *k* in the word *sick* [sɪk] may be formed so briefly that acoustically it seems omitted [sɪ].
6. Too slow a release from the contact may give an aspirate quality to the utterance. "Kuheep the cuhandy" [kʰip ðə kʰændɪ] is an example of this.
7. The lowering of the tongue tip prior to recall of the tongue as a whole can produce such an error as "tsen" for "ten" [tsɛn] for [tɛn]. In this error the case is not inserting an *s* so much as releasing the tongue from its contact in a peculiar fashion.
8. Occasionally the direction of the air stream is reversed and the plosion occurs on inhalation. Try saying "sick" with the *k* sound produced during inhalation, and you will understand this error.
9. The person who says "back" for "bag" illustrates a sonancy error.

Most of the errors in making the *continuant* sounds are caused by: (1) use of the wrong channel for the air stream (using an unvoiced *l* for the *s*); (2) use of the wrong construction or constriction ("foop" for "soup"); (3) use of the wrong aperture (a lateral lisp); (4) use of the wrong direction of the air stream (nasal lisp, inhaled *s*); (5) too weak an air pressure (acoustically omitted *s*); (6) the presence of nonessential movements or contacts (*t* for *s*, occluded lisp); and (7) cognate errors (*z* for *s*, or vice versa).

Most of the errors in making the *glide* sounds are produced by combining the types of errors sketched above. They may be generally classed as movement errors. They include: (1) use of the wrong beginning position or contact ("yake" for "lake"); (2) use of the wrong ending postion [frʊ] for [fɪr]; (3) use of the wrong transitional movement in terms of speed, strength, or direction [rweɪd] for [reɪd]; (4) the presence of nonessential contacts or positions [tjɛloʊ] for [jɛloʊ]; (5) cognate errors [wɛn] for [hwɛn].

It is necessary to analyze any given articulation error according to the above scheme so as to understand its nature. It is not sufficient merely to start teaching the correct sound. We must also break the old habit. Many of our most difficult articulatory cases will make rapid progress as soon as they understand clearly what they are doing wrong. Insight into error is fundamental to efficient speech correction.

To show you how we would record the results of a *kinetic* analysis, let us present the summary report of both the phonetic and kinetic procedures:

Name of case: P. T.   *Examiner:* Wensley   *Date:* 2/5/63

Rapport: Good

Summary of errors:	*Phonetic*	*Kinetic*
k/g	(I,M,F)	Confusion of voiced and un-
t/d	(I,M,F)	voiced sounds; cognate or so-
f/v	(I,M,F)	nancy errors.
s/z	(I,M,F)	Ditto: Vocal cords silent.
θ ə	(I,M,F)	" " " "
w/r	(I,M)	" " " "
— r	(F)	Uses lip glide instead of tongue glide. The r position was made but it was unvoiced.

This case mastered all of his errors at once except the w/r. He was taught the concept of cognates: that there are pairs of sounds, articulated in much the same way, but one is voiced or sonant while the other is unvoiced or surd. He learned that the *v* was made by having his vocal cords vibrate as he made the lip-teeth position for an *f*. He found out that the *s* was a whispered *z*. By feeling both his own and his clinician's throat as the pairs of sounds were produced, he learned to discriminate between them. By holding his fingers in his ears as he shifted from a prolonged *ssss* to a prolonged *zzzz*, he learned to recognize one sound from its twin.

Under What Conditions Do the Articulation Errors Occur? In studying any articulation case it is also necessary to discover the circumstances in which the errors occur. Some of our lispers have difficulty with their sibilants only when emotional. We worked with an exasperating case who never made an error when speaking at a normal rate of speed, but who became unintelligible when hurried. Some children can utter words perfectly when repeating from a model and yet substitute, omit, and distort their speech sounds in spontaneous speech. Some children who can produce every consonant correctly in isolation or in nonsense syllables will seem to be unable to use them in meaningful words. All of these observations point to the necessity for studying the articulation errors in terms of the type of communication being used. The importance of these factors in therapy is obvious. It would be silly to spend a lot of time drilling a child to produce the *r* sound in nonsense syllables if he has always been able to do so. For these reasons, we examine each error in terms of the following: (1) type of communicative situation, (2) speed of utterance, (3) kind of communicative material, (4) discrimination ability. Here is a typical summary report:

> Our analysis of the conditions under which articulation errors occurred is as follows: Jackson substituted θ/s (I,M,F) and ð/z (I,M,F) consistently in swift, emotional speech, swift nonemotional speech, when carefully trying to speak correctly in oral reading, and when repeating single words after the examiner. One exception occurred: he said "six" correctly when repeating it carefully. He made the same errors on nonsense syllables when they were spoken at fast speeds, but had good final *s* sounds occasionally when the nonsense syllables were spoken slowly. He prolonged good isolated *z* sounds when prolonged with teeth closed. The *s* was only occasionally good in isolation, even with strong stimulation by examiner. He was always able to hear the error in another's speech but did not seem to be able to hear his own except on isolated words.

The only reason for such diagnostic procedures is that they may help us in therapy. In the above case, the therapy plan called for the teaching of the *z* sound prior to the teaching of the *s*. A great deal of discrimination ear training was used. Recordings and auditory training units, which enabled Jackson to hear his own *z* and *s* at high amplification, were used. The *s* sound was first taught by isolating it from the key word *six*, and no attempt was made to have oral reading or conversation employed in therapy until the new sounds were thoroughly habituated. The *s* sound was used in the final position of nonsense syllables (*ees-oss-oos*) and in the final position of familiar words (*house, glass, ice*) before it was taught in the initial position (*see, sandwich, sick*). By analyzing the conditions under which errors occur, we are able to treat our cases much more efficiently.

Now let us present a complete articulation test report that will combine the *phonetic* analysis, the *kinetic* analysis, and the conditions under which errors occur.

A Typical Articulation Test Report

Name of case:	*Examiner:*	*Date:*

Summary of errors: t/k (I,M,F) Except in slow nonsense syllables repeated after examiner. Wrong location of contact.

d/g (I,M,F) Same as above, but said "go" correctly. The case can hear these errors when imitated by examiner at both slow and fast speeds, but cannot hear his own errors except in slowly spoken nonsense syllables.

t/s (I,M) Except in slow production of isolated sound after strong stimulation by examiner. Can always hear own error except in fast conversation. Doesn't realize no contact is needed.

— s (F) Makes no attempt to produce it. Evidently does not hear it as a part of the word when it comes in the final position.

Organic factors: High narrow palatal arch, but teeth are normally placed and tongue assumes good lateral contact with the teeth in making the *z* sounds. Makes the contacts for defective *k* and *g* sounds too far forward and with blade of tongue. When he tries to produce a genuine *t* or *d* he uses the tongue tip against the upper teeth.

Motor coordinations: Excellent in every respect.

Emotional factors: Not particularly sensitive. Will try persistently to follow instructions even when failing. Mother says he will try to say a word correctly for his father but not for her. "I'm too impatient, I guess." Boy seems to be mature for his age.

Developmental factors: Had been seriously ill the majority of the first year and a half. Onset of speech at thirty-two months.

Perceptual deficiencies:	Very poor phonetic discrimination except for isolated sounds. Auditory memory span OK. Poor ability to analyze component sounds of words. Could not recognize "mouth," "shirt," or "nose" when they were sounded out phonically.
Prognosis:	Good.

Varieties of Articulation Tests. Although some speech therapists construct their own test materials, we now possess several widely used instruments for determining proficiency in articulation. Of these, the *Templin–Darley*,[3] the *Laradon*,[4] the *Photo–Articulation Test*,[5] and the *Goldman–Fristoe*[6] tests are probably most representative. All of them employ pictures of common objects to elicit spontaneous speech. (Those of the Photo–Articulation Test are actual color snapshots of the objects, while the stimulus materials in the other tests consist of line drawings in black and white or in color.) The *Goldman–Fristoe* also uses a film-strip test as a supplement. The pictures are chosen to test the accuracy of each of the English phonemes in the various positions within the word. In addition, most of these tests provide either sentences to be read or repeated or stories to be retold, and they include other materials that will elicit samples of consecutive speech. Test forms for recording whether the errors are substitutions, omissions, or distortions are also available.

Another articulation test instrument, the McDonald *Deep Test of Articulation*, has a different format in that the test pictures and stimulus materials are presented in pairs, the child being asked to link their names together without pausing.[7] McDonald feels that a person tends to misarticulate certain sounds only in certain contexts, and that deep testing will reveal many instances in which a usually defective sound will be produced correctly. He therefore devised stimulus materials that would present any given sound so that it precedes or follows each of the other sounds.

---

[3] M. C. Templin, and F. L. Darley, *The Templin–Darley Tests of Articulation* (Iowa City, Iowa: Bureau of Educational Research and Service, Extension Division, State University of Iowa, 1960).

[4] W. Edmonston, *Laradon Articulation Scale* (Beverly Hills, Calif.: Western Psychological Services, 1963).

[5] K. Pendergast, S. Dickey, J. Selmar, and A. Soder, *Photo–Articulation Test* (Danville, Ill.: Interstate Publishers, 1968).

[6] R. Goldman, and M. Fristoe, *Goldman–Fristoe Test of Articulation* (Circle Pines, Minn.: American Guidance Service, 1969).

[7] E. T. McDonald, A *Deep Test of Articulation* (Pittsburgh: Stanwiz House, 1964).

For example, if the therapist desired to know whether a child could say the *th* sound correctly in a certain phonetic context, he would ask him to "See if you can make a 'funny big word' out of these two little words," and then show the child the paired pictures of *teeth* and *sheep* so that he will say "tee*th*sheep" and with *tub* to make "tee*th*tub," and again and again with a large number of other words. McDonald insists that the accuracy with which a sound is articulated varies not only with the type of consonant produced but also with the kind of overlapping movements characteristic of ordinary utterance. He says that the basic acoustic and physiological unit of speech is not the isolated sound but the syllable, and the consistency of an articulatory error will vary according to its role in arresting or releasing that syllable. One of the disadvantages of such a deep test lies in its length. To test every speech sound in every phonemic context would take far too much time to be practical. Therefore McDonald advises that the therapist check the spontaneous speech in conversation or in memorized material to locate the obvious errors before doing the deep testing. Deep testing will then locate the combinations in which the usually defective sound might be produced correctly as well as incorrectly. He has also devised a shorter form that deep tests for only those sounds which are usually misarticulated.[8]

Screening Tests. Most of these tests may also be used not only to determine articulation proficiency and type of error, but also as screening tests—i.e., to locate the children in a given school system who may need speech therapy. A screening test is used, as Winitz says, "to provide a comparison of a child's articulatory performance with that of his peers." In the public schools where large numbers of children enter the elementary grades each year, the speech therapist has found that she must screen the children to find those with speech problems. Most of those she does find have articulation errors and so, as quickly as possible, she examines them, not at this time to analyze the articulation problems presented, but merely to locate them. She must identify those children from the others with normal speech or other types of speech disorders. Analysis will come later.

Some of the common methods used in this initial screening are these: (1) The naming of objects or pictures selected so as to include all the most difficult speech sounds. (2) The repetition of test sentences such as "This girl thinks that the cowboys on the television are real," or a series of sentences, each designed to test the errors on just one sound such as the following: "This is my thumb. I put it in my mouth; but I don't bite it with my teeth." (3) Serial speech responses such as counting, naming the

[8] E. T. McDonald, A *Screening Test of Articulation* (Pittsburgh: Stanwiz House, 1968).

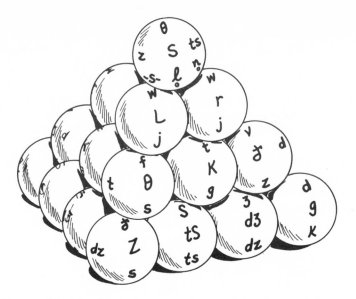

Figure 20: *The Most Common Types of Consonantal Errors*

days of the week, naming the colors on a chart. (4) Repeating nonsense syllables or sounds in isolation or nonsense words. (5) Conversation and questioning. There are other methods, but one or a combination of those mentioned will serve as a quick method for finding those children who have articulation errors.

Prognostic Tests.   Since there are large numbers of children who seem to be able to master their defective sounds without therapy, it would be a waste of time to treat them. The problem is to know which ones they are. This is a problem frequently encountered by the public-school speech therapist who often has case loads so large that she must always put certain children on waiting lists. Several attempts have therefore been made to determine whether or not articulation tests could be made prognostic, i.e., whether they could discover and identify those misarticulating children who will be able to master their standard sounds without therapy. The *Laradon Articulation Scale* yields a prognostic score, but to date no data are available to indicate its reliability or predictive validity. Since several studies had indicated that such a predictive test was possible, Van Riper and Erickson (1969) devised the *Predictive Screening Test of Articulation* (*PSTA*), an instrument which, when applied to first-grade children with articulation errors, seems able to predict fairly well those children who will "outgrow" their misarticulations by the time they enter third grade.[9]

Summarizing the Diagnostic Examination. To illustrate how we bring all the test and interview data together to give an overall picture of an articulation problem, we provide the following illustrative report:

Case: John Smith   *Age:* Ten   *Grade:* Fifth   *Referral:* Mrs. K. Jones

Informant: Mother   *Examiner:* Madrid   *Date:* April 2, 1970

Previous Therapy: None   *Type of Disorder:* Articulation

Case History Data: No foreign language background; parental speech and attitudes toward child, good. No evidence of imitation as a factor. Birth history normal. Developmental history: child experienced great difficulty in sucking; bottle fed with large opening in nipple required; digestive troubles during first two years of life; much crying, "little babbling." Normal physical development. Usual childhood diseases were mild. Cut tongue tip with paring knife at 22 months; no permanent injury or scar tissue; intelligence normal: Binet IQ at eight years was 108; good student and excellent reader (silently); well-adjusted child with no pronounced emotional conflicts or behavior problems; interests normal for his age; first words spoken at 13 months and was speaking in "long sentences" by his second birthday; parents tried to correct child by demanding he repeat his difficult words after them, but this method failed and no further attempts have been made except by the kindergarten teacher, who also had no success. Child is aware of the fact that he does not talk correctly but is not too concerned. Some teasing to which he reacted by laughing and making his speech even worse.

Hearing: Audiometric examination reveals no hearing loss.

Organic Examination: No abnormalities. Palatal arch fairly high but with normal variation. No frenum interference.

Motor Coordinations: Large muscular coordinations adequate for his age norm. However, child seems unable to move tongue independently of jaw except at very slow speeds. Tongue thrust and strength seem normal. Tongue-curling and lifting are accomplished with great difficulty. Cannot sustain half-lifted tongue tip in a fixed position. It always returns to lower gum ridge, or teeth.

Perceptual Deficiencies: Auditory memory span normal; cannot discriminate *w* from *l* and made one error on *t* and *k*; cannot locate or recognize own errors in conversation or in single words; vocal phonics

---

[9] C. Van Riper, and R. Erickson, "A Predictive Screening Test of Articulation," *Journal of Speech and Hearing Disorders,* XXXIV (1969), 214–19.

very poor: could integrate only two stimulus sounds (sh-oe); failed consistently in trying to integrate three sounds. Has little conception of words as sound sequences. Poor rhyming ability. Hears words as "chunks of sound."

Articulation Test Results: The *Templin-Darley Articulation Test* was first administered. Child cooperated fully. Of the screening test items, forty were produced correctly and ten defectively, thus showing that the child was performing at about the seven-year level at best. Three single sounds were misarticulated, the *k*, *g*, and *l*. Error types were as follows:

t/k (I. M. F)   — k (F)
d/g (M. F)   — g (F)
w/l (I. M)   — l (F)
o/l (F)

All *l* blends (sl, pl, etc.) have the *l* omitted. All *kr* and *gr* blends defective. Occasionally defective *r* (I) distorted by lip protrusion.

Following stimulation, John could correctly articulate the *k* and *g* sounds in isolation and in nonsense syllables but not in blends of words. The final *l* was never uttered correctly, but stimulation produced it normally in consonant vowel (CV) syllables but not in words.

McDonald's *Deep Test of Articulation*, supplemented by other word combinations, was then given to John, using the cards for *k* and *l*. These sounds were correctly articulated in the following context: /uk/; /ok/; /nk/; and /tl/; /lt/; /nl/. We also discovered several key words in which the usually defective sound was employed correctly. They were: "OK"; "Go"; and "li-" (Like).

Manner of Error Production: This case tends to anchor the tongue tip on the lower gum ridge and produces the acoustically correct *t*, *d*, and *n* as well as the defective sounds by raising the blade of the tongue instead of the tip.

Conditions Under Which Errors Occur: Case can produce the *k* in isolation [kə], but only with strong stimulation and at slow speeds. The *g* can be produced in isolation and in nonsense syllables in all positions by repeating after the examiner and without need for strong stimulation. Case also uses *g* occasionally in his conversation. Fails consistently if excited or hurried. Omissions of both these sounds in the final position are most prominent in swift conversation. Discrimination of correct versus incorrect sounds as made by examiner is good. Self-discrimination is poor. Child cannot produce or discriminate a good *l* sound even with strong stimulation. Error on this sound always occurs.

Intelligibility: Generally good. Occasionally when speaking swiftly or excitedly, some difficulty in understanding a word or two was experienced by examiner. Other children and his parents and teacher understood him readily.

Attitude Toward Prospective Therapy: Fifteen minutes of trial therapy were administered in which discrimination of *t* from *k* was attempted. Child seemed interested. Cooperative. Rapport easily established. Should be a good case if motivation can be achieved.

TREATMENT OF ARTICULATORY DISORDERS

Although the profession of speech pathology is a very young one, its history shows that the treatment of the various disorders with which it is concerned has been marked by progressive change. Fifty years ago, all the emphasis was upon drill. The person with an articulatory disorder was exhorted and commanded to practice sentences such as these over and over again: "Rover ran further than Rex" or "Samantha slowly sewed the seam." When errors occurred, they were "corrected," the correction consisting of an impatient "Don't say it that way; say it like this!" A bit later on came the era of appliances. Curiously contrived forks, spoons, probes, and tongue-pushers filled the mouths of little children as they attempted to produce the sounds they could not say. Some years later, in 1931, we find Travis protesting against the use of these instruments:

> If a child used *p* for *f* from pressing the lips too tightly together, a thick stick or finger was struck between the lips so that they could not close tightly. As far as the child is concerned, he is still making *p* regardless of whether a stick or finger was stuck between the lips or not. A sound cannot be broken into its component parts, as into lip movements or tongue movements. It is a unit, a whole, and can be learned only as such.[10]

To replace these devices Travis recommended strong stimulation using the whole syllable. He told his students to flood the person with such stimulation: "See-Saw-Say-So-Sue." Now say "say." "See, saw, say, so, sue." Now say "Say." "See-saw-say-so-sue." Now say, "So!" So it went for hours at a time, and we can testify that some of our cases did learn to correct their defective sounds by this technique, though it was boring murder for the therapist.

---

[10] L. E. Travis, *Speech Pathology* (New York: Appleton-Century-Crofts, 1931), p. 193.

Indeed, we still remember observing with astonishment a young girl with an unrepaired complete cleft of the hard and soft palate who produced one perfect, nonnasalized syllable without any trace of nasal emission after an hour of such repeated stimulation. She failed at least one hundred times, but finally she said "Sue" correctly and begain to cry, but her therapist was triumphant. "If we can just stimulate them long enough and vividly enough, they'll say it right!"

This belief, which doubtless reflects the usual naïve parental opinion and practice of commanding a child not to "say it wrong; say it right!", assumes that the use of the error is voluntary, that misarticulation is identical with mispronunciation, a proposition which is simply untrue. Most children with articulation errors have difficulty recognizing their errors, more trouble in discriminating the characteristics of the standard sound, and still more difficulty in learning to produce it. Though such massed stimulation does not appear to be sufficient, nevertheless we still find therapists relying on it almost exclusively today. Milisen, for example, suggests that very intensive stimulation (integral stimulation) is the basic tool for helping a person to acquire a new sound.[11] He recommends that the models presented by the therapist should be produced by increasing the loudness of the sound, the visibility of the focal articulation points, and the tactile aspects of the model. All of the sense modalities are employed in this intensive stimulation.

We have previously mentioned the Motokinesthetic Method invented by Edna Hill Young as one of the approaches used in teaching a child with delayed speech to talk. It has also been used in the elimination of misarticulations. Essentially, this method is based upon intensive stimulation; however, the stimulation is not confined to sound alone but to tactile and kinesthetic sensations as well. The therapist, by manipulation and stroking and pressing the child's face and body as she utters the stimulus syllable, helps him recognize the place of articulation, the direction of movements, the amount of air pressure, and so on. Watching an expert motokinesthetic therapist at work on a lisper is like attending a show put on by a magician. The case lies on a table with the therapist bending over him. First she presses on his abdomen to initiate breathing as she strongly makes the *s* sound; then to produce a syllable from the patient, her fingers fly swiftly to close his jaws, spread the lips, and tap a front tooth, thereby signaling a narrow groove of the tongue or the focus of the air stream. Then her magical fingers squeeze together to draw out the sibilant hiss as a continuant.

One therapist, when working with a child, used to "draw out" the *s*,

[11] R. Milisen, *The Articulation Disorder: A Coordinated Program for Testing, Diagnosing and Designing Therapy* (Bloomington: Speech and Hearing Clinic, Indiana University, 1967).

wind it around the child's head three times then insert it into her ear, thus insuring that it would be prolonged enough to be felt. Each sound has its own unique set of deft manipulations, and considerable skill is required to administer motokinesthetic therapy effectively. Viewed by the cold eye of the modern speech scientist, many of the motokinesthetic cues seem inappropriate; and a therapist would need sixty fingers and thirty arms to provide sufficient cues to take care of the necessary integration and co-articulation. Moreover, much of our research has indicated that standard sounds are produced in different ways by different people, and that their positionings vary widely with differing phonetic contexts. We suspect that much of the effectiveness of this method is due to its powerful suggestion (the laying on of hands), to its accompanying auditory stimulation, or to the novelty of the situation, which may free the case to try new articulatory patterns. We have used it successfully with some very refractory cases, but we always have felt a bit uncomfortable when doing so, as though we were the Magical Monarch of Mo in the Land of Hocus Pocus.

Rebelling against the intensive drill and stimulation with nonsense syllables, Backus and Dunn (1947) insisted that articulation therapy should be group therapy and be done in the normal communicative situation, that conversational patterns should always be used rather than isolated sounds or even words. They insisted that good interpersonal relationships would facilitate the maturation of articulation and that there was no need to concentrate on defective sounds.[12]

Others more recently have also stressed the need for corrective methods which stress meaningful utterance as the vehicle for therapy.[13]

There are various reasons for this emphasis upon communication-centered therapy. It avoids all drill; it makes error recognition important; the successful conquest of misarticulation in a meaningful context transfers readily, and the carryover is said to be excellent. The rewards and punishments are less artificial. Speech is more than an auditory-motor skill; it involves not only thinking and feeling, but also the self-concept and many other aspects of the person's functioning. Nevertheless, although most modern therapists try as much as possible to work with misarticulation in contexts involving all these components of the communicative act, there are many times when we must deal directly with the auditory and motor characteristics of the standard sound and its error.

---

[12] For students interested in this point of view we recommend the following reference: O. L. Backus, "Group Structure in Speech Therapy," Chapter 33 in L. E. Travis, ed., *Handbook of Speech Pathology* (New York: Appleton-Century-Crofts, 1957).

[13] E. Hahn, "Indications for Direct, Nondirect and Indirect Methods in Speech Correction," *Journal of Speech and Hearing Disorders*, XXVI (1961), 230–36; S. Goda, "Spontaneous Speech, A Primary Source of Therapy Material," *Journal of Speech and Hearing Disorders*, XXVII (1962), 190–92; E. Smathers, "Speech Play Therapy," *Journal of Speech and Hearing Disorders*, XXIV (1959), 59–61.

More recently, we find an emphasis upon structuring articulation therapy in terms of learning theory—particularly that represented by operant conditioning. Most of the work has been experimental rather than clinical, but it has been clearly shown that a child can learn to discriminate the correct from the incorrect sound by appropriately programming the contingent reinforcement. By beginning with paired sounds, syllables, or words that are widely different, then gradually shifting to those that are more similar and ending with the correct sound and its error, children become able to discriminate the essential differences. Such procedures have been used for years by experienced clinicians, but the programs devised by advocates of operant conditioning have systematized and objectified them.

In contrast to its use in facilitating discrimination, the application of operant conditioning methods in helping a person acquire a new sound has been less successful. Although some individuals are able to produce the correct sound as soon as they can tell the difference between it and its error, this is not usually the situation. Far too many persons just cannot discover by themselves the necessary coordinations that will produce it. If a lateral lisper, for example, never emits a normal sibilant, it is obvious that we have nothing that can be reinforced. Punishing such a person for his errors usually just makes the matter worse. In such a situation, programs are designed which involve what is called "shaping." A chain of target responses is set up, beginning with a sound the person can already produce, and then gradually progressing through a series of slight modifications which more and more resemble the standard sound. At each stage in the sequence, the patient is reinforced for successful production until that particular component sound in the chain is learned. Then this production is no longer reinforced and the patient gets his reinforcement only when he varies his attempts enough to achieve the next transitional target sound. By working through this series of transitional sounds, the standard sound is finally acquired. We shall discuss and illustrate this shaping process later under the heading of "progressive approximation."

Recent interest in linguistics has also been reflected in articulation therapy. Articulatory errors are viewed as failures to perceive the significant contrasts between the standard sound and its error. Therapy is structured so as to emphasize the distinctive features of the standard sound and the error, and to help the person realize that the differences are really vital. Weber describes some of this linguistically based therapy thus:

(1) The main difference from traditional therapy was that an entire pattern was worked on by involving all the sounds in that particular category. In other words, the immediate goal was to correct a deviant pattern, not to correct one sound at a time. The child who had used

stops for fricatives, was taught in one session to make [s, ʃ, f, θ]; then in subsequent sessions these sounds were worked on as a group of sounds in order to teach and reinforce the common fricative element in each sound. (2) The second important difference stemmed from the use of contrasting sounds in the phonemic and auditory discrimination analyses. Therapy was based on pairing contrasting features. The child was taught not only to make voiceless fricatives but to contrast these sounds with the voiceless stops which he usually substituted for them. Throughout every stage of therapy the child was asked to make both the erred feature (e.g., voiceless stops) and the correct feature (the voiceless fricatives) one after the other.[14]

This review of the various ways of doing articulation therapy may leave the student wondering which one to use. Is one better than another? Our answer is that, since the problems presented by our articulation cases are so diverse, a competent therapist needs to have more than one arrow in his quiver. Each of these approaches has merit. We have found value in all of them as the description of our therapy will indicate. We use strong stimulation in all of the modalities; we use phonetic placement techniques; we stress the distinctive features of the standard sound and its error; we employ the principles of learning theory including those characteristic of operant conditioning. Our verbal illustrations will demonstrate our concern that therapy be structured whenever possible in terms of real communicative interchanges. And, above all, we seek to establish a relationship between the clinician and his client that will permit and encourage personal growth in all directions. Unless a therapeutic climate can be created in which such change is possible, all methods fail.

The Design of Therapy.   Whatever approach we use, it is always necessary to have in mind an overall therapy plan based upon the unique problems presented by our client. In devising such a plan, we must first take into account those causal factors which may prevent the acquisition of normal speech. If, for example, a twin is speaking the same way as his misarticulating brother, we may need to make a change in the environment so that he will have other models. If there are significant organic abnormalities such as a gross overbite, we may have to teach compensatory ways of producing the standard sounds. If the child desires to remain an infant because of emotional conflicts in the home, we may have to deal with the parent-child relationship. Somehow we must minimize those causal factors which seem to maintain the disorder. In most of our cases, however, we are unable to find any of these, and therefore we proceed directly to the therapy process.

[14] J. L. Weber, "Patterning of Deviant Articulation Behavior," *Journal of Speech and Hearing Disorders*, XXXV (1970), 140.

Convincing the Child that He Does Not Speak Correctly.   One of the first things we must do is to convince the child that he has a problem which he should solve and can solve. This is not so easily done. Owing to sheltered environments and the tolerance of associates who have become accustomed to the speech difference, many speech-defectives grow to adulthood without ever having been made aware of their speech disorder, although it may be so noticeable that it shrieks its presence whenever its possessor opens his mouth. If friends and acquaintances will not mention it, certainly the average stranger will not. We seldom hear ourselves speak. Instead, we listen to our vocalized thinking. And so the speech-defective himself has little chance of becoming fully aware of the nature or frequency of his errors.

Although many articulatory cases are thoroughly aware of their speech disorder, they do not seem to recognize all of their errors; and there are other cases who seem totally unaware of any speech difficulty. Small children, especially, need to be convinced that they have sound substitutions, additions, omissions, or distortions before they will cooperate or respond to treatment. The older ones must learn to recognize error whenever it occurs. A vague, generalized feeling that something is wrong with the speech will not provide sufficient motivation for the type of retraining that is necessary.

Teachers frequently ask whether or not it is advisable to work upon the child's speech in view of the self-consciousness and embarrassment which might be produced. The answer to this question is that the quickest way of getting rid of these errors is to make the child aware of them. The habits should be broken before they become fixed. Moreover, it is perfectly possible to work on a speech defect without shame; and if the teacher makes the child understand that a certain skill is to be learned and a problem is to be solved, no insecurity will be created. If she adopts a calm, unemotional attitude herself, empathic response will ensure a similar attitude in the child.

There are various ways of teaching an articulatory speech defective to recognize his errors, and some of them are given in the next paragraphs. One mother patiently corrected her child on every mispronounced word for three successive days, and he responded by refusing to talk at all for a week. With small children, no such nagging is necessary or advisable. The teacher should select five or six common words in which the child uses the error and should try to create in the child the feeling that in these words he is doing something incorrectly. She may tell him that there are other troublesome words, but she should set up as the first definite project the correction of these five or six. By narrowing the disorder to such a slender nucleus, the task is made easier and specific. The child must learn to recognize these words as "wrong words" and must come to realize that in these words he is likely to use "wrong sounds."

Here is an example of how one therapist sought to convince a seven-year-old lisper that he did have errors:

> Joe asked me why he had to come to "thpeech clath." Although his misarticulations were obvious and consistent, it was very clear that he did not know that he lisped. (I found out later that his mother also lisped.) Somehow I had to find some way of helping him recognize his errors without, at the same time, making him upset about them. I answered his question directly but gently. I told him that he some-times didn't say his *s* and *z* sounds right. I told him that many people made these mistakes but never knew that they did. I told him that it was easier to hear mistakes in the speech of others than in oneself, and then I asked him if he could find my mistakes and to correct me before I could correct myself. Then I told him a story about the goose that could hiss and deliberately put in some lisping on some of my words, correcting each error after a pause.

> Every time he was able to catch one of my mistakes before I corrected it, I gave him a salted peanut, and soon he was catching all of them. In doing this, at first I made the errors fairly obvious and prolonged, but later I speeded them up and made them very casually. He learned very fast. But I knew that recognizing the errors in another's speech is far different from identifying them in your own, so as a next step I asked him to listen to another older boy who was already at the stage where he was correcting his defective sibilants. (I did not use a tape recorder because the one I have doesn't have enough fidelity to help a listener recognize the distinctive contrasts between *th* and *s*.) This older boy was able to catch and correct most of his mistakes when reading, but he still missed a good many of them in conversational speech. So again I used the peanut reinforcement, giving one to Joe if he could identify any error that the older boy failed to notice. The activity was good for both of them. Finally, I took a chance and re-versed the routine, asking Joe to name various objects in the room, and the older boy got the peanut when Joe showed his lisp. I had to be a little careful because I noticed Joe became a bit anxious, so we ended the session by having both of them competing to see which one could catch me as I put some of them in my own speech. Both of them won enough peanuts and were delighted. I distracted them sufficiently by talking about something very interesting so that I slipped in one or two defective sibilants which they didn't notice, whereupon I ate the peanut and they had none. It was a fun session, and it was obvious that I had made my point. From that time on, Joe knew that he wasn't saying certain sounds correctly.

The Learning Process. Articulation therapy is a process involving both learning and unlearning. In cases of misarticulation, calling attention to the error and getting the person to recognize that he has a problem is not enough. We must help the individual to unlearn his error; we must teach him to produce the standard sound. We cannot merely demand that he do so, for he cannot produce the correct sound at will. He may try to do so, but the result is unacceptably far from the normal standard. He has habituated a wrong sound; he must learn a right one. Thus, in mastering an articulation error such as the substitution of a *th* for an *s*, we are forced to deal with the revision of movements and sounds. New patterns of muscular coordination that produce new sounds must be mastered. Old patterns must be extinguished. Accordingly, the learning process requires goal-setting in terms of target sounds or movement patterns. The clearer the perception of the goal, the faster the learning. But locating targets is not enough. We must also try to hit the bull's-eye; we must try and try again. But this, too, is not sufficient. We must know, after we shoot, how far away from the center our arrows have hit. We must be able to scan our misses if we are to correct our aim. We must know the *amount* of error if we are to reduce that error. We may need help in varying our postures or the speed and direction of our movements so that we won't continue to make the same mistake. Finally, we need rewards, not only for the final hitting of the bull's-eye, but also for shooting, for coming closer. We also need to learn to hit the target consistently. All of these operations require the application of the laws and principles of learning. The therapist's skill lies in his ability to motivate, to define goals and subgoals, to program reinforcements contingently, and to make those reinforcements meaningful. Old responses must be weakened and extinguished; new ones must be acquired and strengthened.

Operational Levels. The mastering of a new sound so that it can be used in all types of speaking may be viewed in terms of four successive levels: (1) the isolated sound level, (2) the sound in a syllable, (3) the sound in a word, and (4) the sound in a meaningful sentence. This is the staircase our patients must climb. Once they have reached the top step of this staircase they find a wide platform on which they must explore the communicative, thinking, social control, and egocentric functions of speaking, using the newly mastered sound in each.

With such a concept, it is possible for both therapist and case to know just where the latter is at each moment during therapy, and to know what has been achieved and what remains to be accomplished. There is no excuse for unplanned therapy, for random activity or busy-work when a child or adult is unable to talk as others do. The therapist has many responsibilities when working with an articulation case. She must establish a close relationship, provide many rewarding reinforcements, create situations in which learning can occur, and provide models not only of the correct utterance but also of scanning, comparing, varying, and correcting processes. But she has one other responsibility of paramount importance: she must know where the case is, where he has been, and where he has to go in therapy. And she must help the case to know too.

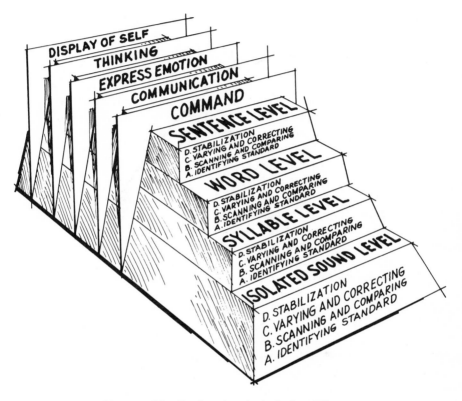

FIGURE 21: *Design for Articulation Therapy*

The Focus of Therapy. Since the essential error consists of a defective sound, it is upon this that we must focus our therapy. Let us repeat: It is the defective *sound* which is in error. It is the misarticulated, nonstandard sound that spoils the syllable, spoils the word, spoils the sentence, and spoils whatever type of speech is being used. In whatever context it occurs, the acquisition and use of a standard sound must be our goal. The child's playmates say to him, "What's the matter with you? You talk funny. Say it this way!" and they provide him with an entire sentence to attempt. The child fails. Parents and teachers focus their therapy on the word level. "Don't say wabbit," they command. "Say rabbit!" The child fails again, or if, by chance, he does say it correctly, there is no transfer to any other *r* word and there are thousands of *r* words he must use. The speech therapist usually focuses her efforts on the sound first, and then on the syllable, for she knows that these are the foundation stones of standard speech. Once a lisper can make a good *s* in isolation, in various nonsense syllables, and has learned how to incorporate it in a few words, he has acquired the tools needed to conquer all *s* words. He need not learn each one individually.

As we have seen, some controversy exists as to whether the new sound should be taught in isolation, or in a syllable, or in meaningful sentences. Our own practice has been to begin with the level which seems most appropriate for the individual case. For example, if our client can make the correct sound at will in words and sentences but fails to do so consistently, we would probably begin at the sentence level. Thus we would even find the sort of treatment used by Marshall in treating an adult with an unrecognized and mildly inconsistent interdental lisp to be quite appropriate. What he did was merely to have the person talk spontaneously and to give him an electric shock every time he made an error. As the author states, "The patient understood the reasons for the use of punishment and was not overtly disturbed by the mild shocks administered during the conditioning segments of each therapy session." [15] It is quite possible in such a case that the shock or the threat thereof served as an efficient alerting device as well as a punishment. But most of our cases do not present so easy a problem.

One of the reasons for the deep testing we described in the preceding section of this chapter is to identify those words (key words) in which the usually defective sound is used *correctly*. When there are a good many of these words, it is often possible to begin therapy by merely increasing their number and finding ways of implanting enough of them in the person's habitual speech until, through the process of generalization, the misarticulation disappears. Many normal children probably master their infantile misarticulations in this way. Again, if this testing reveals that a substantial number of certain syllables containing the sound in question are spoken correctly, we may begin immediately by working on syllables rather than isolated sounds. Some persons find it very difficult to break words into syllables or to recognize isolated sounds. With these we would probably begin at the word level. We also find persons with so many articulatory errors that their speech is almost unintelligible. It would be folly to begin treatment by concentrating on only one of so many defective sounds. Such persons need concrete evidence that they can indeed say something right, and they need it in a hurry. We would try to give them some intelligible words and phrases or sentences as soon as possible so that they can have

[15] R. C. Marshall, "The Effects of Response Contingent Punishment Upon a Defective Articulation Response," *Journal of Speech and Hearing Disorders*, XXXV (1970), 236–40.

some hope of being able to communicate. Nevertheless, most therapists prefer to begin therapy by teaching most of their cases to produce the new sound in isolation. We feel that immediate and direct focusing upon the isolated sound or syllable has much to recommend it. It defines the target immediately. A new sound when mastered can spread very quickly to many syllables, many words, and not just those used in structured conversation. A child who learns to use the *th* sound in "Thank you" in a pretended picnic in the therapy room may remember to say the phrase correctly when his father gives him a dime to spend; but he may have more trouble saying "birthday" or "think" or "bath" than those who have learned immediately to say "th." There are transfer problems in all types of articulation therapy.

THERAPY AT THE ISOLATED SOUND LEVEL

All of the continuant sounds such as *s, l, r,* or *th* can be produced in isolation since they are easily prolonged. Plosives such as *k* and *g* and affricates such as *ch* can be uttered only syllabically; and so when we teach these in isolation, we begin usually by using the *schwa* (or neutral vowel), *uh* [ə], or [ʌ] to create syllables such as *kuh, guh,* and *chuh.* We work on only one or two target sounds at a time. When too many quail flush at once, most marksmen miss. We shoot better when we have our sights focused on a single target. Nevertheless, there are times when we do work with a group of sounds at once. If a child's multiple errors seem to be due to the fact that he has failed to distinguish between stops and fricatives, we would begin by helping him learn the contrasts between these features. Thus one of our children was almost unintelligible because (except for the nasals) the only consonants he used were the *p* and *b,* the *t* and *d,* and the *k* and *g.* Instead of saying "We went swimming yesterday and I saw a fish," he said something like this: "Me met timmun tettaday and I taw a tit." With this boy we did not single out one sound as the nucleus of therapy. We began by teaching him to recognize the contrasts between sounds that "popped" and were made suddenly, and those that were prolonged. We showed him that he could prolong the *f* and the *sh* and *v* as he walked all the way across the room, but that this was impossible for the *t, d, p,* or *k.* We also rewarded strongly all words that he did say correctly.

The First Targets. Those children who have but one sound error present no difficulty so far as targets are concerned, but those who have many errors do. With which sound or sounds shall we begin? No set rules can be offered, but the following items should be considered when selecting the target sound. Of several defective sounds, we would select the one which (1) would have the most key words, (2) have the simplest coordinations, (3) is mastered earlier by most children in their speech development, (4) can be spoken correctly after a bit of trial therapy, (5) have been especially penalized by others. The therapist has to use her judgment as to the importance of each of these factors. At times it is possible to work on pairs of similar sounds such as the *s* and *z* or the *k* and *g* at the same time, since they are cognates that have similar motor patterns. The lateral lisping errors and distortions of the *l* and *r* sound seem to be the most difficult. If the person can produce the sound as a *single* (*l* as in *lack*) but not as a blend (*bl* as in *black*), we might begin with this blend if there is much need to give the child some early success.

Identifying the Characteristics of the Sound to be Taught. As Milisen has shown clearly, the task of learning to correct an articulation error is much more difficult than one might think.[16] The stimulus sounds that a child must learn are very brief, and they vary with the phonetic context; different sense modalities are involved in the discrimination process. Their perception depends upon the sort of stimulation provided by others. Comparison of the standard sound with the error poses many problems. Many a child has persisted in his articulation errors simply because he has never really recognized the distinctive features of the standard sound. He has never heard it in isolation. At best the only help he has had is when others have said it to him, "Don't say fumb, say thumb!" The memory traces of sounds fade fast. Usually the sound he must learn has always been buried in the fast-flowing words, sentences, and communications of other people. The child, consumed by his need to listen for meanings, not for sounds, may hear the standard sounds flicker by, but he does not attend to them. Hidden as these sounds are in the fast torrent of speech, they have little stimulus value. Somehow we must make the characteristics of the sound vivid enough to be mastered. The task of the speech therapist is to aid the child to recognize the distinctive features of the correct sound and to know the contrasts between it and its error. We must help him know how it looks, and especially how it sounds. If the child already has some key words in which the usually misarticulated sound is spoken correctly, we can even help him pay attention to how it feels, and we can use tactile and kinesthetic cues to identify the target sound he has always been able to use correctly in these few words.

Discrimination of the Target Sound from Other Sounds. Here is an account of how a clinician tried to help a child who had a consistent interdental lisp to know the characteristics of the sibilants he had to learn:

> Peter was a fast-talking child, and he talked freely and almost constantly. So far as I could tell, he was completely unaware of his con-

16 R. Milisen, "Articulatory Problems," Chapter 11 in R. W. Rieber and R. S. Brubaker, eds., *Speech Pathology* (Philadelphia: J. B. Lippincott, Co., 1966).

sistent substitution of the voiced and unvoiced *th* for the *z* and *s* sounds. My first job was to get him to recognize these latter sounds as the ones he had to learn. Using a variety of activities in which he had to do something as soon as he heard me make an *s* or *z*, I helped him to discriminate these from other sounds. For example, I covered him up with a towel which he could throw off; and he could "scare" me whenever he heard me make one of these sounds as I pronounced a series of isolated sounds, syllables, words or finally when I spoke to him in sentences. He missed some of these at first, but he learned rapidly. Next, I taught him to tell when the *s* sound occurred at the beginning or at the end of a syllable, first using nonsense syllables, then monosyllabic words, then longer words. I would pronounce a series of these, and it was his task to shout "Head" or "Tail," depending upon whether the *s* occurred at the beginning or the end; and if he got the discrimination right, both of us would have to waggle our heads or tails. He enjoyed seeing me do this and learned swiftly when he made a misjudgment and I didn't do what he expected. When he got so he could locate these sounds in my speech pretty well, I then spent some time in showing him just what the *s* sound looked like —that my teeth were together and my lips retracted—and also that in it there was a high-pitched hiss. By pantomiming isolated sounds, syllables, and words, some of which contained the *s* sound and some did not, I taught him this visual discrimination. Then I put big paper sacks over our heads and repeatedly said the name of an object in the room which began with the *s* sound, but he was not to throw off his sack and run to get the object until he heard the high-pitched hiss that I had set up as the signal. I fooled him a few times using *th* and *sh* sounds and laterally emitted sibilants before he got so he could recognize the high-pitched hiss of the correct *s* sound; but again he soon mastered the discrimination. Finally, I gave him a good dosing with some isolated and prolonged *s* sounds. I got behind Pete and made a continuous *s* sound shifting my mouth from side to side. He was to indicate in which ear he heard it loudest. I varied the intensity. Then I told him his left ear was for the *th* sound and the right ear for the *s*, and he was to point to the one which represented the sound I was making as I made a series of them in isolation—syllables, words, and sentences. I did all of these activities in a forty-minute session, and at the end of the time I felt Pete had learned pretty well the characteristics of the sound he had to learn to make.

This account of a single therapy session illustrates very clearly how we can help a person define a sound he must learn to make. The speech clinician aided Peter to locate the sound, to isolate it, and to discriminate it from other sounds. She pointed out and demonstrated its distinctive features—how it looked and how it sounded. Instead of hiding it in the swift flow of her speech, she prolonged it and intensified it so that it had some stimulus value. She helped the boy to know the differences between the *s* and the *th* sound he was using habitually to replace it. She could have used many other activities to attain the same goals, but those she used were evidently very appropriate to his needs. If a child fails to perceive the characteristics of his target sound, all the therapy in the world will not help him to acquire it. If a child is to know what his target is, he must learn to cock his ears in such a fashion that he can locate and identify the standard sound he must learn to make. He must learn to analyze the speech he hears in terms of its sounds rather than meanings. He must come to know the characteristic features of this new target sound. The lisper must learn to listen with strange ears, to recognize the high-pitched hiss of his therapist's *s*, to observe how she makes it. He must know when it is distorted and when it is right. In helping such a person to acquire the concept of a standard sound, one against which he may later match his own utterance, we have four basic sets of techniques: (1) isolation, (2) stimulation, (3) identification, and (4) discrimination. All these are designed to define the target. They provide the model which he must match. Without such a model, how can he correct himself?

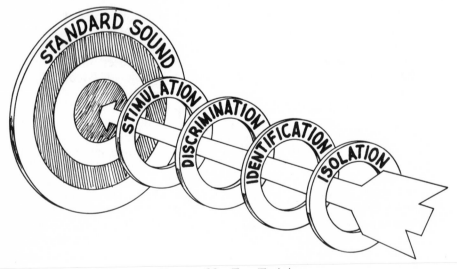

FIGURE 22: *Ear Training*

Please note that this is ear training, not mouth training. In this necessary perceptual defining of a standard pattern, the ear training period, we do not ask the child to attempt the new sound. Not yet. First let us be sure that he internalizes the model. In this first phase of therapy for articulation cases, the emphasis is all on listening. It is ear training.

The student is asked to write down the symbol corresponding to the sound used.

1. *Matching.* The teacher slowly reads a newspaper article, occasionally using the student's error. The student is asked to name each correct and incorrect sound, using the names taught in the identification exercises. He must interrupt the teacher to do this naming.

2. *Signaling.* The student is asked to raise his right hand the moment he hears the correct sound and to raise his left when he hears the error. The teacher pronounces a series of nonsense syllables, slowly at first, but with a gradual increase of speed.

3. *Signaling.* The teacher reads tongue twisters, occasionally using the error. The student is asked to rap on the table the moment he hears the error. If his response does not occur until after the teacher has said the next two words, he has failed. The procedure is continued until he collects five successes.

Scanning and Comparing.   The second major phase of therapy also involves ear training but now the case is to listen to himself. It is training in *self-hearing* rather than in listening to the speech of others. By this time, he should have acquired a clear concept of the target sound. Now he must scan his own speech so that the differences between his own utterance and the standard sound will be made clear. Most of our cases have no idea of how they sound. Many of them do not even hear their errors. This is quite natural. When we speak we have to use our ears to find out what we are saying. Only rarely do we think before we speak. When we were babies, babbling in the crib, we listened to the sounds we were making and found joy therein. But once we learned the magical power of speech in sending messages, in formulating thoughts, in controlling others, we stopped listening to the sounds that emerge from our mouths. We had to keep our ears relatively free for receiving the *thoughts* of others and for scrutinizing our own meanings to see if they were well expressed. Perhaps this is why articulation errors persist. We do not hear them.

Somehow we must open up the invisible channel between the person's ear and his own mouth. We must help him to locate his errors whenever they occur. We must give them new vivid stimulus value. When the laller says a defective *r* sound, some hidden signal must be triggered off somewhere within the skull. Usually the therapist has to do the signaling first, pointing out when the error has occurred. We have found that it is wise to make these therapist signalings pleasant experiences to prevent the child from hearing echoes of past penalties. Here is one example:

Therapist: Today we're going to try to help you know whenever you lisp because you've got to know when you do if you are to stop lisping.
Case: OK.
Therapist: Fine. Here's a gong. It makes a fine sound when you bang

it like this. . . . Now tell me what I'm doing as I'm doing it and if you ever hear yourself lisp like *thith*, instead of like *thissss*, you can give it a wallop. All right. Here we go. Tell me what I'm doing.

Case: You're putting the penthil in your mouth.

Therapist: Huh?

Case: Oh, you're putting the penthil (*bangs the gong*) in your mouth. Wow, what a big noith!

Therapist: (*Takes hammer away and rings the gong herself*): Noith . . . (*banging gong*). It should have been noise. No, don't try to say it right yet. Just bang it when you hear it wrong.

The preceding example illustrates how we can use this training in self-hearing at both sentence and word levels. The following one illustrates the process at the syllable and sound levels.

Therapist: Let's play a follow-the-leader game. Do what I do and say what I say, and if you can notice when you say a sound wrong and can clap your hands before I can say, "Oops! Hey nonny nonny!" I'll go over and put my head in that wastebasket. Understand?

Case: (*Enthusiastically*): Sure.

Therapist: (*Raises hand*): Bah-bah.

Case: (*Raises hand*): Bah-bah.

Therapist: (*Shakes her foot*): Moogie-moogie.

Case: (*Shakes his foot*): Moogie-moogie.

Therapist: (*Touches nose*): Nnnnnnnnnnnnnnnn.

Case: (*Touches nose*): Nnnnnnnnn.

Therapist: (*Wiggles fingers*): Sobba-sobba.

Case: (*Wiggles fingers*): Thobba-thobba.

Therapist: Ooops! Hey nonny nonny. Hah, I didn't have to put my head in the basket then.

Case: I catch you nekth time.

Therapist: (*Raises hands above head*): Allee-oh.

Case: (*Raises hands above head*): Allee-oh.

Therapist: (*Pulls ears*): Fff-a-sss.

Case: (*Pulls ears*): Fff-a-th . . . There one. (*Claps hands.*)

Therapist: (*Puts head in basket*): You got me. You said fff-a-th instead of fff-a-sssssss.

It is possible to teach a child to recognize his own errors most easily when the process is pleasant rather than distasteful.

Recalling, Perceiving, and Predicting Errors.   In this training in self-hearing, we operate in a time dimension. At first the child recognizes his errors only after they have occurred; next, when they are occurring; finally he can predict them. The wise therapist understands this natural sequence of recognition and uses it. She signals her perception of the child's error at first only after an interval sufficiently long to let him listen to what his mouth has produced. Here are some examples:

Therapist: Repeat each of these sounds twice before telling me if you've made a mistake: mmm. . . .
Case: Mmmm . . . mmmmmm . . . it's OK.
Therapist: Right! Now this one: rrrrr.
Case: Rrrrr . . . rrrrr . . . it's OK too.
Therapist: Yes. Now this one: ssss.
Case: Th . . . th . . . no, thath wrong.
Therapist: Now let's do it in a syllable. Try this one: lllee.
Case: Llleee . . . lllee. Thath all right.
Therapist: Now this one: oossss.
Case: Ooosss . . . oooossss. Thatth wrong. Hey, wait! ooosss. It ith OK. . . .
Therapist: Now this word: coop.
Case: Coop . . . cooop. Good one.
Therapist: Now this one: soup.
Case: Thoup . . . thoup. . . . I got that wrong.
Therapist: Now this sentence (*illustrating the action*) I pat my face.
Case: I pat my fayth. . . . I pat my fayth. Hey, I thaid fayth wrong.
Therapist: Yup. You're beginning to catch almost all your mistakes. Pretty soon we'll teach you how to say that *sss* sound correctly.

In the simultaneous perception of the error as opposed to this delayed perception, one very effective device is to have the therapist read or speak in unison with the case with her mouth to his ear. If at the moment he makes an error, she signals by making the correct sound very loudly, or by stopping her own speaking, or by some other stimulation, he will be brought to notice it instantly. Another device is to have the child record some sounds, syllables, words, or sentences, a few of which contain the target sound, and then to require the child to say them again in unison with his own recorded speech. The therapist turns up the volume of the playback very loudly at the moment of error. There are many other ways.[17]

In predicting errors, the therapist provides sample utterances on each of the various levels and then asks the child to predict whether or not he will make an error on them when he says them. Here is one example:

Therapist: I'm going to say three sounds: first, *mmmmmmmmmmm*; second, *ssss*; third, *ffff*. In a moment I'm going to ask you to say them but first you tell me on which one you think you might make a mistake: *mmmmm* . . . *sssss* . . . *fffff*.
Case: On the latht one.
Therapist: OK, let's see. Try them.
Case: Mmmm . . . *th* . . . *ffff*. Oh it wath the thecond.

[17] Further examples of delayed, simultaneous, and predictive recognition of errors may be found in Van Riper and Irwin, *Voice and Articulation*, pp. 134–41.

Therapist: All right. Now let's try these syllables: *eepoo . . . ommee . . . issah.*

Case: Oh, it wath on the latht one.

Therapist: Right! Now try these words: *house . . . ham . . . heavy.*

Case: Houth ith the one.

Therapist: Good. It should have been "house."

All the various exercises for isolating, identifying, and discriminating the correct sound in the therapist's speech can also be used to help the child recognize the errors in his own speech once he has a clear concept of how the correct sound is spoken.

Teaching the New Sound.   Once we have been able to establish a clear perception of the standard sound and have opened up the circuit of self-hearing so that the child can recognize and identify his errors, we are ready for the next step: learning to produce the new sound. As we have said earlier, this mastery of a new sound must be accomplished on all levels: isolated sound, syllable, word, sentence, and function, but we have found it most efficient to teach it first in isolation by concentrating on its motor and acoustic aspects. There are five different ways of approaching this task. The new sound may be taught by (1) progressive approximation, (2) by auditory stimulation, (3) by phonetic placement, (4) by the modification of other standard sounds already mastered, or (5) by using key words. Each of these will be described in detail.

Varying and Correcting.   Whichever approach is used—and there are times when we must try first one then another—the person must go through a process of varying his utterance. Change must occur in the way he shapes his tongue, in the acoustic patterns which emerge from his mouth. One of the basic problems confronting the therapist at this stage of treatment is to provoke such variation. Long-practiced habits are very resistant to change. Often before we can hope to get our case to have a fair chance of hitting his target, we must get him to try new postures, new attacks, new movement patterns. Variation must precede approximation. By this we mean something similar to what happens when a person learns to shoot an arrow at a target. When he shoots and misses, he first must know where the arrow has hit, and next he must vary his aim or stance so 'that his second shot will have some chance of hitting a different part of the target, preferably a spot closer to the bull's-eye. But he must vary and he must try to correct. This same process occurs in articulation therapy. We must get our lisper to try and try again, but to try differently each time so that he comes closer and closer to producing the desired standard sound. Variation must precede approximation.

Progressive Approximation.   This method is a trail-blazing method. The therapist joins the case and makes the same error the case makes. She then shows the case a series of transitional sounds each of which comes

a bit closer to the standard sound until finally the standard sound is produced. Each little modification the case makes that comes a bit closer to
the goal is rewarded. Those variations that move away from the target
sound are ignored. Through this process, the *degree* of error is constantly
determined; and new attempts are aimed at reducing the amount of deviation. The uniqueness of this approach is that it resembles the way that
infants seem to acquire normal articulation. They do not suddenly shift
from saying *wabbit* to *rabbit;* instead they seem to proceed through a series
of gradual and progressive approximations as McCurry and Irwin have
described.[18] This also is the process known to psychologists as "operant
conditioning." Instead of asking the person to exchange a correct sound for
his incorrect sound, we help him to shift gradually from where he is to
where he has to go. Let us observe some progressive approximation therapy.

> *Therapist:* Now cup your hands like this so they make a channel from
> your mouth to your right ear. I'm going to talk into your left ear
> like this. (*Therapist cups her hands and speaks a sound into the
> person's left ear.*) Now we're going to try to make the new sound.
> Say *ssssssss.*
> *Case:* Thththththththth. Thath no good.
> *Therapist:* (*Still talking into his left ear*): OK, let's do it again. This
> time I will join you and make the same sound so that we're in tune
> even if it is wrong. But then I'll change it just a bit and you try to
> follow me. I'm not going to change it all the way to the correct *sss*
> but I'll pull back my tongue a little and that will make a different
> sound. Try to follow me. But we'll start with your sound. Say *sssss.*
> *Case:* Thththththththth.
> *Therapist:* (*In unison*): Thththth. (*And then she makes a slight varia-
> tion in the direction of the standard sound, and the case varies
> his sound also.*) Start with your old sound and let's try to shift a bit
> further like this. . . . (*Therapist illustrates the change the case has
> already made and a second change that comes even closer to the* sss.)

We feel that progressive approximation is the best of the five main
methods for teaching a new sound. It permits reward for modification
instead of reserving it for final attainment of the goal. It helps the identification of therapist and case. It reduces the task. It encourages variation.
Even very resistant cases seem to move under this regime. We have found
it very efficient.

Nevertheless there are times when other methods are to be preferred.
For example, if a child can make the new sound fairly easily with direct

[18] W. H. McCurry and O. C. Irwin. "A Study of Word Approximations in the
Spontaneous Speech of Infants," *Journal of Speech and Hearing Disorders,* XVIII
(1953), 133–39.

stimulation, we find it easier merely to ask him to imitate us as described in the auditory stimulation method. Again, some cases are unable to perceive tiny variations in auditory experience. They are not at all ear-minded. They have better visual or proprioceptive imagery than auditory imagery. With these we prefer to use the phonetic placement techniques. Finally, there are some children who have been defeated for so long in attempts to correct themselves that it is better to use the modification of sounds they have already mastered.

Auditory Stimulation.   This method relies upon simple imitation and demand. An example might run as follows:

> *Therapist:* Now, Johnny, I'm going to let you have your first chance to make the snake sound, *sss.* Remember not to make the windmill sound, *th-th.* This is the sound you are to make: *sss, sss, ssssss.* Now you try it.

If the ear training has been adequate, this simple routine, in which the wrong sound is pronounced, identified, and rejected, then followed by the correct sound given several times, will bring a perfect production of the correct sound on the first attempt. Occasionally it will be necessary to repeat this routine several times before it works, and the student should be encouraged to take his time and to listen carefully both to the stimulation and to his response. He should be told that he has made an error or that he has almost said it correctly. He should then be encouraged to attempt it in a slightly different way the next time. No pressure should be brought to bear upon him; and a review of discrimination, stimulation, and identification techniques should preface the new attempt. He should be asked to make it quietly and without force. The procedure may be slightly varied by asking the child to produce it in a whisper. After the sound has been produced, the teacher should signal the child to repeat or prolong it and to sense the "feel" of it. The attempt should be confined to the isolated sound itself or to a nonsense syllable beginning with it.

Phonetic Placement.   The phonetic placement method of enabling a speech defective to produce a new sound is the old traditional method. For centuries, speech correctionists have used diagrams, applicators, and instruments to ensure appropriate tongue, jaw, and lip placement. Children have been asked to watch the teacher's tongue movements and to duplicate them. Observation of the teachers mouth in a mirror has also been used. Many very ingenious devices have been invented to adapt these techniques for children, and often they produce almost miraculous results. Unfortunately, however, the mechanics of such phonetic replacement demand so much attention that they cannot be performed quickly or unconsciously enough for the needs of casual speech. At best, they are vague and difficult to sense or recall. The positions tend to vary with the sounds that precede or follow them, and to teach all of these positions is an almost impossible task. Frequently dental abnormalities will make an exact repro-duction of the standard position inadvisable. Many speech correctionists produce the sounds in nonstandard ways, if, indeed, there is a standard way of producing any given speech sound. Despite all of these disadvan-tages, the phonetic placement methods are indispensable tools in the speech therapist's kit; and when the stimulation method fails, they must be used. They are especially useful in working with the individuals with hear-ing defects, and they certainly help to identify the sound.

Excellent diagrams and descriptions of the various speech sounds may be found in the texts to which references are given at the end of this chap-ter. The speech correctionist should have these texts available and should know the mechanics of articulation thoroughly enough to interpret the diagrams and assume the positions illustrated and described. The teacher should be able to recognize any sound from its description and diagram.

In using methods of phonetic placement, it is necessary that the stu-dent be given a clear idea of the desired position prior to speech attempt. If an adult, he should study diagrams, the clinician's articulatory organs in position, when observed both directly and in a mirror, palatograms, models, and the written descriptions of the mechanics whereby the sound is produced. Every available device should be used to make the student understand clearly what positions of tongue, jaw, and lips are to be as-sumed. It is frequently advisable to have the student practice other sounds that he can make easily, using diagrams and printed descriptions to guide his placement. This will familiarize him with the technique of translating diagrams and descriptions into performance.

Various instruments and applicators are used to help the student attain the proper position. Tongue depressors are used to hold the tip and front of the tongue down, as in the attempt to produce a *k* or *g*, or they may be used to touch certain portions of the tongue and palate to indicate positions of mutual contact. Tooth props of various sizes will help the student to assume a proper dental opening. Thin applicators and wedges are used to groove the tongue. Curious wire contrivances are occasionally used to insure lateral contact of tongue and teeth. Small tubes are used to direct the flow of air. In our experience, they are more dramatic than useful. Enforcing a certain tongue position through some such device produces such a mass of kinesthetic and tactual sensations that the appropriate ones can seldom be attended to. Usually, the moment the instrument is removed the old, incorrect tongue position is assumed.

If these devices and instruments have any real value, it seems to be that of vivifying the movements of the tongue, and of providing a large number of varying tongue positions from which the correct one may finally emerge. Many individuals have difficulty in realizing how great a repertoire of tongue movements they possess, and instruments frequently enable them to attempt new ones. When the correct sound has been produced (and frequently a lot of trial and error must be resorted to before it appears), the student should hold it, increasing its intensity, repeating it, whispering it, exaggerating it, and varying it in as many ways as possible without losing its identity. He should focus his attention on the "feel" of the position in terms of tongue, palate, jaws, lips, and throat. He should listen to the sound produced. Then he should be asked to leave the position intact but to cease speech attempt, resuming it after a long interval. Finally he should let the tongue assume a neutral position on the floor of the mouth and then attempt to regain the desired position. Sounds produced by phonetic placement are very unstable and must be treated very carefully or they will be lost. Strengthen them as soon as possible and keep out distractions. After a successful attempt, one should insist that the student remain silent for a time before taking part in conversation. This will permit maturation to become effective.

Modification of Other Sounds.   Another special method of teaching a speech defective a new sound involves the modification of other sounds, either those of speech, those that imitate noises, or those that imitate other functions such as swallowing. These methods are somewhat akin to those of phonetic placement, but they have the advantage of using a known sound or movement as a point of departure for the trial-and-error variation which produces the correct sound. The modification method may take many forms, but in all of them the sequence is about the same. The student is asked to make a certain sound and to hold it for a short period. He is then requested to move his tongue or his lips or jaws in a definite manner while continuing to produce his first sound. This variation in articulators will produce a change in the sound, a change which often rather closely approximates the sound that is desired. An illustration of this method may be given. A lateral lisper is told to make the *th* sound and to prolong it. Then, while continuing to make the sound, he is required to draw in the tongue tip slowly and to raise the whole tongue, slowly scrape its tip upward along the back of the upper teeth, and finally bring it to rest against the alveolar ridge. The *th* sound will change as the tongue rises, and a rather good approximation to the desired *s* will be produced. If this is combined with ear training and stimulation, it will be found to be very effective.

Key Word Method.   As we have seen, one of the items in both the voice and articulation tests requires the examiner to record all words in which the usually defective sound is made correctly. Many teachers of speech correction fail to realize the value of these words in remedial work. They may be used to enable the student to make the correct sound at will and in isolation. They are also extremely valuable in getting the student to make clean-cut transitions between the isolated sound and the rest of the word. Finally, they serve as standards of correctness of sound performance. Speech defectives need some standard with which to compare their speech attempts at correct production of the usually defective sound. Although occasional cases are found who never make the sound correctly, the majority of speech defectives have a few words in which they do not make the error. The teacher should be alert enough to catch these when they do occur. Often these words are those which have the usually defective sound in an inconspicuous place—that is to say, the sound occurs in the medial or final position, or is incorporated within a blend; seldom is it found in an accented syllable. The teacher must train her ear to listen for it in the student's speech or it will escape her. At times it occurs in words in which an unusual spelling provides a different symbol for the sound. To illustrate: A child who was unable to make a good *f* in any of his words using that printed symbol, said the word *rough* with a perfect *f* sound. This was probably due to the strong stimulation given by the child's spelling teacher.

These words are worth the trouble needed to discover them, for they simplify the teacher's work tremendously, since it is possible to use that sound as a standard and guide and to work from it to other words in which error normally occurs. The experienced teacher greets these nuclei words as veritable nuggets. Similarly, even when the student is highly consistent in his errors, there comes a stage in his treatment when he is saying a few words correctly. These words may be used to serve the same ends as those mentioned in the preceding paragraph.

The procedure used in this method is roughly as follows: The teacher writes the word on one of several cards (or uses a picture representing it). Then she asks the student to go through the series one at a time, saying the word on each card ten times. Finally, the special word to be used is repeated a hundred times, accenting and prolonging if possible the sound which in other words is made incorrectly. Thus the lingual lisper who could say *lips* correctly repeated the word one hundred times, prolonging the *s*. He was then asked to hold it for a count of twenty, then thirty, then forty. Finally, he was required to hold it intermittently, thus; *lipssss.ssss..sss*. The purpose of such a gradual approach is that the sound must be emphasized in both its auditory and its motor characteristics to prevent its loss when the student becomes aware of it as his hard sound. For example, one baby-talker made the initial *r* in *rabbit* perfectly until told that he did. Immediately the child changed to the *w* substitution and was unable to make the initial *r* again.

After the child has emphasized the sound a great many times, has listened to it and felt it thoroughly, and can make it intermittently and in a repetitive form, he may be asked to think the word and to speak the sound. It is often wise to underline the sound to be spoken, asking the student to whisper all but the letter underlined. Other sounds and other words may be similarly underlined if a careful approach is necessary. Through these means, the child finally can make the sound in isolation and at will.

Stabilizing the New Sound.   One of the greatest causes for discouragement in treating an articulatory case may be traced to the parent's or teacher's ignorance of a very important fact. A new sound is weak and unstable. Its mechanics are easily forgotten or lost. Its dual phases of auditory and motor sensation patterns are easily confused. Many people believe that a complicated skill (such as that involved in a speech sound) once achieved is never lost, although any musician or tennis player will tell us that a new stroke or fingering sequence must be practiced and strengthened a great deal before it can be used in competition or concert. Many speech therapists become discouraged and blame the speech defective for his frequent relapse into error or his sudden loss of the sound he had been taught to make. Many children who can make the correct sound at will never learn to incorporate it within familiar words. All of these unfortunate occurrences are due to the fact that a new sound must be strengthened before it can win the competition with the error in the speaking of common words. A lisper who has said "yeth" for "yes" several thousand times cannot be expected to say the latter as soon as he has learned to make the *sss* sound in isolation. Perhaps that sound has been performed only three or four times. Yet parents and teachers constantly ruin all of their preliminary work by saying some such sentence as this: "Fine, Johnny. That was fine! You said *sss* just as plainly as anyone. Now say 'sssoup.'" And Johnny, ninety-nine times out of one hundred, will say triumphantly, "thoup." Most speech therapists have to train themselves to resist this urge to hurry. When the child has been taught to make the new sound, the utmost patience and restraint are needed.

When a new sound has just been born, it is a tender thing and must be carefully treated. It should be repeated or prolonged as soon as possible, but there should be no great hullabaloo over the achievement or it may be lost again.

During this repetition and prolongation, the student should be told to keep a poker face and to move as little as possible. A sudden shift of body position occasionally produces a change in the movements of articulation as well. As soon as the new sound tends to loose its clear characteristics, the teacher should insist upon some rest and should then review the procedure used to produce the sound. Rest should be silent in order to let maturation take place. Little intensity should be used; and when working with a pair of sounds such as *s* and *z*, the unvoiced sound is preferable. Often sounds such as *l* and *r* should be whispered or sung.

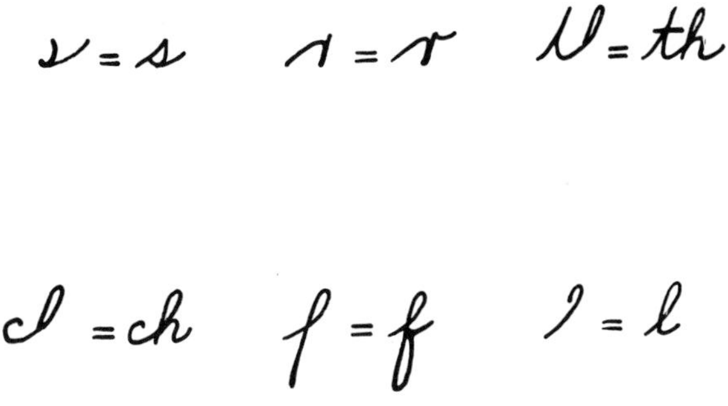

$\mathcal{V} = \mathcal{A}$ $\mathcal{A} = \mathcal{r}$ $\mathcal{N} = \mathcal{th}$

$\mathcal{d} = ch$ $\mathcal{f} = \mathcal{f}$ $\mathcal{l} = \mathcal{l}$

FIGURE 23: *Nonsense Symbols*

After the speech defective is able to produce the sound readily and can repeat and prolong it consistently, the therapist can ask him to increase its intensity and exaggerate it. He should be asked to focus his attention on the "feel" of the tongue, lips, and palate. Shutting his eyes will help him to get a better awareness of the tactual and kinesthetic sensations thereby produced. Ask him to assume the position without speech attempt and, after a short period of "feeling," to try the sound. Many other supplementary devices will occur to the teacher.

After the student reaches the stage where he has little difficulty in producing the new sound, he should be encouraged to shorten the time needed to produce it. A sound which the student takes too long to produce will never become habitual. This speeding up of the time needed to initiate it may be accomplished by demanding fast repetitions, by alternating it with other isolated speech sounds, and by using signals. In this last activity, the student should keep his articulatory apparatus in a state of rest or in certain other positions, such as an open mouth; and then, at a certain sharp-sound signal, he should react by producing the new sound immediately.

One of the most effective methods for strengthening a new sound is to include it in babbling and the student should attempt to incorporate the new sound within the vocal flow as effortlessly as possible. It should not stand out and there should be no pausing before it. Doublings of the sound should be frequent. These babbling periods should be continued daily throughout the course of treatment.

The most important of all strengthening devices is the use of simultaneous talking-and-writing. In this procedure, the student writes the script symbol as he pronounces the sound. The sound should be timed so that it will neither precede nor follow the writing of the symbol, but will coincide exactly with the dominant stroke of the letter. Since this dominant stroke varies somewhat with different persons, some experimentation will be needed. At first the teacher should supervise this talking-and-writing very carefully to ensure clear vocalization of the new sound and proper timing. Later the student can be assigned to hand in several pages of this talking-and-writing every day. The continuant sounds should be pronounced by themselves (*sss, vvv, lll, mmm*), and the stops should use a lightly vocalized neutral vowel (*kuh, puh, duh*). Simultaneous talking-and-writing techniques not only provide an excellent vehicle for practice of the new sound, but also give a means of reinforcing it by enriching the motor aspect of the performance. They also improve the identification and, as we shall see, make possible an effective transition to familiar words. For children who cannot write, the sound may be tied up with a movement such as a finger twitch or foot tap. In this case, as in writing, the timing is very important.

ARTICULATION THERAPY AT THE SYLLABLE LEVEL

As soon as the person has learned to produce the new sound in isolation whenever he tries to do so, we move immediately to get him to use it in syllables. You will recall that the second operational level is that of syllabic utterance in the sequence: isolated sound, syllable, word, and sentence.

Beginning with the Syllable.   Some speech therapists prefer to start with this syllabic level—to teach *ree* and *ra* and *roo* rather than *rrr*, because they feel that the syllable is the basic unit of motor speech. They also point out that many sounds such as the plosives *k* and *g* can only be produced syllabically and that prolonging an isolated sound distorts its pattern in time and creates unnecessary difficulty in shifting from sounds into syllables and then into words. Why not begin immediately with the syllable and teach *la-lee-lie-lay-lo-loo* instead of the isolated *llll* sound? We will not argue the point with any real vigor, for we have often begun therapy with the syllable in certain cases where the person seemed to produce the sound more easily therein than in isolation. For example, we have known several children who could produce the *l* sound more easily in a syllable such as *lee* than they could in saying the isolated *llll*.[19] However, since we begin with acoustic ear training rather than with the motor aspect of speech, the basic unit of auditory perception is not the syllable but the phoneme, the sound. It provides one target rather than several. It transfers easily to many syllables once it is mastered in isolation so that there is no need to teach each syllable in turn. Moreover, when we have begun with the syllable, we

---

[19] These two sounds, however, are not identical. The *l* sound at the beginning of a syllable is more fricative and less vocalic than one used in isolation or at the end of a syllable such as *ol*.

notice that unconsciously we kept prolonging and stressing the sound anyway. It is the sound, not the syllable, which is our first target's bull's-
eye.

However, when therapy begins with the syllable, the therapist follows
the same basic sequence we have outlind for the isolated sound. The standard acoustic and motor patterns of the various syllables as they occur in
the speech of others are defined through ear training. Next, self-hearing
of the person's own syllable production is scanned and compared with the
features of the correct syllable to define the syllabic errors. Next, the
same techniques of progressive approximation, auditory stimulation, and
phonetic placement are used to teach the isolated syllables. The process is
the same; it is the target that differs initially. Moreover, once we have
trained the person to make the new sound in syllables, we usually return
to the isolated sounds, pointing them out within the syllable so that the
person comes to recognize the correction he has made.

Strenghtening and Stabilizing the New Sound in Nonsense Syllables.
Whether we begin with the syllable or the sound, our next major step
in therapy is to help our case to use the new sound in all phonetic contexts.
This is very important since any sound changes slightly whenever it is preceded or followed by other sounds. The *s* in the nonsense syllable *seeb*,
for example, is acoustically higher in pitch than the *s* in *soob*. Also the
contour of the tongue varies a bit with differing phonetic contexts. Since
we must be able to produce the new sound in all possible combinations,
we must have some means of teaching these variations. The nonsense
syllable provides us with such a vehicle.

Types of Nonsense Syllables. There are three main types of nonsense syllables: CV (consonant-vowel syllables such as *la*), VC (vowel-
consonant syllables such as *al*), and CVC (consonant-vowel-consonant
combinations such as *kal* or *lod*). These syllables can be readily constructed
by combining the new sound with the fourteen most common vowels and
diphthongs. The first nonsense syllables to be practiced are those in which
the transitional movements from consonant to vowel involve the fewest
and simplest coordinations. For example, *ko* involves less radical transitional movements than does *kee*. The next nonsense syllables should be
those which use the new sound in the final position (*ok*); and, finally, those
in which the new sound is located in the medial position (*oko*) should be
practiced. Double nonsense syllables may also be used, but simple doublings
are preferred (*kaka*).

These nonsense syllables should be practiced thoroughly before
familiar words are attempted. The talking-and-writing technique can be
used to facilitate their production if any difficulty is experienced. The student should speak the new sound as he writes the symbol until he gets
to the end of the line, then should add the vowel, thus: *s s s s s s saaa*.

Signal practice such as that described later in this section can also be used to form the nonsense syllable if it is needed. Generally, however, a simple request by the teacher to repeat the nonsense syllable he pronounces will produce the desired results. This repetition from a model is the usual way in which the syllables are used. They may also be written by the teacher and read by the student. They may be used to precede each sentence of conversation or used as substitutes for such words as *the* or *and*. Lists of them may be used for practice, and all the various vowel combinations should be employed. The student should practice them finally at high speeds.

Although most young children have no difficulty in using the standard letter symbol for the sound in these nonsense syllables or talking-and-writing, many adults and some young children who have read and written the letter while pronouncing it incorrectly will have difficulty. The letter *s*, for example, means *th* to such a lisper, and he cannot use the usual syllables in talking-and-writing. For these cases, it is wise to use a nonsense symbol in place of the standard letter. In general, the symbols should be parts of the standard symbols, though the student should not realize this fact until later. These symbols should be used for identification techniques and for all strengthening techniques. After the student has finally begun to use them in regular words, he may be shown that the nonsense symbol is really a part of the true symbol for the sound.

Nonsense Words.   The big advantage of using nonsense syllables rather than words is that no unlearning is needed. Were we to use familiar words for this stabilizing, we would immediately find trouble because of the competition of the old error. A child who has said *thoup* for *soup* all his life will find it easier to say the nonsense syllable *soub* than *soup*. Moreover, by giving meanings to nonsense syllables or combining them to form nonsense words we can facilitate transfer to communication and the other functions of speech. The fingers and toes may be given nonsense names. The doorknob may be christened. The teacher can make nonsense objects out of modeling clay, giving them names which include the new sound. Nonsense pictures may be drawn and named. Card games using these nonsense pictures seem to be peculiarly fascinating to almost all cases. Through talking-and-writing techniques, repetition from a model, reading, conversation, questioning, and speech games, these nonsense names can be used repeatedly. The various sound combinations are thereby practiced, and remarkable progress will soon occur. Examples of some of the nonsense pictures are given in Figure 24.

Once we have given meanings to nonsense words, we can immediately begin to use them in the various functions of speech. The child can command us to put the *sooba* in the basket. We can ask him how many red *soobas* are in the box. He can even vent his hostility by calling us a dirty, low-down *poos*. Children enjoy these activities and they are much more effective than drill.

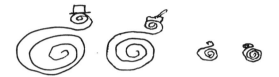

Figure 24: *The Sooba Family*

Articulation Therapy at the Word Level

We are now ready to move onward to our third operational level—the word level. The new sound has now been sufficiently strengthened so that it has a fair chance to hold its own in competition with the error if we can make sure that the odds are in its favor. We must remember that the articulation case has used his old error in meaningful words thousands of times and that it would be unreasonable to expect him suddenly to be able to speak them correctly. We therefore need new techniques to insure the successful incorporation of the newly-acquired sound into his words.

Beginning Therapy at the Word Level. There are times when we even begin our therapy at the word level. We have already discussed how we use key words to provide in-the-mouth samples of the correct sound, and we have emphasized the point that inconsistency of error is much more common than we realize until we do some deep testing. These observations indicate that it might be possible to start therapy immediately by teaching correctly spoken *words* instead of isolated sounds or nonsense syllables. Indeed, most children seem to acquire correct articulation from this type of teaching. This is how parents normally teach a child to speak correctly. The fact that his method has failed with this particular person may not mean that the approach is all wrong, but perhaps merely that it was not correctly administered. Although we have already stated our preference for beginning with the isolated sound for the majority of our cases, we are not prejudiced against using any approach that might be more useful with a particular case. We have taught many children to achieve correct articulation by starting at the word level.

The Key Word as a Nucleus. We suspect that the failure of the traditional parental method of teaching a child words instead of sounds is due primarily to their use of too many words with too many different sounds as stimuli. When the speech therapist begins with the word level approach, she concentrates on teaching only a *few* important words, all of which contain the *same* desired sound. Parents, on the other hand, demand correction of many words containing many different errors. This confuses the child and he gives up trying to conform. The speech therapist tries to create nuclei of standard words and to insert them into the main functions of speech. We try to implant little colonies of these key words within messages, commands, emotional expressions, and even in thinking. Once planted and tended, these nuclei can attract other phonetically similar words. It is vitally important that the child *know* that these key words are ones that he can speak correctly and without error, that when he says these, he is speaking just as well as any other person, big or little. These are his yardsticks. These are his mouth models of correct utterance. He must know that when he says "Yes" he is not lisping. Only those of us who have worked long in the vineyard with discouraged children can realize how important it is that such a child can come to be completely certain that he can say at least a few words perfectly. Once he has such a nucleus, he can start a collection.

Creating Key Words. How do we get these key words? Some of them we can find, as we have said, by deep testing, by searching through the child's spoken vocabulary, by checking the lists of assimilation words we can assemble, by varying the conditions of communication. Others we must create out of the sounds and syllables that compose them, using the isolated-sound or nonsense-syllable approaches. Thus, we see that no matter where we begin, we find ourselves sooner or later at the point where we must operate on the word level, creating and collecting key words to serve as nuclei for correct utterance. With most children we find it best to begin with the isolated sound, then move into the syllable and then into key words; with some children, we start with the syllable and move into key words; with a few special children we start with the key words themselves.

Creating Key Words from Sounds and Syllables. We have two main techniques for creating key words once the child has mastered the sound in isolation and in the nonsense syllable: reconfiguration training and signaling.

Reconfiguration Techniques. Frequently the reconfiguration techniques must be carried out rather gradually. Their purpose is to teach the individual that words are made up of sound sequences and that these sound sequences can be modified without losing the unity of the word. If, for convenience, we use a lingual lisper as our example, the reconfiguration techniques would follow somewhat the same sequence: (1) the student reads, narrates, and converses with the teacher, substituting the sound of *b* for that of *f* whenever the latter occurs in the initial position. He reads, for example, that "Sammy caught a bish with his hook and line." The purpose of using these nonerror sounds is to make a gradual approach. (2) The student substitutes his new sound for other sounds, but not for the error. Thus: "Sammy sssaught a fish with his hook and line." (3) The student substitutes another sound for the *s* in the same material. Thus: "Bammy caught a fish with his hook and line." (4) The student omits the *s* in all words beginning with it. Thus: "—ammy caught a fish with his hook and line." (5) The student "substitutes" his new sound for the *s*. Thus: "Ssssammy caught a fish with his hook and line." Many similar techniques are easily invented. It may seem to the young speech therapist that such techniques are far too laborious and detailed. But, after he has met with persistent error in his articulatory cases, he will appreciate the fact that careful and thorough training will produce a thoroughgoing and permanent freedom from error. Sketchy and slipshod training will enable a speech defective to make the correct sound and perhaps to use it in a few words when he watches himself carefully, but this is far from the goal that should be set. Too many speech therapists have blamed the student for failure when they should have blamed themselves.

Another group of reconfiguration techniques requires the use of writing or drawing simultaneously with the utterance. For children who can read and write, these techniques are often very useful.

Simultaneous Talking-and-Writing. The simultaneous talking-and-writing techniques previously described will be invaluable if used properly. The student should talk-and-write the symbol alone for one line, and then, on the next line, talk-and-write the first letter, the first syllable, and, finally, the whole word. Thus: *s s s s s s s s s s; s si sick s si sick*, and so on. Later he can alternate the symbol and the word, and finally he can write only the symbol as he says the word. Assignments can be given for home practice. Frequently such a gradual approach is not necessary, and the student need write only the symbol and say any *s* word.

We also ask our cases to draw on paper or trace in the air various figures. The case is trained to associate certain sounds with certain parts of the figures and then to trace continuously through the whole figure, thus producing a word.

Signaling Techniques. This group of activities uses preparatory sets to integrate the sound or syllable into the words. Signaling can generate many key words. In this, the student prolongs or repeats the new sound and then, at a given signal, instantly says the prearranged vowel or the rest of the word. The student should be given a preparatory set to pronounce the rest of the word by preliminary signal practice. During this practice he waits with his eyes closed until he hears the sound signal which sets off the response. Thus, during the student's prolongation of *sssssss*, the instructor suddenly raps on the table, and the syllable *oup* is automatically produced. With a preparatory set, the response is largely automatic and involuntary, and thus the new sound is integrated within the word as a whole. Often it is wise to require the student to say the word twice. Thus:

sssssss(rap)*oupsoup*. Signal practice can also be used with repetition. Thus: *kuh-kuh-*(rap)*atkat*. After some training with this type of signal practice, the student may use other signals, such as those provided by the timing of a rhythm. Thus: *s-s, s-s-soup* or *s-s-soup, s-s-soup*. The student may also be required to repeat over and over some nonsense syllable which he can make well, suddenly saying the new word when the signal is given. Thus: *ssi-ssi-ssi-ssi*(tap)*ssip*. The nonsense syllable and the new word may also be used alternately. The isolated sound may be used in the above exercise in place of the nonsense syllable. Various other combinations may easily be invented.

Difficulties in Forming Key Words from Isolated Sounds or Syllables. At times difficulty will be experienced in making the transitions into the words. The student will say *rwabbit* and be confident that he has pronounced the word correctly. The error must be brought to his attention by the therapist's imitation and by the student's voluntary production of the error. Signal practice will help a great deal to eliminate this error.

Another invaluable technique is provided by a signal used in a slightly different way. The student is asked to form his mouth for the vowel which begins the rest of the word; i.e., for the vowel *a* in *rabbit*. He may whisper a prolongation of this vowel. Then, at a given signal, he is to say *rabbit* as swiftly as possible. This preformation of the vowel will often solve the problem. Similarly, the practice of pairs of words, the first ending in the vowel of the second, will be effective. Using pairs of words in which the first word ends with the new sound and the second begins with the same sound is occasionally useful, although the student should be cautioned to keep out all breaks in continuity.

Still another method of eliminating this error is to use some nonsense symbol to represent the part of the word which follows the new sound. Thus, one individual was asked to say *oup* every time he wrote a question mark (?), and after ten minutes of this, he was told to read the following symbols, *t?, kr?,* and *s?*. The last symbol was pronounced *soup* rather than *sthoup,* and no further difficulty was experienced.

Creating Key Words Directly. When we decide to forego the isolated-sound or syllable approaches and to begin immediately by teaching key words, we use the same basic methods described for the other approaches. We must make sure through ear training that the person comes to realize how the *word* sounds when uttered by the therapist. He must also be made to *scan* his own utterance of the word and to *compare* it with that of the therapist. Finally he must be taught to *vary* his attempts until the correct word is uttered. All the methods used for teaching the isolated sound or syllable can be used also for the word as a whole. Here is an excerpt from an ear-training session in which the therapist is operating at the word level:

The child and therapist are seated at a table. There are a number of little plastic objects on the table and two glass jars, one full of water and one empty.

Child: Put the kitty in the water. (*Therapist does so.*)
Child: Put the baby in the water.
Therapist: OK. Baby have bath.
Child: No, baby drown. All dead.
Therapist: OK. Baby dead now.
Child: Take baby out the water. (*Therapist does so.*)
Child: Baby OK now. You thpank baby bottom. Baby naughty.
Therapist: If you ask me to ssspank her I will, but you didn't. You asked me to thpank her. What's that? (*She holds baby up high.*)
Child (reaching): Thpank her! Thpank her! Thpank her! (*Slaps hand hard on table.*)
Therapist: Thpank her? . . . Oh, you mean . . . sspank her? (*Child nods*). OK. Here goes. (*Therapist spanks baby.*)

Now let us see how we would continue, but using the word level for the therapeutic process of establishing the standard pattern for two key words.

Therapist: No, that's no penthil.
Child: It ith too a penthil.
Therapist: Nope, you said it wrong. You said "penthil" . . . th . . . penth . . . penthil. That's not the same as sss, pensss, pencil. Look, here's a penthil. (*Therapist takes out of the desk a pipe cleaner with two knots and a bolt on it.*) OK, this is your "penthil." Look, it sssinks. The pencil swims.
Child: Oh.
Therapist: Shut your eyes again. I'm going to put the penthil (listen now, I said *penthil*, not *pencil*) I'm going to put the penthil in the water. Can you tell me if it swims?
Child: No. It thinks.
Therapist: You're right. It isn't swimming. But you didn't say *sssssssinks* right. It's *sss, sssih, sssinksss*, not *thinks*, but *sssinkss*. You can't peek until you can guess whether I'm saying it right or wrong. OK. Here we go: Which is right, the first or second: The *penthil thinks*, or the *penthil sinks*.
Child: The penthil *sssssssinks*. . . .
Therapist: And the pencil . . .
Child: Sssssswims.

Not all children make such rapid progress.

We have already indicated in our play-by-play description of this interchange between therapist and child that it is possible to use several operational levels in the same activity. In these stimulation, identification, and discrimination activities, the focus of therapy has been at one time on the sentence, at another on the word, on the syllable, and even on the isolated sound. Sometimes, as our illustration suggests, the child needs little help in producing the correct sound or in incorporating it into words, sentences, and functional speech. A child who gets the words *pencil, swim,* and *sink* in this five-minute period can be taught to use them immediately in commentary, communication, and control, and he should be given opportunity to do so in the interests of stabilization. Here is how it was done in the situation described above.

> *Therapist:* OK. I'll close my eyes, and see if I can guess which one you'll pick up and play with.
> *Child:* I'll pick one up.
> *Therapist:* I bet it's a penthil.
> *Child:* No, it a pensssssil.
> *Therapist:* Is it the yellow one?
> *Child:* Yeth.
> *Therapist:* What are you going to do with it?
> *Child:* I going put it in water.
> *Therapist:* What's it doing now?
> *Child:* It thwims.
> *Therapist:* Thwims? What's that?
> *Child:* It sssssssswims. You want to look?
> *Therapist:* Good for you. That's right. It's the pencil, not the penthil and it's swimming all right. Now you be the teacher and boss me around with the pencil and the penthil. Tell me what to do.
> *Child:* Put penthil in mouth. (*Therapist does so with pipe cleaner.*)
> *Child:* Put pencil in water. (*Therapist does so.*)
> *Child:* Give penthil a bath. (*Therapist puts pipe cleaner in water.*)
> *Therapist:* Which one do you think will get dry the faster?
> *Child:* The pencil.
> *Therapist:* How many penthils have I in my desk drawer here? (*Child looks.*)
> *Child:* FF . . . no, no. You got none. But four pensssils. I almost forgot. SSS. Pencil!
> *Therapist:* Finish this sentence: I can write with a . . .
> *Child:* Write with a pencil.
> *Therapist:* The only one that sinks is the . . .
> *Child:* It's the penthil.
> *Therapist:* The penthil is heavier than the . . .
> *Child:* Pencil.

ARTICULATION THERAPY AT THE SENTENCE LEVEL

Once we have taught our case a group of key words which contain the new sound in the initial, medial, and final positions, and he can now correct

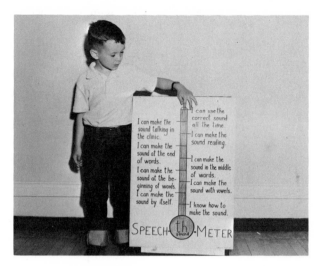

FIGURE 25: *Checking Progress*

his misarticulations when he is being careful, we move on to the next operational level: the sentence. Again, we find here some new techniques, but before we describe them, let us tell how sometimes we begin our therapy, not at the sound, syllable, or word levels, but immediately at the sentence level.

Beginning at the Sentence Level. When we *begin* therapy at the sentence level we do so primarily to provide motivation and hope for those who have never felt they could talk normally. Usually, this sentence level therapy is carried out only after the child has mastered the new sound in isolation, nonsense syllables, and key words. However, careful exploration sometimes reveals not only key words but key sentences, or rather key utterances, in which the usually defective sound is always spoken correctly. A child with whom we worked recently and who could not make a *th* sound in isolation, syllable, or word, was able immediately to say "shut *the* door!" as a command. He could not say the word "the" or the sound of *th* or the nonsense syllable *shuthoo*. We found that by using other commands of a similar nature, "Shut the window," "Shut that box," in slow motion and echoed speech, we could procure a nucleus of correct utterance from which we could isolate the words, sounds, and syllables and still have them articulated correctly. Most speech therapists, if they *begin* treatment at the sentence level, do so for two reasons: to convince the child immediately that the correct production of the target sound is not as difficult as he had believed, and secondly, to help him analyze the correctly spoken sentences to locate the target sounds, syllables, or words which he must use in the rest of his speech.

Thus with the lisper who can say "Oh, you're nuts!" perfectly, we want him to scrutinize this sentence level expression of emotion to know that the final *s* sound of the last word was said as well as any other person on earth could say it; that he has said the syllable *uts* and the word *nuts* perfectly, and most important of all, that the whole insulting utterance was spoken without error. We pair these key sentences with other sentences in which errors exist and ask the case to scan them when we say them right or when we say them wrong, and to scan them again when he speaks them. Thus we locate the error and target the correct standard pattern.

Creating Key Sentences. As we have said, some of these correctly spoken sentences can be discovered by careful exploration and deep testing. It is also possible to create them, not only synthetically by incorporating sounds into syllables, syllables into words, and words into key sentences, but as sentence wholes. We have several techniques for doing this: slow-motion speech, echo speech or shadowing, unison speaking, cumulative speaking, and the corrective set. Each of these attempts to teach sentences as wholes.

Slow Motion Speech. In this technique the therapist and child say the error sentences in unison, but in extreme slow motion. For example: "Iiiiiz-thththththe-pennnnnnsssssillll-wwwet?" The therapist should precede this with other slow-motion behavior such as walking, arm-lifting, head-scratching. She sets the tempo and the child follows her slowly shifting model. Often it is important that the therapist sit behind the child with her mouth slightly above his head so as to make the two sound fields similar, and so, by putting her mouth close to the child's ear for the difficult sounds or words, he can be stimulated more vividly.

Echo Speech. There are two forms of this. In the first, *shadowing*, the child tries to repeat instantly and automatically what the therapist is saying, word by word. The child's utterance should follow immediately on the heels of the therapist. For example:

Therapist: Let's play an echo game today. Try to say what I say just as soon as I say it. Don't wait. Say each word just as soon as it comes out of my mouth. Ready?
Child: OK.
Therapist: One.
Child: One.
Therapist: Two . . . seven . . .
Child: . . . Two . . . seven . . .
Therapist: Quicker, say it quicker.
Child: Quicker . . . Oh, I thee. You mean right away.
Therapist: Yes.

Child: Yes.
Therapist: I'm . . . going . . . to show . . . you . . . a picture.
Child: . . . I'm . . . going . . . to show . . . you . . . a picture.
Therapist: Good!
Child: Good!
Therapist: The dog is chasing . . . the cat.
Child: . . . The dog is chasing . . . the cat.
Therapist: Good! You said chasing, not chathing.
Child: Good! You said chasing, not chathing.

This shadowing, or echo speech, seems to be more easily learned by children than adults, and it is curious to find how faithfully they can do it. Once he has learned how to shadow automatically (almost as in echolalia), the child's voice follows not only the words but also the inflections with surprising fidelity.

In the second form of echo-speaking, which they have called "long-echo talk," the child repeats not single words, but a *series* of words or phrases or sentences after the therapist when she pauses and signals for him to catch up and give back the echo. This should be done with a gestural or postural or behavioral accompaniment which the child must also duplicate as closely as possible. For example:

Therapist: All right, now we're going to play follow the leader, and I'll be the leader this time. You do what I do and say what I say, but wait till I stop before following me. Do and say just exactly what I do and say. If I sing, you sing. If I stand up while talking, that's what you have to do. If I scratch my nose, you've got to do so too. Ready?
Child: OK.
Therapist: (*begins to shiver*): On a coooold winter night . . . (*signals*)
Child (*shivering*): On a cooooold winter night . . .
Therapist: a little boy (*therapist huddles in a crouch and signals*)
Child (*squats*): a little boy . . .
Therapist (*puts hands over face*): had a bad dream. . . .
Child (*covering face*): had a bad deem. . . .
Therapist: He thought he was out in the sssssssssssssssssnow. (*Therapist claps hands on each word of this except for* snow. *On the prolonged* s *she pretends to pull a string of sound out from between her closed teeth and winds it around her ear.*)
Child (*does the same action*): He thought he was out in the sssssssnow.
Therapist (*sings*): And he sssssssaid, "I'm cooooooooooooooold as aissssssssssss." (*ice*)
Child (*sings*): And he sssaid, "I'm coooold as ice."
Therapist (*laughs*): He didn't have any covers on his bed.
Child (*laughs*): An' he waked up.

In both types of echo speech it is important that the child try to follow the therapist as automatically as possible. Children who have never produced standard sounds or who cannot do so under direct stimulation in their speech are able to make them easily when doing this automatic kind of echo-speaking. We also teach them to echo themselves.

Unison Speech. In this the child and therapist speak some previously formulated utterances together. It is important that again the child follow the therapist's movements, speech tempo, pitch, and intensity patterns. For this purpose, each utterance is spoken several times. Often the therapist cups her hands and directs her voice into one of the child's ears, while the child listens with the other ear to his mouth with cupped hands, a speech shoe, or auditory training unit. This binaural listening permits a simultaneous comparison of correct and incorrect forms. Hand-tapping signals are used to time the moment of attempt and to insure unison speaking. Often, as the same utterance is spoken each time, it is wise to have the child accompany it with a certain head or body movement so that it can be stabilized thereby when the child must speak it alone. We also taperecord some of the child's own speech which is spoken without error and ask him to say it again in unison with himself. Here is an example of such unison speech, this time based upon self-expression or egocentric speech. (You will have to remember that the child's utterance will be spoken in unison with that of the therapist.)

> *Therapist*: Now we're going to play a game in which we can grow up and be awfully big. You've got to say what I say at the same time I say it. And do what I do. We'll do and say everything at least twice, before we change. Ready?
>
> *Child*: Uh-huh.
>
> *Therapist (puts her head down by her knees)*: Oh, I'm ssso ssssmall. (*Then whispers*) OK, when I touch you, say it with me, just like I do.
>
> *Child*: OK.
>
> *Therapist (in a tiny voice)*: I'm sssso ssssmall. (*Touches child.*)
>
> *Child (very softly)*: I'm so ssmall.
>
> *Therapist*: I'm so small, so ssmall.
>
> *Child*: I'm so ssmall, so small.
>
> *Therapist (rising up and stretching out arms)*: I'm getting bigger. I'm getting bigger. (*She speaks in a low voice.*)
>
> *Child (duplicates behavior)*: I'm getting bigger, bigger too.
>
> *Therapist (climbs up on chair and shouts)*: I'm the king of the cassstle! I'm the king of the castle.
>
> *Child (climbs up on his chair and yells)*: I'm the king of the cassstle!
>
> *Therapist*: No, *I'm* the king of the castle; *I'm* the king of the castle!
>
> *Child (in unison)*: I'm the king of the castle.

Therapist: And you're a dirty rassscal; and you're a dirty rascal; and you're a dirty . . .

Child (*chiming in*): . . . rascal; and you're a dirty rassscal.

In this illustration, the first two sentences had previously been practiced in unison with the therapist, using a binaural auditory training unit. However, if error had occurred in the acting out, the sentences could have been then worked upon as unit utterances until they were spoken in standard fashion.

Cumulative Sentences. In this technique, the therapist has an opportunity to work on the sound or syllable or word within the sentence without losing the sentence wholeness or gestalt. Essentially, it consists of having the child and therapist, working in unison or alternately in echo speech, build sentences and utterances word by word cumulatively. An example follows which is based on emotional expression.

Therapist: See these blocks. We're going to block-talk. I bet you never heard of that game, did you? Well, you and I must pile one block on top of another and say something at the same time until it all falls down. I'll show you. We're going to talk about things we don't like.

Child: OK.

Therapist: You see, you have to say one word for each block, and start over again with each new block. OK. I'll start with I (*puts out a block*) . . . I don't (*puts another block on first one*) . . . I don't like . . . (*piles on third block*) . . . I don't like . . .

Child: Baby thiththerth. I don't like baby thiththerth.

Therapist: You mean baby sssssssisterssss. OK, now you do it with me, and say it with me every time we put on a new block. You put on the blocks.

Both: I . . . (*one block*)

Both: I don't . . . (*two blocks*)

Both: I don't like . . . (*three blocks*)

Therapist: Now, let's just say "baby" this time.

Both: Baby . . . (*fourth block wobbles*) I don't like baby . . .

Therapist: Now remember, it's I don't like baby sssisssterssss, not I don't like baby thiththerth. (*Therapist says it very loudly in the child's left ear as they speak in unison.*)

Both: I don't like baby sisters. (*Fifth block teeters but holds precariously.*)

Therapist: Now let's say, "I don't like baby sisters very much."

Child: I don't like baby sssisters at all. (*Blocks come tumbling down as he smashes them.*)

The Corrective Set. We have also found that often a child with an articulation problem can be able to produce his usually defective sound correctly in a whole sentence when he is given a corrective set. The way we usually do this is by saying or doing many things in which our error is obvious and asking the child to correct us and to set us straight. We begin with mistakes which are so apparent that any person would be likely to recognize them. Once the child is thoroughly enjoying our stupidity and mistakes, we slip in some utterance containing his own common errors. Over and over again we have been surprised to find how easily he can show us how to say the sentence without error. Here is an example:

> *The teacher and child are seated at a table. The child lisps and has other defective sounds. The teacher has a bag with various articles in it.*
>
> *Therapist:* I'm going to say and do some things all wrong, and I want you to show me and tell me how to do or say them right. Understand?
> *Child:* Uh huh.
> *Therapist:* See, here's a comb. I brush my teeth with a comb. (*Pretends to do so.*)
> *Child (laughing):* No, No. You comb you heh.
> *Therapist:* Show me. (*Child does so.*) Oh, I see, I comb my hair. (*Reaches into bag and pulls out a plastic spoon.*) See, here's a thpoon.
> *Child:* Yeth.
> *Therapist:* Oh ho! I fooled you that time. I said something wrong and you didn't catch me. I said *thpoon,* not ssspoon. OK. Watch me fool you again.
> *Child:* No, you can't.
> *Therapist (points to her mouth):* I open my mouf.
> *Child (scornfully):* You open your mouth, MOUTH! not mouf.
> *Therapist (pretends to cry):* OK, you caught me that time. Oh look, here's a picture of a horth. See the big horth.
> *Child:* No, no. Horsssssssssss! Not horth. Horssssssssey, and it is a little horse, not a big one.

Role-playing. A most curious discovery to many speech therapists is that some children, when completely immersed in some other person's role, can speak almost perfectly the same sentences that they cannot possibly say without error in any other situation. We use fantasy, children's theater, and creative dramatics to establish these roles and much suggestion and coaching to make them vivid enough so that the child can throw himself completely into them. Identification must be very thorough. Here is a short illustration:

> *Therapist:* All right, let's play bank robbers. Who am I?
> *Child:* You the man at the bank. Thit there at the table with the money.

Therapist: Where's the money?

Child: Here! (*Tears up some paper and gives it to the therapist.*) I'm going out and come in with gun.

Therapist: Don't shoot me when you come in.

Child: Oh hoh. I'll thcare you. You be thcared now when I come in.

Therapist: OK.

Child (*goes out, then enters with handkerchief over mouth and pencil in hand. Points it at therapist who pretends to be afraid*): Stick em up!

Therapist (*lifts two fingers*): Like this?

Child (*returning to his own role*): Naw. Look, when I thay "Stick em up" you've got to thtick em up like thith. (*Demonstrates.*)

Therapist: Oh I understand. Let's start again.

Child: Stick em up now!

Scanning, Comparing, Correcting at the Sentence Level.   It is one thing to acquire the ability to use a new sound correctly in isolation, syllable, word, or sentence; it is another to be able to use it habitually and automatically. A person who has thought, commanded, sent messages, expressed himself in lisping speech for years needs special help in making the new unlisped speech habitual. Somehow we must build in this person a control system which will continuously scan the utterance and notice and correct the errors automatically. No one can continually listen to the output of sound from his mouth. We need our ears to hear our thoughts and the thoughts of others. How can we automatize this corrective process? We have three main methods for doing so: (1) enlarging the therapy situation, (2) using the new sound in all types of speaking, (3) emphasizing proprioceptive feedback.

Enlarging the Therapy Situation.   First of all, we must expand the therapy room to include the person's whole living space. He must be given experiences in scanning, comparing, and correcting in school, on the playground, on the job, and at home. Here are some of the ways we do this:

Speech Assignments.   Some typical speech assignments to illustrate methods for getting the child to work on his errors in outside situations are:

> (1) Go downstairs and ask the janitor for a dust rag. Be sure to say *rag* with a good long *rrr*. (2) Say the word *rabbit* to three other children without letting them know that you are working on your speech. (3) Ask your father if you said any word wrongly after you tell him what you did in school today.

The teacher should always make these assignments very definite and appropriate to the child's ability and environment. He should always ask for a report the next day. Such assignments frequently are the solution to any lack of motivation the child may have.

Checking Devices and Penalties.   Checking devices and penalties are of great value when properly used. Typical checking devices are:

(1) Having child carry card and crayon during geography recitation, making a mark or writing the word whenever he makes an error. (2) Having some other child check errors in a similar fashion. (3) Having child transfer marbles from one pocket to another, one for each error. Many other devices may be invented, and they will bring the error to consciousness very rapidly.

Similarly, penalties are of great service when used properly. It should be realized, however, that painful and highly emotional penalties should not be used, for they merely make the bad habit more pronounced and cause the child to hate his speech work. Penalties used in speech correction should be vivid and good natured. Typical penalties used with a ten-year-old lisper were: put pencil behind ear; step in wastebasket; pound pan; look between legs; close one eye; say *whoopee*. Let the child set his own penalties before he makes the speech attempt.

Nucleus Situations.   Many parents and teachers make the mistake of correcting the child whenever he makes speech errors. It is unwise to set the speech standards too high. No one can watch himself all the time, and we all hate to be nagged. As a matter of fact, too much vigilance by the speech defective can produce such speech inhibitions that the speech work becomes thoroughly distasteful. Fluency disappears, and the speech becomes very halting and unpleasant. Then, too, the very anxiety lest error occur, when carried to the extreme, increases the number of slips and mistakes themselves. Other errors sometimes appear.

Therefore, we recommend that the parents and teachers of the speech defective concentrate their reminding and correcting upon a few common words and upon certain nuclei speech situations. Use a certain chair as a good-speech chair. Whenever the child sits in it, he must watch himself. Have a certain person picked out who is to serve in the speech situation where the child must use very careful speech. Use a certain speech situation, such as the dinner table, to serve as a nucleus of good speech, and when errors occur in these nuclei situations, penalize them good naturedly but emphatically. You will find that the speech vigilance and freedom from errors will spread rapidly to all other situations.

Finally, we recommend that after a child has mastered a new sound and several words in which it occurs, he be required to say it occasionally in the wrong way. This is called negative practice, and it has no harmful effect. Indeed, it merely emphasizes the distinction between the correct and incorrect sounds.

Negative Practice.   By negative practice we mean the deliberate and voluntary use of the incorrect sound or speech error. It may seem some-what odd to advise speech defectives to practice their errors, for we have always assumed that practice makes perfect, and certainly we do not want the student to become more perfect in the use of his errors. Nevertheless, modern experimental psychology had demonstrated that when one seeks to break a habit that is rather unconscious (such as fingernail-biting or the substitution of *sh* for *s*), much more rapid progress is made if the possessor of the habit will occasionally (and at appropriate times) use the error deliberately. The reasons for this method are: (1) the greatest strength of such a habit lies in the fact that the possessor is not aware of it every time it occurs. All habit reactions tend to become more or less unconscious, and certainly those involved in speech are of this type; consciousness of the reaction must come before it can be eliminated. (2) Voluntary practice of the reaction makes it very vivid, thus increasing vigilance and contribut-ing to the awareness of the cues that signal the approach of the reaction. (3) The voluntary practice of the error acts as a penalty.

The use of negative practice is so varied that it would be impossible to describe all the applications which can be made of it. Variations must be made to fit each type of disorder and each individual case. There are, however, certain general principles which may be said to govern all dis-orders and cases. Make the individual aware of the reasons for his use of the incorrect sound, for unintelligent use of the error is worthless. Never ask the student to use the error until he can produce the correct sound whenever asked to do so. Negative practice is a technique for getting the correct sound into the student's speech; it is used to make the correct sound habitual.

Set up the exact reproduction of the incorrect sound as a goal. The use of mirror observation, teacher imitation, and phonograph recording is invaluable. This is a learning process and does not come all at once. The therapist should confine all negative practice to the speech lesson until the student is able to duplicate the error consistently and fairly accurately. One should begin the use of this technique by asking the student to dupli-cate the error immediately after it has occurred—that is to say, the student should stop immediately after lisping on the word *soup* and attempt volun-tarily to duplicate his performance.

Work constantly to make the negative practice serve the purpose of comparing the right and wrong sounds. It is often well to provide lists of words for the students to work with, speaking each of them in this se-quence: correctly, incorrectly, correctly, correctly. Work first on individual sounds, then on words, then on certain words in sentences containing two words which begin with the difficult sound, one of which is to be said correctly and the other incorrectly. Have the student read material in which certain words are underlined for negative practice.

Make speech assignments for the student's use in outside situations. Examples are:

(1) Collect (write down on cards) ten words on which you have used negative practice. (2) Write down on a card two words on which you have used negative practice during each hour of the morning. (3) Write the first sentences of five phone calls, underlining the words on which you are going to use negative practice. (4) Collect, during the day, twenty words which you have said wrongly and in which you have become aware of your error, have made a retrial and said them correctly, and then have made a second retrial using negative practice.

The preceding list of examples merely indicates the type of assignments that may be used. It is vitally important that no assignment be made that does not call for an objective record of some kind. The teacher must ask for the card and discuss the fulfillment or nonfulfillment of the assignment. Assignment plus checkup will work wonders in the treatment of any speech defective. Vary the assignments to fit the case, and always make them purposeful, never a matter of routine or drill.

In concluding this section on articulatory disorders we wish to point out that in very few instances will it be necessary to spend more than five or ten minutes of individual work each day on any speech defective. Most of the work can be carried on in connection with the regular school activities, and so it should be if the new habits are to be made permanent. Any teacher can see the possibilities for combining speech work with the language activities. In the names of the numbers themselves, arithmetic presents almost all of the speech sounds. Geography and science activities may be arranged so as to give the lisper recitations in which he is responsible for all new *s* words. Questions may be phrased so as to demand responses that involve the sound in which error occurs. The teacher and student may have a secret signal for correction. The student should check all errors in a notebook. At times it is wise to post on the board a list of five words with which the student has trouble unless he watches himself. Occasionally, some other student may be asked to check on the speech defective's errors. Class recitations should be used not for teaching a new sound, but for building up the strength of the new sound after the student can make it correctly.

Using the New Sound in All the Various Types of Speaking. In stabilizing and automatizing the new sound, we find it wise to provide systematic training which incorporates the new sound into real live message-sending, social control, thinking, emotional, and self-expressive types of speaking. Again we must make deliberate nucleic implants of good speech in all these various functions. First in the therapy room, and then in all the person's living space, we must make sure that our case can use his new standard sounds in all the *kinds* of talking he must do. When the lisper commands his dog, he must say "Sit down!" When he responds affirmatively to a question he must say "Yes!" When he must mentally add four and three, he must think "seven," not "theven." In expressing his fear, he must say "I'm scared" not "thcared." He must be able to use good sibilants in his speech of self-display. Until certain correctly spoken sentences are used automatically in each of these forms of speaking, we cannot feel our task as a therapist is over.

Emphasizing Proprioceptive Feedback. Proprioceptive feedback is a term which refers to the perception of contacts and movements and postures. If we place a finger on our lower lip, the felt contact is proprioceptive; if we cock our head to the left or move a foot, the sensations of posture and movement are proprioceptive. We know what has happened without seeing or hearing. In much the same way, we can know what is happening in our own speech even when we cannot hear ourselves speaking. It is quite possible to talk correctly in a boiler factory. We do not need self-hearing if our proprioceptive senses are operating well.

We believe that once a person has left babyhood, the most important automatic controls for monitoring articulation are proprioceptive. These controls see to it that we use the right movements, the right postures, the correct contacts. We feel that when the baby first learns to talk, self-hearing is most important. That is why he babbles so much and does so much vocal play. But after he begins to use language and to understand the meanings of others, self-hearing is given a less important role. Proprioceptive thus becomes much more important, so important, indeed, that obvious errors can persist for years without the person recognizing them auditorally. In articulation therapy, we must first reopen the self-hearing circuits and put more energy into them so that these errors can be distinguished. But we must not stop here. We must return to proprioceptive controls if the child is to use the new sound automatically. No one can listen to himself constantly. The burden is too great. Too many other functions interfere.

Accordingly, in terminal therapy with the articulation case, we teach him to use the new sound correctly by feel and touch alone. We put masking noise in his ears so he cannot rely on self-hearing. We ask him to speak correctly with his ears plugged. We ask him to speak in a soft whisper and in pantomime. All these activities decrease the monitoring of speech by self-hearing and emphasize its proprioceptive control. We have found these techniques invaluable in automatizing the new sound.

REFERENCES

Articles

1. Altshuler, A. W. "A Therapeutic Oral Device for Lateral Emission." *Journal of Speech and Hearing Disorders*, XXIV (1961), 179–82.
    Describe the appliance and how it was used.
2. Aungst, L. F. and Frick, J. V. "Auditory Discrimination Ability and Consistency of Articulation of [r]." *Journal of Speech and Hearing Disorders*, XXIX (1964), 76–85.
    What are the implications of this research for articulation therapy?
3. Black, M. and Ludwig, R. A. S. "Analysis of the Games Technic." *Journal of Speech and Hearing Disorders*, XXI (1956), 183–87.
    Compare this presentation with the criticism in Mowrer, D. E. "An Analysis of Motivational Techniques Used in Speech Therapy." *ASHA*, XII (1970), 491–93.
4. Curtis, J. F. and Hardy, J. C. "A Phonetic Study of Misarticulation of the [r]." *Journal of Speech and Hearing Research*, II (1959), 244–57.
5. Engel, D. C., Brandreit, S. E., Erickson, K. M., Gronhovd, K–D, and Gunderson, G. D. "Carry-Over." *Journal of Speech and Hearing Disorders*, XXXI (1966), 227–33.
    Why is it sometimes hard to transfer the gains made in the speech clinic to outside situations, and how can this be facilitated?
6. Goda, S. "Spontaneous Speech. A Primary Source of Therapy Material." *Journal of Speech and Hearing Disorders*, XXVII (1962), 190–92.
    Find a quotation in the present chapter which illustrates Goda's point of view.
7. Hahn, E. "Communication in the Therapy Session." *Journal of Speech and Hearing Disorders*, XXV (1960), 19–23.
    What material in the present chapter reflects Hahn's beliefs?
8. ———. "Indications for Direct, Nondirect, and Indirect Methods in Speech Correction." *Journal of Speech and Hearing Disorders*, XXVI (1961), 230–36.
    Describe the indirect methods for helping children with speech disorders.
9. Hawk, S. S. "Motokinesthetic Training for Children with Speech Handicaps." *Journal of Speech Disorders*, VII (1942), 357–60.
    Describe the motokinesthetic method.
10. Jenkins, E. and Lohr, F. E. "Severe Articulation Disorders and Motor Ability." *Journal of Speech and Hearing Disorders*, XXIX (1964), 286–91.
    What evidence indicates that persons with severe articulation disorders are poorer in motor coordination?
11. Johnson, W., Brown, S. F., Curtis, J. F., Edney, C. W. and Keaster, J. *Speech Handicapped School Children.* 3d ed. New York: Harper & Row, Publisher, 1967.
    What differences are there in the discussion of the causes of articulatory disorders in this book (pp. 120–35) with that of the present text?
12. Larr, A. L. *Tongue Thrust and Speech Correction.* San Francisco: Fearon, 1962.

How does tongue-thrusting tend to produce articulatory defects, and how can it be treated?

13. Low, G., Crerar, M., and Lassers, L. "Communication-Centered Speech Therapy." *Journal of Speech and Hearing Disorders,* XXIV (1959), 361–69.
    How can the therapist structure articulation therapy so that it involves live communication?

14. Marquardt, E. "Carry-over with 'Speech Pals.' " *Journal of Speech and Hearing Disorders,* XXIV (1959), 154–56.
    How did this clinician manage the transfer?

15. Massengill, R., Maxwell, S., and Rickrell, K. "An Analysis of Articulation Following Partial and Total Glossectomy." *Journal of Speech and Hearing Disorders,* XXXV (1970), 170–73.
    What happens to speech when a person loses all or a part of his tongue, and what can be done?

16. Milisen, R. "A Rationale for Articulation Disorders." *Journal of Speech and Hearing Disorders,* Monograph Supplement, IV (1954), 6–17.
    What are Milisen's beliefs about how articulation therapy should be organized?

17. Mims, H. A., Kolas, C. and Williams, R. "Lisping and Persistent Thumbsucking Among Children with Open-bite Malocclusions." *Journal of Speech and Hearing Disorders,* XXXI (1966), 176–77.
    What are the findings of this research?

18. Morley, M. E. and Fox, J. "Disorders of Articulation: Theory and Therapy." *British Journal of Disorders of Communication,* IV (1969), 151–65.
    What differences are there in the approach presented by these authors and that of this text?

19. Mowrer, D. E., Baker, R. L., and Schultz, R. E. "Operant Procedures in the Control of Speech Articulation." In Sloane, H. N. and Macaulay, B. B., eds., *Operant Procedures in Remedial Speech and Language Training.* Boston: Houghton Mifflin Company, 1968. Pp. 296–321.
    How did the authors apply operant conditioning methods to eliminate a lisp?

20. Pendergast, K., Soder, A., Barker, J., Dickey, S., Gow, J., and Selmar, J. "An Articulation Study of 15,255 Seattle First-Grade Children With and Without Kindergarten." *Exceptional Children,* XXXII (1966), 541–47.
    What were the findings of this research?

21. Prins, D. U. "Relations Among Specific Articulatory Deviations and Responses to a Clinical Measure of Sound Discrimination Ability." *Journal of Speech and Hearing Disorders,* XXVIII (1963), 382–87.
    What are the implications of this research for the treatment of articulation errors?

22. Renfrew, C. E. "Persistence of the Open Syllable in Defective Articulation." *Journal of Speech and Hearing Disorders,* XXXI (1966), 370–73.
    Children with this sort of articulation errors do not respond to the usual kind of therapy. How should they be treated?

23. Slipakoff, E. L. "An Approach to the Correction of the Defective [r]." *Journal of Speech and Hearing Disorders,* XXXII (1967), 71–75.
    What is the essence of this clinician's method for teaching this sound?

24. Snow, K. "Articulation Proficiency in Relation to Certain Dental Abnor-

malities." *Journal of Speech and Hearing Disorders,* XXVI (1961), 209–212.
What were the author's findings?

25. Sommers, R. K. "Factors in the Effectiveness of Mothers Trained to Aid in Speech Correction." *Journal of Speech and Hearing Disorders,* XXVII (1962), 178–86.
What were these factors?

26. Spriestersbach, D. C. and Curtis, J. R. "Misarticulation and Discrimination of Speech Sounds." *Quarterly Journal of Speech,* XXXVII (1951), 483–91.
What is the relationship between discrimination of articulation errors and their production?

27. Templin, M. C. and Darley, F. L. *The Templin–Darley Tests of Articulation.* Iowa City, Iowa: Bureau of Educational Research, 1960.
Describe this test.

28. Van Riper, C. "Binaural Speech Therapy." *Journal of Speech and Hearing Disorders,* XXIV (1959), 62–63.
Why is it lucky that our articulation cases have two ears?

29. Van Riper, C. and Erickson, R. A. "A Predictive Screening Test of Articulation." *Journal of Speech and Hearing Disorders,* XXXIV (1969), 214–19.
Describe the test and its uses.

30. Webb, C. E. and Siegenthaler, B. M. "Comparison of Aural Stimulation Methods for Teaching Speech Sounds." *Journal of Speech and Hearing Disorders,* XXII (1957), 264–70.
Which methods were most effective?

31. Winitz, H. and Lawrence, M. "Childrens' Articulation and Sound Learnin Ability." *Journal of Speech and Hearing Research,* IV (1961), 259–68.
Summarize their findings.

32. Young, E. H. "The Motokinesthetic Approach to the Prevention of Speech Defects Including Stuttering." *Journal of Speech and Hearing Disorders,* XXX (1965), 269–73.
Describe the motokinesthetic method and its applications.

Texts

33. Carrell, J. A. *Disorders of Articulation.* Englewood Cliffs, N.J.: Prentice-Hall, Inc., 1968.
This book provides basic information on the nature of articulation and misarticulation and on the structural, functional, and neurological causes of articulatory disorder. Treatment is subordinated to understanding.

34. McDonald, E. T. *Articulation Testing and Treatment: A Sensory Motor Approach.* Pittsburgh: Stanwix House, 1964.
The author's methods for deep testing are presented, along with his view that since speech consists of overlapping movements, it would be preferable to use the syllabic approach.

35. Nemoy, E. M. and Davis S. *The Correction of Defective Consonant Sounds.* Magnolia, Mass.: Expression Co., 1954.
Presents the common errors of articulation with suggestions for their elimination.

36. Van Riper, C. and Irwin, J. V. *Voice and Articulation*. Englewood Cliffs, N.J.: Prentice-Hall, Inc., 1958.
The first six chapters of this book present the causes of defective articulation, methods of testing, symptomatology, and a model for therapy based upon cybernetic feedback theory.

37. Winitz, H. *Articulatory Acquisition and Behavior*, New York: Meredith, 1969.
This text reviews all the significant research on the development of articulation and misarticulation, and offers some suggestions concerning the programming of therapy from the operant point of view. The contributions of linguistics are stressed.

38. Young, E. H. and Hawk, S. S. *Motokinesthetic Speech Training*. Stanford, Calif.: Stanford University Press, 1955.
This text describes and illustrates the motokinesthetic method.

7

Stuttering

Of all the types of disorders with which the profession of speech pathology must deal, stuttering is certainly one that intrigues and fascinates students, researchers, and practicing therapists alike. Many writers have commented on the many unsolved problems that cluster about this ancient human affliction, and one of them, C. S. Bluemel, having entitled his book *The Riddle of Stuttering*, thought that he had solved the riddle, and yet failed to get the acceptance he had expected.[1] An incredible amount of research has been devoted to the disorder, and a host of widely varying forms of treatment have been devised, but we still need to know much more about its nature and to find better ways of treating it. In this chapter we shall assume the role of a guide so that the newcomer to this field will not be completely lost in the labyrinth.

The Nature of Stuttering

We have seen that the other disorders of speech reflect deviancy in certain of the fundamental characteristics of speech. Speech involves phonation; therefore we find voice disorders. Speech is articulated; therefore some persons have articulation problems. Speech also has a time dimension; some of the movements which produce the sounds of speech occur simultaneously and others sequentially. In stuttering we find mistiming in both the simultaneous and successive programming of the components of speech. The stutterer may open his mouth to speak, but fail to phonate at the precise instant when he should start the utterance. Or he may hold

[1] C. S. Bluemel, *The Riddle of Stuttering* (Danville, Ill.: Interstate, 1957).

the first sound of a syllable longer than he should, or he may introduce a gap between a consonant and a vowel, or repeat a syllable when he should say it only once. When these behaviors occur, the forward flow of speech is interrupted; and when they occur so frequently or conspicuously that they interfere with communication, we find the disorder called *stuttering*. Stuttering is therefore a disorder of the time aspect of speech. At its core we find broken sounds, syllables, and words. They are broken because they are disrupted temporally and temporarily. A moment of stuttering does not last forever. The failure in timing is intermittent, not permanent. No one dies of a moment of stuttering. It passes, and the flow of speech moves forward again. Nevertheless this very inconsistency and intermittency is one of the most aggravating features of the disorder. One of our cases said this: "Sometimes I envy the person who is blind or deaf or deformed because they're always that way. Bad as these handicaps are, those who have them are forced to get used to it and make the best of it. But with me, the stuttering comes and goes. I can't adapt. I can't get used to it."

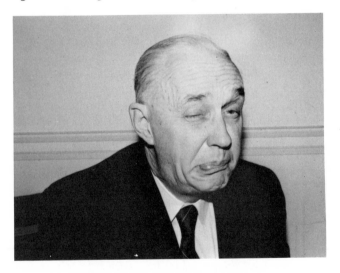

Figure 26: *An Old Stutterer*

While there are almost as many definitions of stuttering as there are writers on the subject, let us attempt a simple one. *Stuttering occurs when the forward flow of speech is interrupted abnormally by repetitions or prolongations of a sound, or syllable, or articulatory posture, or by avoidance and struggle reactions.*[2] In examining this definition, we note that the inter-

[2] For a further consideration of the problem of definition, see the article by M. E. Wingate, "A Standard Definition of Stuttering," *Journal of Speech and Hearing Disorders*, XXIX (1964), 484–89.

ruptions are abnormal ones. Are these interruptions abnormal in frequency, duration, or form; and who then sets the norms?

The research shows rather conclusively that stutterers have more syllabic repetitions and sound prolongations than normal speakers. They have more syllabic repetitions per hundred words, and they have more of them per word. We examined one stutterer who repeated one syllable forty-three times on a single word. Normal speakers occasionally hang onto a sound or posture only briefly, but stutterers show a longer duration on their prolongations. The author once had a silent prolongation on the posture of the first sound of the word "pass" that lasted six minutes by a schoolroom clock, though it was interrupted several times by the need for the intake of air for survival. Normal speakers do not have these experiences. There also seem to be differences in the form of the repetitions and prolongations which distinguish the stutterer from the normal speaker. When a normal speaker repeats a syllable (and he does so only rarely) he uses the correct vowel and he repeats it at the regular tempo of his other syllables. He says "Sa-Saturday." The stutterer tends to say "Suh-Suh-Sih-Suh-Suh-Seh-Sa-Saturday," and the variable repetitions occur irregularly and often with tension. Also the syllables in the stutterer seem to be arrested; they are terminated suddenly; the breath is interrupted. These phenomena do not seem to be characteristic of the few syllabic repetitions shown by normal speakers. We say "few" because they are rare. When a normal speaker repeats, he tends to repeat words and phrases, not syllables or sounds. All of us repeat and hesitate and filibuster at times as we utter our thoughts. None of us is completely fluent in every communicative situation. Knowing this, we do not consider the repetition of a word or phrase or the use of pauses, um's and er's, or reformulations as abnormal. We even accept a few repetitions of a syllable. But when a sound or syllable is repeated not once or twice but many times, and when this behavior occurs too frequently, then we prick up our ears and say to ourselves that the speaker stutters. We tend to say the same thing when a sound is prolonged, as in this example: "I think that mmmmmmmmmmmy mmmmmmmmm-mother wwwwwon't let me go." The tolerance for such prolongations of a sound seems to be much less than for repetitions of a sound or syllable. We have also used the word *posture*. Not all these repetitions and prolongations are vocalized. The stutterer often makes several silent mouth postures before the word is spoken, or he may assume a fixed position and struggle silently with it before blurting out what he wants to say. These fixed postures may be located anywhere in the speech structures. One stutterer may hold his breath with both true and false vocal cords closed tightly. Another may protrude his tongue or twist his lips to one side. Since these silent postures take time, they break up the normal time sequence of speech. Finally, we have included in our definition the terms "avoidance" and "struggle." Although most beginning stutterers show little struggle or avoidance, in the advanced stages of the disorder these reactions may constitute the major part of the problem.

Perhaps some descriptions of these struggle reactions would be useful here. In our speech clinic at the present time, we have a young man who speaks fluently most of the time; but when he does stutter he usually protrudes his lips grossly, makes sucking and clicking noises, then suddenly throws back his head and says the word. This is his characteristic behavior when attempting words beginning with stop consonants; but when he begins a word that starts with a continuant sound such as *s* or *th* or *v*, he protrudes not his lips but his tongue, and this vibrates tremorously. Occasionally he may also simply repeat a syllable several times automatically and without forcing. We also have another man who shows no facial contortions at all but whose stuttering moments are marked by sudden gasps. Sometimes these are so deep that his shoulders jerk upward. A third man shows none of these reactions. He opens his mouth widely agape and neither sound nor air emerge as he exerts a powerful abdominal thrusting in his attempt to break a blockade. These are only a few of the wide variety of struggle reactions to be found in adult stutterers.

We also have some stutterers who show very little of this overt struggle. They duck and dodge their feared words and speaking situations. They have a host of strategies for hiding their difficulty. They may substitute nonfeared words for feared ones. They may just stop talking and pretend to be thinking. They may interject "ah" or "um" or "well" to postpone their expected misery as long as possible. Some of these persons become very skillful in the use of these avoidance tricks but at a great cost of anxiety and tension. Often called interiorized stutterers because most of their stuttering is hidden, they live in a state of constant vigilance lest their disorder be exposed. They scan and plan, trying to anticipate every eventuality. They carry a heavy burden.

Physiological Reactions.   Certain important features of stuttering are difficult to see with the naked eye, and yet they can be revealed by instrumentation. Severe stutterers in the advanced stages of the disorder show abnormalities in heart and pulse rate and in breathing. Investigations have revealed changes in blood composition and distribution, states of general or localized tension, tremors, odd brain waves, dilatation of the pupils, and many other abnormal reactions. However, these do not seem to form the core of the disorder. All severe stutterers do not show all of them. These reactions occur during the moment of stuttering or during its anticipation. They are especially vivid during the stutterer's efforts to escape from the fixations or oscillations. They are probably no more than the reflection of the stress he feels. They are the physiological correlates of his struggle or fear. They do not occur on the shorter unforced stuttering. They do not appear in the young stutterer whose automatic repetitions and unforced prolongations do not seem to bother him. But for the older, more severe stutterer they form a major part of his internal distress. They contribute much to his feeling that something terrible is happening to him. The brain that controls the mouth is flooded with static from the viscera. The normal automaticity and monitoring of utterance is thus doubly beset. It is more difficult to talk.

THE ORIGINS OF STUTTERING

It is difficult to find the true source of a river; too many streams flow into it. Many explorers have attempted to trace the course of the river of stuttering to what they thought were the lakes of its origin. It should not surprise us to learn that different explorers found different lakes.

At one time, the poor student of speech therapy had to be able to describe fifteen different theories concerning the nature and treatment of secondary stuttering, and there were others they might have included in their study. While there is still disagreement and confusion among therapists with respect to their explanations of this disorder, the arguments are not so strident, and large areas of mutual thinking prevail. Formerly there tended to be various schools, each holding a definite and rigid theoretical dogma. Modern research has made available new sources of information. Cooler heads have examined the evidence again and have been able to reconcile opposing points of view. Probably the most important factor was the giving up of the belief in a *single cause* for stuttering. The fallacy of the *single cause* has been responsible for confusion in many fields, and it certainly caused plenty of difficulty in speech correction.

Nevertheless, there are still explorers who insist that the lake they have found is the only true source of the river of stuttering. Let us not argue with them; they may all be correct; let us look at their lakes. There seem to be three of them, since the many different points of view concerning the origin of stuttering can be grouped into three major theories: the *learning* theories; the *neurotic* theories, and the theories of *constitutional difference*. Each has its advocates.

How shall we understand this mysterious disorder? Where shall we find the "impediment"?

Many people have tried to find the answers to these questions. Many have been sure that they knew the answer to the stuttering problem, but the honest speech therapist knows that he is still confronted with a disorder which retains much of its age-old mystery. Most of the past and present explanations contain some truth; none of them is entirely satisfactory. Many beginning students are so disturbed when they discover such a state of affairs that they tend to lose interest in the subject. But there is a similar mystery in many of the other disorders that afflict mankind—heart disease, tooth decay, asthma, and cancer, to name only a few. If there are conflicting theories concerning the nature of stuttering, there is also the ever-present fact that stutterers are with us and need help. And we can do much to help them.

Stuttering as a Neurosis. This point of view is held by many psychiatrists and some psychologists, perhaps because their clinical practice brings them, not the garden variety of stutterers, but those with deep-seated emotional problems. If you stuttered but were also deeply disturbed by emotional conflicts, to whom would you go for help—to a speech therapist or to a psychiatrist? In exploring *their* cases of stuttering, these workers therefore come to have a firm belief in the neurotic origin and character of the disorder. Stuttering behavior is viewed as the outward symptom of a basic inner conflict. Some statements of this position should be provided:

> Psychoanalysis regards stuttering broadly as a neurotic disorder in which personality disturbance is in part reflected in disturbance in speech.[3]
>
> . . . stuttering is a defense created with extraordinary skill and designed to prevent anxiety from developing when certain impulses of which the stutterer dares not become aware, threaten to expose themselves.[4]
>
> When a stammerer attempts to talk, the mouth movements are the persistence into maturity of the original sucking and biting lip-nipple activities of infancy. . . .[5]
>
> Sometimes he is in constant fear lest he inadvertently reveal something he would rather his elders did not hear.[6]
>
> Stuttering is by far the most important of all neurotic speech disturbances.[7]

These are but a few of the formulations of the neurotic theory. In essence, the professional workers who hold these beliefs feel that stuttering is the outward manifestation of repressed desires to satisfy such inner needs

[3] Peter Glauber, "The Psychoanalysis of Stuttering," in Jon Eisenson, ed., *Stuttering: A Symposium* (New York: Harper & Row, Publishers, 1958), p. 73.

[4] Lee Edward Travis, "The Need for Stuttering," *Journal of Speech Disorders*, V (1940), 193–202.

[5] I. H. Coriat, "The Psychoanalytic Conception of Stuttering," *The Nervous Child*, II (1943), 167–71.

[6] K. Dunlap, "Stammering: Its Nature, Etiology and Therapy," *Journal Comparative Psychology*, XXXVII (1944), 187–202.

[7] H. Freund, "Psychopathological Aspects of Stuttering," *American Journal of Psychotherapy*, VII (1953), 689–705.

as these: to satisfy anal or oral eroticism, to express hostility by attacking and smearing the listener, or to remain infantile.

We are pretty sure that some stutterers have this type of causation; some of our cases cannot be reasonably understood in any other way. These are in the marked minority, however. In them the stuttering is symptomatic of a primary neurosis. But there are many more stutterers in whom the neurosis, if any, is secondary. The stutterer develops the stuttering he has acquired from other sources into a defense mechanism. As one of our cases said, "Sure, I get some good out of it. If I have to stutter, I might as well use it to dodge some of the pain of living. It's not good for anything else." Most normal people are neurotic some of the time, and so are most stutterers, in this sense. A few, however, have compulsive symptoms which can only be understood in terms of psychopathology. In them, the stuttering starts in a neurosis and remains in one.

Learning Theories.   Other explorers of stuttering have traced its main flow to another source. Perhaps they worked the other side of the river— i.e., the stutterers who came to them were not those who went to the psychiatrist. At any rate, according to these theories—and there are several which may be included in the category—stuttering is learned behavior. The child is so conditioned that he learns a truly broken English—or Swahili or Japanese. Beginning, as most stuttering does, in the very early years of life, it often seems to coincide with the period of speech learning and development. According to this theory, stuttering has its origin in the early fumblings and hesitancies and interruptions which seem to be a natural and common phase of the speech learning process. We have already seen what a complicated business is this speaking we take so much for granted. We must master complicated muscular coordinations, use the right sounds, formulate our thoughts aloud, express the glandular squirting of our emotions, control others, and use it for the communication of messages. Any of these may present many difficulties.

Rigmor Knutsen, a Danish speech therapist, said to us, "In Denmark we find a great many children who begin to stutter after the speech therapist has treated them for their delayed speech. Do you not also find this true?" We answered that we had known several cases who bore out her observations and told her about Carlene.

Carlene, at four, had no intelligible speech. She used a few vowels and grunts with her gestures to make her wants known. She was referred to us by the psychological clinic who had found her IQ on the performance tests to be so low that they were considering suggesting commitment to a state school for the feeble-minded. By imitating her behavior until she imitated us, we were able to go about getting her to produce almost all of the isolated speech sounds. By avoiding all requests to name objects, and through the use of self-talk and parallel talking, we evoked enough vocalized and whispered words to accept her for therapy. At the end of three months of daily work, she was speaking in short phrases, and retests in the psychological clinic showed her to be of normal intelligence. Her parents were very proud of her achievement; but during the summer vacation, they worked too hard upon her speech production, and she began to stutter very markedly. Advised to give up all therapy, the parents cooperated willingly and within two more months the symptoms disappeared completely. The burden of trying to master her articulation and fluency skills had been too great. It was interesting that she regressed to simpler phrases and sentences as the stuttering disappeared, and for a time her articulation became worse.

Many children who do not have delayed speech go through a similar period of non-fluency when, urged by parental approvals, they try to master the adult patterns of speech too quickly. It is a long step from the single-word utterance of the one-year-old to the multiple-word phrases and sentences of adult speech. Children who try to dance before they have learned to walk trip themselves, and the same thing occurs in speech. We tend to think of penalties as being provocative of stuttering, but excessive approvals at the wrong times can create such a demand as to produce speech hesitation as well. Many children from happy homes can start to stutter in this way.

As we have seen in our section on how children learn to talk, some parents fail to make speech learning easy for their children. They do not listen. They demand answers which the child may not be ready to give. They may command verbal confession. They set standards of fluency and articulation that may be far beyond the capabilities of the child. Siblings may interrupt excessively. When the communicative interchange is broken either at the sending or receiving end, or when speaking becomes disrupted by emotion, there are only three things a person can do. He can repeat; he can fixate; or he can give up the attempt to speak. Some children choose the latter course and develop voluntary mutism. Others deny the parental demands to conform and talk a gibberish of fluent, but distorted sounds. The stutterer keeps on talking, but he falters. Driven by his urge to talk, all he can do is to repeat or prolong, to oscillate or fixate when these disrupting influences are present.

However, we have not explained why in stuttering the stoppages occur on the sound or its silent posture, nor why the repetition is of the syllable and sound rather than of the whole word or phrase. Wingate's critical review of the research seems to show fairly conclusively that the child who is called a stutterer shows different *kinds* of hesitancies than the one who is presumed to speak normally.[8] The one child mainly responds to

[8] M. E. Wingate, "Evaluation and Stuttering," *Journal of Speech and Hearing Disorders*, XXVII (1962), 106–15, 244–57, 368–77.

these communicative pressures by behavior our culture calls stuttering; the other primarily by hesitating or filibustering. They show both types of nonfluencies, but the child who becomes a stutterer has many more difficulties with the sound and syllable rather than with the word or phrase.

Why do some of these hesitaters become stutterers? We do not know the answer to our question. Perhaps the difference lies in the amount and intensity of the communicative stress. With minor stress, repetitions of sentences or phrases occur; with more stress, words are repeated; with even more pressure, the oscillating occurs on syllables. When complete disruption occurs but the urge to speak still remains, first prolongations of an audible sound (mmmmmother) are shown, and finally even this breaks down to a silent posture. The syllable and sound are the smallest motoric and acoustic elements into which speech can be broken.

Perhaps the normally speaking child has, for one reason or another, developed his formulative and fluency skills in speaking to such a degree of stability that only occasionally will he show the small percentage of syllabic and sound repetitions and prolongations. The stuttering child, perhaps because of constitutional difference, interpersonal relationship problems, or other reasons, may be more vulnerable to the same stress which normal speaking children handle with word and phrase repetitions. We do not know. Wyatt has suggested that when breakdown occurs, a child regresses to an earlier stage. She points out the resemblance of early stuttering to the reiterative babbling of the infant.[9] We do not know the answer to our question.

The Semantic Theory.   According to Wendell Johnson, chief exponent of the semantic theory, stuttering begins, "not in the child's mouth, but in the parent's ear." He lumps all types of repetitions and prolongations into the category of nonfluencies, which he feels are quite normal reactions and common to all children. The difficulty, Johnson believes, arises when a parent hears these normal nonfluencies and reacts to them by anxiety or penalty. Johnson feels that even when the repetitions and prolongations are excessive, they are merely normal reactions to the abnormal conditions of communicative stress operating at the moment. He insists, therefore, that the source of the real problem lies in parental misdiagnosis and misinterpretation. He points out that when parents become anxious or punitive about these normal hesitancies, the child, reflecting their attitudes, will begin to fear, avoid, or struggle to inhibit them.

Ricky, aged five, illustrates Johnson's theory of stuttering. We first met the child at the age of three. He was brought to us by his mother, a former college speech teacher. She was tense and anxious about the

[9] G. Wyatt, "A Developmental Crisis Theory of Stuttering," *Language and Speech,* I (1958), 250–64.

boy, claiming that he was beginning to stutter. In three hours of observation, play, and parent conversation, we were unable to find anything but an occasional repetition of a phrase or whole word, usually under conditions of word choice which would have made any adult hesitate. Each time one of these occurred, she would roll her eyes or tug at our sleeves to point out the stuttering. Knowing that stuttering is intermittent, we even introduced some experimental stress, hurrying the child, interrupting, rejecting his statements, and averting our attention. He was remarkably fluent, much more so than most children of his age.

Recognizing the mother's anxiety, and being as careful as possible, we tried to reassure and educate her concerning the prevalence of repetition and hesitation in most children's speech. We made available some parental counseling to help her face her own problems, but she refused to participate. Said she, "You're just like everyone else. Every doctor and speech therapist I've taken Rickey to has said the same thing. You can't fool a child's own mother. He's stuttering and you know it."

A year later she brought the child back to the clinic, and sure enough, he was stuttering with all the abnormality of an adult. "See!" she said triumphantly, "I told you he was a stutterer all the time."

Frustration Theory.   But stuttering need not necessarily begin in the *parent's* ear; it may also begin in the ear of the *child*. The need to communicate a message, to verbalize one's thoughts, to control another person, to express an emotion—these can be powerful drives. Besides, there are children whose appetites for speech for one reason or another are almost monstrous. They must be heard! When such speech-hungry children find these drives blocked by the repetitions and prolongations produced by listener loss or other fluency disrupters, they experience much frustration. If you have had to use a typewriter or piano on which the keys stick occasionally, you will understand. The urge to consummate the response is blocked and impeded by the delay occasioned by the repetitions and prolongations. Interruptions frustrate, whether they come from others or from one's own mouth. Too many of the young stutterers we have studied do not appear to have the origin of their difficulty in parental mislabeling of normal nonfluencies for us to accept blindly Johnson's thesis. Some parents actually deny the existence of any problem. Usually, stuttering has had a gradual history of growth in frequency and severity before it ever gets labeled. We feel that the role of frustration in the development of stuttering must receive the attention it deserves. Not only can frustration account for the initial breaks in the flow of speech; it also can help us understand why children eventually begin to struggle and avoid.

Frustration is unpleasant; we avoid unpleasantness and we fear it. Frustration also leads to aggression, and so we struggle.

> Jimmy, aged four, was in most respects a rather ordinary normal child. But he differed markedly from other children his age in his outstanding inability to tolerate frustration. This was not inborn, but the result of poor handling by his parents, his uncle, and his older sister. The whole family loved to tease each other, to play practical jokes, to upset apple carts and egos. Even as a baby, Jimmy was teased with the bottle being held tantalizingly to the lips, or withdrawn, or waved from side to side. The adults liked to pretend to drop him; they put obstacles in the way of his crawling; they greatly enjoyed seeing him become purple with rage. At the age of two he was holding his breath until his face became blue. Toilet training was slow and his family interpreted his occasional urinary lapses upon those who held him as a sign of his family-belongingness. As is obvious from the foregoing description, a good amount of hidden hostility permeated the entire family living, but it appeared only in joking and teasing forms. The approved culture pattern was to be a good sport, to be able to take it and dish it out.

> Jimmy, however, never quite managed to adopt these values. He fought back; he threw temper tantrums; he kicked and bit and howled. They called him a poor sport, and since they despised poor sports, they worked hard to toughen him to their teasing. He had spoken well and without any nonfluency until his fourth birthday when his sister began to kid him about his pronunciation of words beginning with the *s* blends which he had not mastered.

> At this point they gave him, for the first time, a nickname "Twaberry Bwonde" since his hair was that color and he pronounced the words in that way. He reacted by going berserk, and so more teasing occurred, this time focused primarily on speech. The sister learned that he would tend to make more articulatory errors if she interrupted him, finished his sentences, or hurried him, and she went to work. Within one week he was stuttering severely, though in a repetitive fashion. Two weeks later, he was showing facial contortions and severe struggling in breathing. At this point the parents became alarmed and brought the child to the speech therapist.

> Although the parents and family changed their policies and all teasing was eliminated, the stuttering persisted. It was not until a lot of release therapy through play was administered and a course of training in frustration tolerance was instituted that first the struggle, and later the repetitions, subsided and disappeared.

Conflict Reinforcement.   The "conflict reinforcement" theory of stuttering treats the disorder from the viewpoint of modern learning theory.

The primary symptoms are seen as the result of competitive and opposing urges to speak and not to speak. When these tendencies are approximately equal, oscillations and fixations in behavior occur. These are the repetitions and prolongations of the primary symptoms. The conflicting urges may come from many sources. The child may want to speak but may not know what to say or how to say it. He may need to speak at a time when he thinks his listener is not listening or does not want to hear him. He may have the urge to say something "evil" which may receive penalty. He may want to speak like big people, yet not have the fluency or articulatory skills to keep the flow going. He may have an urge to express himself at a time when he feels ambivalent. The lag of a clumsy tongue may oppose a strong need to talk quickly. Any of these and many other situations could produce the opposing forces. All this theory considers is what results when the urge to speak meets a contrary urge not to do so. In essence, this theoretical formulation holds that stuttering occurs when there are conflicting urges to speak and to hold back from speaking. Here is a case study illustrating an approach-avoidance conflict.

> One of our cases began to stutter severely on Christmas morning, repeating sounds and syllables, hesitating, and prolonging vowel sounds so markedly that he was referred to us that very afternoon. We had seen the child the week before and had noticed no speech abnormality, nor had his parents, according to their report. He spoke normally that morning until he asked the question "Dih-dih-dih-dih-dih-didn't I g . . . ggg . . . ge . . . get a-a-a-anything fr . . . om mmmmmmy Da . . . da . . . daddy?" The father was not present, having been on a business trip, and he had expected to return that afternoon, bringing his presents with him. However, he was delayed for three more days, and his return did not allay the problem. Subsequent exploration revealed that the child felt profoundly rejected by his busy father.

These three variants of the learning theory seem to complement one another. Together they provide a description of how stuttering starts and develops. We are certain that each of them explains how certain children began to stutter. We are not sure that all of them explain how all stuttering starts.

Sheehan explains stuttering in terms of conflicting roles. He points out that the adult stutterer. tends to oscillate between the roles of normal speaker and stutterer. Much of his speech is fluent; at times he can "pass" as a normal speaker. Only intermittently is he a deviant. When the stutterer uses a different accent or plays a part as an actor, thereby escaping from his usual roles, he may be very fluent. He has more difficulty when talking to authority figures where he must reluctantly assume a subservient role, and much less trouble when speaking to someone of lesser status.

When caught in false or conflicting roles, the ambivalence leads to hesitancy and stuttering.[10]

Stuttering as Learned Behavior. The semantic frustration and approach-avoidance theories reflect an old belief that stuttering is basically learned behavior—a set of bad habits or maladaptive responses. This is an ancient belief and also one that has many contemporary advocates. Modern writers on the subject of stuttering almost universally feel that some of its features reflect the influence of past learning, though not all would agree that this is the only source of the problem. The agreement is based upon the acknowledged changes in stuttering which occur as the stutterer grows older and on the variations that distinguish one stutterer from another. One can almost see the disorder being learned as the child seeks to avoid or cope with his speech interruptions. One person learns to stutter in one way and another in a different way, but the question remains: were the original speech interruptions also learned? Here we find opposing points of view.

Operant Conditioning Views. Proceeding from the observation that some repetitions are to be found in the speech of most speakers and that they occur more frequently in children and more frequently under communicative stress, there are those who seek to explain the nature of stuttering in terms of reinforcement alone. The repetitions are said to evoke desired parental attention or concern or to enable a child to escape listener-loss. These desired listener reactions then reinforce the repetitive behavior, and so it tends to occur more frequently. Once stuttering has really taken hold, then whatever the stutterer does to avoid or release himself from the habitual repetitions (which now have become unpleasant) will also be strongly reinforced, since the escape from fear or frustration is always rewarding.[11]

Two-factor Learning Theories. Other writers find it very difficult to accept the view that the initial fluency breaks are operantly conditioned. The very consistency of the *core* behaviors of stuttering—the syllabic repetitions and fixations or prolongations—that are found in all stutterers and which in young children seem to constitute most of the abnormality seems to indicate that these are precipitated rather than learned. Accordingly Brutten and Shoemaker and others have held that this core behavior occurs initially as a result of emotionally induced breakdown in coordination.[12] Under stress the smooth sequencing of speech becomes disintegrated.

[10] J. G. Sheehan, *Stuttering: Research and Therapy* (New York: Harper & Row, Publishers, 1970).

[11] For a more detailed exposition of this point of view, read G. H. Shames, and C. E. Sherrick, "A Discussion of Nonfluency and Stuttering as Learned Behavior," *Journal of Speech and Hearing Disorders,* XXVIII (1963), 3–18.

[12] E. J. Brutten and D. J. Shoemaker, *The Modification of Stuttering* (Englewood Cliffs, N.J.: Prentice-Hall, Inc., 1967).

All of us tend to halt the flow of speech, to repeat or fixate when the pressures on communication are too great, and some persons are viewed as being more vulnerable to this breakdown than others. The core behaviors of stuttering, according to Brutten and Shoemaker, are produced in this way; and then they become classically conditioned through the association of stimuli. Fluency failures may result from many kinds of stress; but when they result from conditioned negative emotionality, they result in the special kind of fluency failure called stuttering. These authors do not deny that much of the struggle or avoidance behavior may be learned instrumental responses. They agree with the operant conditioning writers that these coping behaviors are instrumentally learned, but they insist that not all of the behavior called stuttering is due to contingent reinforcement. By attributing the core behavior to classical conditioning and the avoidance and struggle responses to operant conditioning, they therefore support a two-factor theory of the nature of stuttering as a learned response.

Constitutional Theories of Stuttering. Does stuttering ever have an organic basis? Are some stutterers different from their fellows in their neurological functioning? At one time this belief was widely held, and later it was discarded in favor of the explanations in terms of neurotic or learned behavior. Now the pendulum is beginning to swing back again toward some belief in a constitutional difference, at least as shown in certain stutterers. To cite but one study, R. K. Jones, a neurosurgeon, operated on the dominant hemispheres of the brains of some epileptic stutterers to relieve them from their seizures, and found surprisingly that they stopped stuttering.[13] He attributed the dramatic change to the fact that he had thereby reduced the interhemispheric interference with speech production, the stutterers being presumed to have not one dominant hemisphere for speech, but two. We find here an echo of an old theory of stuttering—the cerebral dominance theory based on the concept of *dysphemia*. This word refers to an underlying neuromuscular condition which reflects itself peripherally in nervous impulses that are poorly timed in their arrival in the paired speech musculatures. It was felt to be an inherited problem or one due to a shift of handedness. At the present time few subscribe to the cerebral dominance theory in its original form, but the concept of dysphemia has been broadened to include what Gutzmann called "a weakness in the central coordinating system."

The importance of the concept of dysphemia is that it explains the stutterer's speech interruptions in terms of a nervous system which breaks down *relatively easily* in its integration of the flow of nervous impulses to the paired peripheral muscles. In order to lift the jaw, for instance, nervous

[13] R. K. Jones, "Observations on Stammering After Localized Cerebral Injury," *Journal of Neurology and Neurosurgery*, XXIX (1966), 192–95.

impulses must arrive simultaneously in the paired muscles of each side. In some stutterers these arrival times are disrupted; they are not synchronized. It is very difficult to lift a jaw or a wheelbarrow by one handle. The dysphemic individual is able to time his speech coordinations pretty well as long as the coordinating centers in the brain are not being bedeviled by emotional reactions and their backflow of visceral sensations. He can talk pretty well when calm and unexcited. But his thresholds of resistance to emotional disturbance are low. His coordinations break down under relatively little stress. We have all known pianists and golfers who could play excellently by themselves but whose coordinations were pitifully inadequate to the demands of concert or tournament pressures.

Although it has generated a tremendous amount of research, the concept of "dysphemia" has failed to gain wide acceptance. Nevertheless, the belief in the presence of some constitutional factor in some stutterers stubbornly persists, perhaps because of the disorder's tendency to run in families, plus the sex ratio in favor of more males who stutter, certain brain wave anomalies and coordination difficulties, and perhaps some organically determined perceptual differences which interfere with the monitoring of sequential speech.[14]

With regard to the last of these items, there seems to be some evidence that stutterers may have a defective auditory processing system, especially for their own speech. By delaying the feedback of a normal speaker's voice so he hears himself a fraction of a second after he has spoken, behaviors very similar to stuttering have been produced. Also, by distorting the phase relationships of a normal speaker's voice as heard in the two ears, complete blockages of utterance have been created. These findings still need corroboration and further exploration, but there is enough research showing that stutterers speak better under masking noise and under delayed auditory feedback to lend some support to the theory that a perceptual defect of the auditory system may possibly be present.[15]

Cluttering Origin. Another statement of the constitutional theory that finally is arousing real interest in speech pathology in this country, although it has had a long history elsewhere, is the concept that stuttering is rooted in cluttering, which itself is viewed as the reflection of a constitutional difference. Weiss has called this difference "central language imbalance," and others have used the term "specific language disability." [16] The clutterer is usually late in speaking, has a family history of cluttering

[14] For a review of the research dealing with organicity in stuttering, see C. Van Riper, *The Nature of Stuttering* (Englewood Cliffs, N.J.: Prentice-Hall, Inc., 1971).
[15] *The Nature of Stuttering.* The student may find the following two articles of interest: G. A. Soderberg, "Delayed Auditory Feedback and Stuttering," *Journal of Speech and Hearing Disorders,* XXXIII (1968), 260–67; and J. E. Martin, "The Signal Detection Hypothesis and the Perceptual Defect Theory," *Journal of Speech and Hearing Disorders,* XXXV (1970), 252–55.
[16] D. A. Weiss, *Cluttering* (Englewood Cliffs, N.J.: Prentice-Hall, Inc., 1964).

and stuttering and retarded speech development, speaks very swiftly and in a disordered manner. Speech is poorly organized linguistically, motorically, and perceptually. Reading, writing, and other language difficulties are often present. The articulation is slurred. The onset of speech is delayed. All these features, it is said, point to a basic constitutional difference. Weiss believes that most stuttering begins in the disorganized repetitions of cluttering. It is our clinical impression that some of our cases did show this origin. There are clutterers who do not stutter, stutterers who do not clutter, some stutterers who have cluttered, and some who still do. But when we find this pattern of cluttering coexisting with the stuttering either in the present symptomatology or in the past histories of these individuals, we tend to suspect the presence of an original constitutional difference or predisposition.

Two other final forms of the constitutional theory may be mentioned. Karlin attributes stuttering to delayed myelination of those nerve tracts in the brain which coordinate the muscles used in speech. He explains the fact that there are four times as many males as females who stutter by pointing to the research which shows that myelination in girls is always advanced over that of the boys during the critical age from two to four years, when most stuttering begins.[17] We also have the formulation of Eisenson, who feels that stutterers possess a constitutional difference which shows itself in a tendency to perseverate in motor activity.[18] Again, some research supports this point of view, even as some research seems to support all other theories.

Summing Up. What is a student to believe when so many different explanations exist? Our own resolution of this problem is an eclectic one. We feel that stuttering has many origins, many sources, and that the original causes are not nearly so important as the maintaining causes, once stuttering has started. We can find stutterers who partly fit any one of these various statements of theory and some stutterers who fit several. All stutterers are not cut from the same original cloth. It is important that we know these various explanations because the problems of some of the stutterers we meet can thereby be best understood. The river of stuttering does not flow out of only one lake.

THE DEVELOPMENT OF THE DISORDER

The picture of stuttering at its onset is usually quite different from that shown by the stutterer who has experienced communicative frustration

[17] I. W. Karlin, "Stuttering: Basically an Organic Disorder," *Logos*, II (1959), 61–63.

[18] J. Eisenson, "A Perseverative Theory of Stuttering," in J. Eisenson, ed., *Stuttering: A Symposium* (New York: Harper & Row, Publishers, 1958), pp. 225–71.

and social penalties for years. Although we have often been able to arrest the disorder in its early phases when we had the opportunity, in other cases we have seen it grow in complexity and abnormality as the years went by. We have seen little children stumbling occasionally in their speech, repeating syllables and prolonging sounds quite effortlessly and without apparent awareness; and then we have seen them again some years later with facial contortions, complete blockages of utterance, and deeply troubled by the feeling of stigma. One of the essential evils of stuttering is this tendency toward increasing abnormality. In seeking to cope with the breaks in his speech, the stutterer habituates many coping behaviors which complicate his problem. Under stress, he uses certain tricks of avoidance and postponement to hide or escape his difficulties. When caught in verbal oscillations and fixations, he employs various devices to interrupt them and to release himself from their hold. These coping behaviors soon become automatized components of the stuttering, and the stutterer feels that they are involuntary, that he cannot keep them out.

Different stutterers show different courses of development. The majority seem to run a course in which the initial, effortless syllabic repetitions and sound prolongations become full of tension and struggle and then in turn the interrupter or avoidance reactions begin to develop. Parallelling this overt development, we find a change from unawareness to surprise, to frustration, and finally to fear and shame. This seems to be the most common developmental track, but there are also others. Some stuttering, as we have mentioned earlier, begins suddenly with complete blockages and immediate struggle; and the fears and shame develop swiftly. In other stutterers, the growth is very gradual, and no struggle symptoms appear.[19]

It should be understood that not all beginning stutterers show this morbid growth. Indeed, we have fairly good evidence that about four out of every five children who begin to stutter seem to regain or attain normal speech with or without therapy.[20] Moreover the progressive development even in those who continue to stutter is oscillatory: it is not linear. When we see a child struggling or avoiding, we are concerned; but often a few weeks or months later he may return to the effortless repetitions that characterized his initial difficulty. These swings in developmental severity are usually viewed as indicating a good prognosis. Some stutterers may swing all the way back to normal speech long enough to escape from the clutches of the disorder. Unfortunately, too many do not. They get caught

---

[19] For a detailed description of these patterns of development, see C. Van Riper, *The Nature of Stuttering* (Englewood Cliffs, N.J.: Prentice–Hall, Inc., 1971), Chapter 5.

[20] J. G. Sheehan and M. M. Martyn, "Stuttering and Its Disappearance," *Journal of Speech and Hearing Research,* XIII (1970), 279–89.

in the whirlpool of self-reinforcement; the disorder becomes self-perpetuating.

How does this happen? What is the method by which the disorder becomes self-reinforcing? These are tough questions, and there are many possible answers. Some authorities insist that a neurotic *need for stuttering* is created once the case becomes aware that his symptoms can help him as well as hurt him. They say that often the stuttering serves as an acceptable excuse, as a defense against the exorbitant demands of conscience or culture. Most stutterers reject this explanation, but some secondary gain from stuttering is often to be found, in the adult case at least.

How Situation and Word Fears Precipitate Stuttering. More immediate and probably more important is the fact that the fear of stuttering, like most fears, creates its own hesitancy and tension and ambivalence. These factors are the very ones which create nonfluency in the normal speaker, and they have a more potent effect on the stutterer's speech. Very often, too, feelings of guilt may create the disturbed emotions so disruptive of fluency.

> The fact that I am Chinese is very important in my stuttering. We are trained from infancy never to do anything which would cause our families to lose face. I cannot tell you how strong this need is, but maybe you can understand by my telling you how I cut off part of my tongue when I stuttered in front of my father, when I was only five. I almost bled to death. I don't think at all about my own trouble, only about what a disgrace I am to my family. I fear stuttering more than anyone I have ever known. I am even afraid to talk to myself sometimes. I sleep on my face so I will not speak in my sleep. And the more I think about it, the more I stutter. The more I try to hide it or avoid it, the worse it gets. . . .

The emotions generated during the approach to a feared situation or word are far more powerful than most nonstutterers would suspect. One of our cases with a normal pulse rate of 74 beats per minute found an increase to 87 as he dialed a phone number, a rate of 114 at the moment his listener said "hello," and a final peak of 123 as he attempted his first speech. Intense feelings of panic, frustration, and self-disgust become clustered about the act of talking, and they are bound to interfere with the smoothness of the functioning. Thus, the fear of stuttering produces more stuttering.

Approach-Avoidance Conflicts. Another way of explaining how nonfluency can be increased by word fear is that based on the concept of the approach-avoidance conflict. Suppose the stutterer wants to order a cup of coffee. He starts out: "I would like a cup of. . . ." At this moment, he suddenly becomes highly aware that on the next word his face may become repulsively contorted, that he may find himself frustrated in a long, tremorous prolongation of a tightly pressed-back tongue posture, that his listener may be startled or irritated. Instantly, he feels pulled forward by the need to complete his communication, and he feels a strong urge to utter the word "coffee" as quickly as possible. But at the same time, the expected unpleasantness pulls him backward. A tug of war ensues. Sometimes, when neither force is strong enough to win, oscillation occurs and repetitions, hesitations, retrials, and half-hearted speech attempts reflect the equality of the two competing urges.

To speak or not to speak, that is the stutterer's vital question. At times the struggle shows itself in a complete impasse. The urge to attempt the word "coffee," and the fear of the subsequent abnormality counteract each other to such an extent that the person's mouth is immobilized, frozen in a fixed grimace. Thus, either repetitive (clonic) or prolonged (tonic) symptoms may be created by adding fear to the forward flowing process of communication. Fear is the refrigerant that always congeals action. It inhibits. And when one's fluent utterance is suddenly frozen by fear, hesitancies are bound to occur. It is for this reason that we speak of secondary stuttering as being a disorder infinitely more dangerous and difficult than either primary or transitional stuttering.

How the Stuttering Symptoms Are Reinforced. There is another basic concept which must be understood by those who wish to help the secondary stutterer. It is this very significant fact: the contortions, tremors, and other unpleasant abnormalities which cause the stutterer so much distress are terminated by the utterance of the word. No matter what silly gyrations his mouth goes through, finally the word comes out. When it does, the panicky fear belonging to that word subsides. In essence, what the stutterer does then is to make a very serious error of judgment. He attributes his release to the struggle and the abnormality. He says, "I squeezed my eyes and then the word came out. If I want to have any future word come out, I'll have to squeeze my eyes."

When any bit of behavior in a punishment situation is followed by release from punishment, it gets powerful reinforcement and strengthening. The stutterer is like the cat in a puzzle-box who happens to look under its left leg at the moment its tail hits the lever that opens the cage. The cat will tend to assume the same head position when it is put back in the cage.

In most cases, the actual release from blocking is due to the fact that the stutterer has had sufficient abnormality to satisfy his morbid expectation. Once the fear is satisfied, the tension subsides, and with it, the tremor. The word can now be uttered. If, at this instant, the stutterer by chance happens to gasp for breath, he will tend to feel he must gasp henceforth. The release has rewarded the behavior which preceded it. Why do secondary stutterers show such an amazing variety of bizarre symptoms? The only ones they have in common are repetitions and prolongations. All others are diverse. We would account for this variety in terms of the reinforcement given certain items of struggle behavior occurring at the moment of release. Anxiety reduction is a powerful conditioner. So also is the escape from punishment. Both of these powerful reinforcers play an important part in secondary stuttering. They create new symptoms and help to perpetuate the disorder. Therapy must be so designed as to prevent them from doing their foul work. They cannot be ignored.

How the Fears of Stuttering Develop.   By fear we mean the expectation or anticipation of unpleasantness. The unpleasantness in stuttering can be (1) the experience of frustration, of being unable to communicate, of being unable to move a tongue or lip out of its tremor, of being unable to inhibit facial contortions or abnormal sounds; or (2) it can be the unpleasantness of feeling rejected by one's associates, of being on the receiving end of social penalties, of finding one's speech attempts greeted with anxiety, impatience, pity, or laughter.

Most texts on stuttering stress the fears but ignore the importance of the frustrations which are equally vivid parts of the stuttering experience. The intermittent nature of stuttering makes it all the more unpleasant.

The inability to move or control a part of the body is profoundly disturbing. It has some death threat in it. If suddenly you could no longer raise your arm, you would find yourself terribly frightened. You would struggle and be afraid. You would know frustration of a peculiarly vivid kind. The stutterer feels the same way when he finds his jaws frozen in a tremor or his tongue stuck quiveringly to the roof of the mouth.

This felt inability to move the speech muscles can be explained in many ways: as a manifestation of a latent dysphemia, as a conditioned inhibition, or as a moment of emotional blankness. It may be merely symptomatic of a chronic speech hesitancy which has been practiced so often that it has become habitual. It may be only the result of simultaneous and opposing desires to speak and to remain silent. But introspectively, the dominant feature of the stuttering experience is the feeling of being "blocked" in the forward flow of speech. As one stutterer said:

> What happens is that I can't go on. I can't complete the word I want to say. I'm stuck. I either hang there struggling on a consonant or find my mouth repeating the same syllable over and over again like a broken record. Sometimes I'm talking great guns when bang! I'm hung up higher than a kite. Something seems to freeze my tongue or throat shut, or else it turns it over to an automatic repeater.

In our first chapter we described some of the ways our society reacts to the person handicapped in speech. In it we traced the historical progress from attitudes of rejection, through humor and pity, to the more modern policy of retraining and reeducation. The stutterer knows all these reactions and more, too. Here are some excerpts from autobiographies:

> What hit me worst of all and something I've never forgot or forgiven was how the parents of other kids would yank them away from me when they would hear me stutter. They wouldn't let me come in their yard to play. They told me to go home and stutter somewhere else. They didn't want their kid to get infected.

> Elsie was the worst. She was always teasing me, calling me "stutter-cat" or "stumble-tongue" or mocking me. She was so slick at it that hardly anyone but me noticed it. She'd say it as she went by my desk, under her breathe, so only I got it. I could have killed her if I hadn't been so hurt and helpless. And I couldn't hit her, because boys can't hit girls, not even out on the playground.

> Whenever I'd stutter, Dad would slump down behind his paper, or if he didn't have any, he'd just look away and pretend to think. Sometimes, he'd just drum on the table with his fingers or hum an absent-minded little tune, as though to say, "I'm not listening so it doesn't count." He never teased me or said anything about my stuttering. No one did. It was as unmentionable as Sex. My father, as a small town minister, believed in letting sleeping dogs lie. I grew up feeling that stuttering was somehow pretty sinful.

> My nickname was "Spit-it-out-Joe," or "Spitty" for short. I got it from my third-grade teacher, an impatient, aggressive old dame who couldn't bear to hear me block. Every time I did, she'd yelp, "Spit it out, Joe!" and the kids picked it up and I've carried the tag for years. I still have dreams of killing the old hag.

> My mother only did one thing when I stuttered. She held her breath. She never teased me, punished me, or seemed embarrassed. Her lovely face was always serene. But she held her breath. She was entirely patient, sweet, and understanding. She gave me the feeling that she was proud of me and was completely confident that everything would turn out all right. But she held her breath every time I stuttered. That breath-holding sometimes sounded louder than thunder to me.

It is from experiences such as these that most young stutterers begin to expect unpleasantness in the act of speaking. This expectation may at first be specifically focused on a single word, the one on which the unpleasantness occurred. Or it may start with a more general fear of a certain situation, such as talking over the telephone, or speaking to a hard-of-hearing grandmother. Stuttering fears are of two main types: situation fears and word fears.

Word Fears. The first word fears arise from two main sources: (1) from words which are remembered because of the severe frustration or vivid penalties experienced when uttering them, and (2) from words which, because of their frequent use under stress, accumulate more stuttering memories upon them.

> The question words have always been hard for me to say, ever since I can remember. What? Where? When? Why? How? My folks were always so busy. I always had to interrupt something important they were doing. They either answered without paying any real attention so I had to say it again, or else they told me not to bother them, or they told me to stop asking so many questions.

> My own name is my hardest word. Too many big people have asked me, "What is your name, sonny?" I've had to say it too many times when I got into trouble. I've said it so often and stuttered on it so often that I almost think it should be spelled with more than one *t*, like T-T-T-Tommy.

> I believe I remember the very first time I stuttered or at least it was the first time I ever noticed it. I was in the second grade, in the third row, last seat. The teacher asked me several simple *times* problems in multiplication, and I stuttered and she got irritated and asked me something simpler until finally she said, "Okay, dummy, how much is two and two?" and I couldn't say, "Four." I've been afraid of that number and of all *f* words ever since.

These fears, starting from such simple instances, grow swiftly. Often their growth almost seems malignant, constantly invading new areas of one's mental life. A child begins by first fearing the word *paper*. He has had an unpleasant experience in uttering it. He sees it approaching and expects some more unpleasantness, either frustration or penalty. He finds more difficulty. Soon he is fearing many *p* words besides *paper*. He recognizes *pay* and *penny* as hard words to say. Then the fear generalizes or becomes fastened to other features of the stuttering experience. It spreads to other words having similar visual, acoustic, kinesthetic, tactual, or semantic features.

The visual transfer, for example, may be in terms of spelling cues. Because of his fear of *p* words, he may see the word *pneumonia* as dreaded, even though the actual utterance begins with a nasal sound. Or, to illustrate the acoustic transfer, he may come to fear the *k*, *ch*, and *t* sounds because they, like the *p*, are ejected with a puff of air. Or tactually and kinesthetically, he may soon be fearing all the other lip sounds, starting with the *b*, then spreading to the *w*, *m*, and even the *f* and *v* sounds. The spread of fear can take several directions. The following example illustrates how the cues precipitating fear of stuttering can spread semantically.

I had never, so far as I remember, had any real trouble on words beginning with a *w*. Oh, I might have had some, I suppose, but generally I considered them easy sounds to say. And I had very frequently used the word, "well," as a sort of handle, saying it as a kind of way to get started. Sometimes, of course, I might have to say it three or four times before the next word came out, but, anyway, I could always say "well." It was a handy trick to cover up and postpone. Then one day I had an experience which ruined that word for me forever. To this day, "well" is a very hard word for me to speak without stuttering, and it all happened because of that one experience. It happened like this. I was in a grocery store, asking for five pork chops, and I got blocked in saying the name of the meat. It was a long one with hard sticking in my throat, and I kept trying to break it by saying "well." I must have used too many of them because a man behind me impatiently shouted, "Well, well? You aren't well, young lady. Get out of here and go home to bed. You're sick. Not well, sick! Do you hear, sick!" I fled without the pork chops, but I can never use the word in the sense of healthy without blocking completely. I sometimes can use it as a starter, but if I happen to think of it as the antonym of "sick," I block on it immediately.

Situation Fears.   We have been describing the stutterer's conflicting urges to utter and to avoid the utterance of a given word. Shall he or shan't he attempt it? He scrutinizes the word for cues which might indicate danger, for resemblances to other words formerly provocative of great unpleasantness. The same sort of process occurs on the situation level. Sheehan puts the matter as follows:

> At the *situation* level there is a parallel conflict between entering and not entering a feared situation. The stutterer's behavior toward using the telephone, reciting in class, or introducing himself to strangers illustrates this conflict. Many situations which demand speech hold enough threat to produce a competing desire to hold back.[21]

Often in word fears there occurs an actual rehearsal of some of the expected abnormality. Breathing records show that even prior to speech attempt the stutterer's silent breathing often goes through the same peculiar pattern that he shows when actually stuttering. In situation fears this is not the case. Situation fears are more vague, more generalized, more focused on the *attitudes* of the listener and the stutterer than upon the *behavior*. Situation fears can range in intensity all the way from uncertainty to complete panic. We have known stutterers to faint and fall to the floor in their

---

[21] J. G. Sheehan, "Conflict Theory of Stuttering," in J. Eisenson, ed., *Stuttering: A Symposium* (New York: Harper & Row, Publishers, 1958).

anticipation of a speaking situation. The fear fluctuates in intensity from moment to moment. It is often set off by the stutterer's recognition of certain features of an approaching speech situation as similar to those of earlier situations in which he met great penalty or frustration. Stutterers learn to scan an approaching speaking situation with all the concentration of a burglar looking over a prospective bank. Like word fears, situation fears generalize. They may begin from a simple recognition on the part of the child that he was having much difficulty in talking to a certain store-keeper. Remembering this, he may begin to fear speaking in any store; or to take another tack, he might begin to fear talking to all strange men, or to mention still another, he might fear having to relay any message given him by his mother. Situation fears are like word fears in another way, too. Avoidance increases them greatly. The more the stutterer runs away from a given speaking situation, the more terrifying it becomes.

Both situation and word fears can serve as *maintaining* causes of the disorder. By constantly reinforcing them by avoidance, the stutterer keeps his stuttering "hot." Any therapy worthy of the name must have as one of its basic aims the elimination of this avoidance. Stuttering begins to break down and disappear as soon as the stutterer ceases his constant reinforcing.

Avoidance Behavior. The stuttering picture shown by those who have progressed to this fourth stage in the development of stuttering can best be understood in terms of avoidance and escape. Let us be very clear about what is being avoided and escaped. It is the experience of finding a part of the body mysteriously oscillating or fixating; it is the experience of having communication blocked and retarded; it is the experience of behaving in a way which other people penalize.

No one likes to have feelings of frustration, anxiety, guilt, or hostility. When these feelings appear in conjunction with repetitive or prolonged interruptions in the flow of speech, those interruptions will be viewed as highly unpleasant. The stutterer will seek to prevent, avoid, or escape from repetitions which keep repeating, from prolongations of a sound or posture which persist. It is very important that we understand that, to the secondary stutterer, this repeating and prolonging appears to be involuntary, uncontrollable, mysterious. When this behavior is anticipated, the stutterer tries to avoid it; when it has occurred, the stutterer tries to escape from it.

How the Stutterer Avoids Stuttering. Since, in stage four, the secondary stutterer has learned to scan approaching speech situations for clues that indicate he will probably have difficulty, and since he has also learned to scrutinize the formulation of his sentences for "hard" words and sounds, he naturally tends to avoid these words and situations. One of our child cases just stopped talking altogether; one of our adults became a hermit in the Ozarks. But most stutterers cannot use this drastic solution to their problem. They continue to talk, but they talk as little as possible in these feared situations, and avoid or alter them if possible. It is often difficult for the nonstutterer to realize that much of the abnormality he witnesses in examining a stutterer is due to the latter's efforts to avoid unpleasantness. The desire to avoid stuttering may lead to such jargon as "To what price has the price of tomatoes increased today?" when the stutterer merely wished to say "How much are your tomatoes?" Dodging difficult words and speech situations becomes almost a matter of second nature to the stutterer. He prefers to seem ignorant rather than to expose his disability when called upon in school. He develops such a facility at using synonyms that he often sounds like an excerpt from a thesaurus. He will walk a mile to avoid using a telephone. And the tragedy of this avoidance is that it increases the fear and insecurity, makes the stutterer more hesitant, and doubles his burden.

Postponement.   Procrastination as a reaction to approaching unpleasantness is an ordinary human trait, and the stutterer has more than his share of the weakness. We have worked with stutterers whose entire overt abnormality consisted of the filibustering repetition of words and phrases preceding the dreaded word. They never had any difficulty on the word itself, but their efforts to postpone the speech attempt until they felt they could say the word produced an incredible amount of abnormality. One of them said, "My name is . . . my name is . . . my . . . my . . . my name is . . . my name . . . name . . . name . . . what I mean is, uh . . . uh . . . my name is Jack Olson." Others will merely pause in tense silence for what seems to them like hours before blurting out the word. Others disguise the postponement by pretending to think, by licking their lips, by saying "um" or "er." Postponement as a habitual approach to feared words creates an anxiety and a fundamental hesitancy which in themselves precipitate more stuttering.

Starters.   Stutterers also use many tricks to start the speech attempt after postponement has grown painfully long. They time this moment of speech attempt with a sudden gesture, or eye-blink, or jaw-jerk, or other movement. They return to the beginning of the sentence and race through the words preceding the feared word in hope that their momentum will "ride them over their stoppages." They insert words, phrases, or sounds that they can say, so that the likelihood of blocking will be lessened. One of the stutterers hissed before every feared word, "because I get started with the *s* sound which I can nearly always make." Another used the phrase "Let me see" as a magic incantation. He would utter things like this: "My name is Lemesee Peter Slack." Another, whose last name was Ranney, always passed as O'Ranney, since she used the "oh" as a habitual device to get started. Starters are responsible for many of the bizarre symptoms of stuttering, since they become habituated and involuntary. Thus, the taking of a deep breath prior to speech attempt may finally become a sequence of horrible gasping.

Antiexpectancy. The antiexpectancy devices are used to prevent or minimize word fears from dominating the attention of the stutterer. Thus, one of our cases laughed constantly, even when saying the alphabet or asking central for a phone number or buying a package of cigarettes. He had found that, by assuming an attitude incompatible with fear, he was able to be more fluent. Yet he was one of the most morose individuals we have ever met. Other stutterers adopt a singsong style, or a monotone, or a very soft, whispered speech so that all words are made so much alike that no one will be dreaded. Needless to say, all these tricks fail to provide more than temporary relief, and all of them are vicious because they augment the fear in the long run.

How the Stutterer Tries to Escape. As we have said earlier, the experience of finding one's mouth repeating a syllable uncontrollably or discovering one's tongue or lips frozen in a fixed posture is not only unpleasant but almost terrifying. There is an overwhelming desire to escape from this experience, to "break the block," to "get free from it," to find release. These are the stutterer's own words. Williams has clearly expressed this common experience of the mysterious something which holds the stutterer in *its* mysterious grip.[22] Undesired perseveration in any activity is traumatic. It makes one doubt one's will. It violates the integrity of the self.

Interrupter Devices. The fast little vibrations called tremors which first appear during the third stage are very prevalent in secondary stuttering. They are produced by highly tensing the muscles that form a fixed posture, often an abnormal one. When triggered by a sudden ballistic movement or surge of tension, the tremors come into being. The stutterer doesn't know what they are, or how he sets them off. All he knows is that some part of him is vibrating, and it scares him as it would you. In some stutterers several structures will be vibrating at the same time—the lips, the jaw, and the diaphragm, and often at different rates. The case attempts to free himself from the tremor by increasing the tension or by using some interrupter device similar to the starter tricks he has used to initiate speech attempt after prolonged postponement. He tries to wrench himself out of the frozen vibration of the tremor by sheer force. Even as he closes the articulatory door of the tongue or lips and holds it tightly shut, he strives to blow it open with a blast of air from below. When the opposing forces are equal, nothing happens except the quivering of the muscles. Oddly enough no stutterer tries to open the speech doors voluntarily; he must break them down with a surge of power. As in transitional stuttering, the random struggling often results in out-of-phase movements of the vibrating structures which cause a release from tremor and make possible the utter-

[22] D. Williams, "A Point of View About Stuttering," *Journal of Speech and Hearing Disorders*, XXII (1957), 390–97.

ance of the word. One stutterer may squeeze his eyes shut; another will jerk his whole trunk; another may suck air in through his nostrils. These peculiar reactions have become habituated through their chance presence at the moment of tremor release. The anxiety reduction, the freedom from punishment, give them their compulsive strength. The stutterer comes to feel that only through using them can he ever escape from the dreadful feeling of inability which the tremor creates in him. Even when they do not give release, he will try them over again, sniffing, not once, but twenty and thirty times in his desperate effort to free himself from the mysterious closure that his opposing efforts have produced. There are easier ways to terminate tremors than these, but few stutterers ever find them without the aid of a therapist.

Other Reactions of Escape.   It is obvious that the same devices used to interrupt tremors can also be used to interrupt repetitions or prolongations of sounds, syllables, or postures. A few stutterers split their words, giving up the attempt to produce an integrated word and finishing it after a gap. They would say "MMMMMM . . . other." More frequently the stutterer responds to the experience by ceasing the speech attempt and making a retrial, often only to find himself again in the same predicament. He may stop upon feeling an interruption in speech flow and try the entire word again: he may stop and use some starting device on the retrial, stop and use a distraction, stop and assume a confident behavior, stop and postpone the new attempt for a time, stop and avoid the word, or stop and wait until almost all breath is gone, subsequently saying the word on residual air.

Stuttering as a Self-reinforcing Disorder.   We have said that usually when stuttering develops into its fourth stage, little hope can be held that it will be "outgrown" or disappear. Even when the environment is changed so that it is permissive and free from fluency disruptors, the person continues to stutter. A few individuals are able to escape even after they enter this stage only because their morale is powerfully strengthened through other achievements. But usually, once fear and frustration, avoidance and escape have shown themselves, the disorder becomes self-perpetuating. As a response, it becomes the stimulus to other stuttering responses. It is necessary to understand how this comes about.

The Vicious Circle.   Not only is word fear able to beget stuttering symptoms; it almost seems to be able to reproduce itself. When words or situations are perceived as being full of unpleasantness, the stutterer tends to avoid them. He not only becomes more hesitant in his speech, but also in his general behavior. He escapes from the approach-avoidance misery by refusing to talk, or by using a synonym instead of the word that scares him, or by putting off the speech attempt as long as possible. But the future fear is increased by each successful avoidance. Here is an excerpt from a stutterer's autobiography:

> For years I ducked *k* and *g* words. They were my "Jonah" sounds. They always made me stutter. So I just wouldn't use them. There are lots of ways a stutterer has of hiding his running away from the words he can't say, and I knew all of them and used them. But then, when I was fifteen, my folks moved to Kenmore Street in Greenwood, and I had to give my address using the feared sounds. I would avoid all I could, but there are some times when you can't and you just have to say it. Well, I stuttered harder and longer and more awful on that Kenmore word than any other I've ever said. And even now I'm more afraid of *k* words than of any other. I think it's because I backed away from them so long.

What happens is this: The successful avoidance causes some anxiety reduction. Then, when a similar situation presents itself, the need to avoid is even stronger due to the preceding reinforcement. But now, no avoidance is possible. The conflict becomes even greater. And so several vicious circles (or rather spirals) are set into motion. The more one stutters, the more he fears certain words and situations. The more he fears, the more he stutters. The more he stutters, the harder he struggles. The more he struggles, the more penalties he receives, and the greater becomes his fear. The more he fears, the more he avoids; and the more he avoids speech, the more he fears speaking. And so the stutterer becomes caught in the tangled ropes of his own knotting. Once stuttering creates fear, and this fear, more fear and more stuttering, the disorder can exist on a self-sustaining basis. It can maintain and perpetuate itself even though the original causes may long since have lost all effectiveness and importance. Predisposing or precipitating causes have little importance, once the chain reaction gets going. Perhaps it is for this reason that deep psychotherapy has had but meager success with stuttering. Once stuttering becomes not only a response but also a stimulus, it must be attacked directly.

Personality Changes. In our own clinical studies of stuttering development over the years, it seems that many stutterers begin to show marked changes in personality after they enter the fourth stage of secondary stuttering. Many of them respond to their unpleasant experiences by becoming shy, withdrawn, and aloof. When a group of adult stutterers is compared with a comparable group of normal speakers, the stutterers do appear different, usually more anxious, tense, and socially withdrawn. However, adult stutterers *as a group* are not primarily neurotic or severely maladjusted. Perhaps the wisest course is to assess the degree of maladjustment in any one case. Some stutterers have more traumatic experiences than others. Some are more vulnerable. Some show marked personality changes; others do not. As Murphy and Fitz-Simons write: "A reasonably broad interpretation of the greater number of research findings on the stuttering personality may be that the personalities of stuttering persons can be distributed along a very broad adjustment *continuum* extending from psychotic to normal adjustment." [23]

In our clinical work with severe adult stutterers we find this range described by Murphy. Some of them show obsessive, compulsive behavior and general anxieties, guilts, and hostilities which are far from normal. They show the pattern characteristic of what Freund calls an "expectancy neurosis." This is how Freund describes it:

> The expectancy neuroses represent neurotic disturbances of learned but automatized skills, and also of simple motor or vegetative functions. They are all based on actual traumatic ("primary") experiences of helplessness and failure in the performance of these activities. The activities therefore become dreaded and the anticipation of their recurrence leads, via inhibition, etc., to a repetition of the failure, thus establishing a vicious spiral. [24]

What we are saying is that the experiences of a stutterer in the final stage of stuttering are such that the *possibility* of a marked change in personality can be expected—the possibility, not the certainty. Indeed, in working with these people, we are constantly surprised that so many of them appear pretty normal except in communication. We find the odd ones, but we also find others who seem to have made the best of a bad situation. It is our impression that those whose stuttering seems to stem from constitutional factors make the best adjustment; those of developmental origin, the next best, and those whose stuttering comes from basic emotional conflicts, the worst.

SUMMARY

Perhaps the best way we can summarize this material is to use the picture or map in Figure 27. Stuttering has three sources; the major one represented by the largest, Lake Learning, into which the stream from Constitutional Reservoir flows. Neurosis Pond is also one of the sources of stuttering, but it is smaller. Its contribution to the flow also occurs further down the river's course. Stuttering can come from any of these three sources.

[23] A. T. Murphy and R. M. Fitz-Simons, *Stuttering and Personality Dynamics* (New York: The Ronald Press Company, 1960), p. 153.

[24] H. Freund, "Psychopathological Aspects of Stuttering," *American Journal of Psychotherapy*, VII (1953), 679.

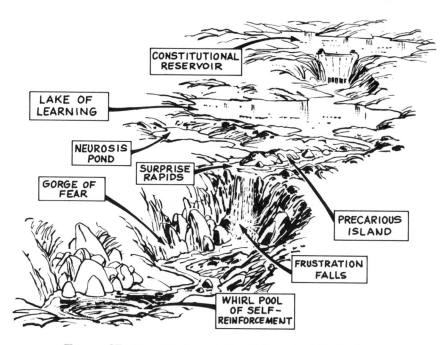

FIGURE 27: *The Origin and Development of Stuttering*

As the stream leaves Lake Learning, it flows slowly and many a child caught in its current may make it to shore by himself or with a bit of parental or therapeutic help. Some of them are cast up on Precarious Island and become fluent for a time, only to be swept away again by the swift-moving emotional currents from Neurosis Pond. The second stage in the development of stuttering is represented by Surprise Rapids, and the stutterer begins to know that he is in trouble. It isn't hard to rescue him, however, if you know how to do it.

Once he is swept over Frustration Falls, however, he takes a beating from the many rocks that churn the stream. Despite their random struggling, a few make it to shore even at this stage, the third, but they usually need an understanding therapist and cooperative parents to help them. The river flows even faster here, and soon it enters the Gorge of Fear. This is the worst stretch of the whole stream of stuttering, for below it lies the Whirlpool of Self-reinforcement. Once the child is caught in its constant circling, there is little hope that he will ever make it to shore by himself. Only an able and stout swimmer who knows not only this part, but all of the river of stuttering, can hope to save him. Where does the river end? King Charles the First knows.

The Treatment of Stuttering

One of the fascinating things about this disorder is that literally hundreds of methods for successfully helping stutterers have been reported. Many of these are mutually contradictory; some of them, on first glance, make no sense whatsoever. Yet we do not doubt the honesty of these reports. Some stutterers have been helped and even cured by each of these many diverse procedures; the same procedures applied to other stutterers have failed.

We know an elocutionist who cures stutterers by drill in mental multiplication. We have seen a few of them before treatment and afterward. There is no doubt that they were helped. We have also seen some of her cases who showed no improvement and who actually got worse. We would explain her successes as the result of the increased motivation. The children who improved were deprived, young, rather dull children. They had few personality assets, and their initial morale was low. They were not severe stutterers. Their situation and word fears were mild and infrequent. Most of the penalty they had received was for their poverty and poor grades in school. They had not reacted very much to their stuttering by frustration, anxiety, guilt, or hostility. No one had expected much of them, nor had they expected much of themselves. Fortunately for them, the elocutionist is an older woman, child-hungry, unmarried, and she gave these children her love and time and faith without measure. She was very patient with them. She believed that they would be cured if they could only learn how to multiply in their heads; and they also came to believe it. She did not penalize their stuttering. She ignored it. As a result of her drilling, they became able to astound and astonish their schoolmates, their parents, and their teachers with their often-paraded ability to solve these problems. Their stuttering decreased and finally disappeared. The elocutionist believed it was the mental multiplication that was the healing agent. Our own belief is that it was the morale, motivation, and self-confidence they had attained.

Two stutterers with about the same amount of stuttering may have completely different problems so far as therapy is concerned. Because of his habitual avoidance of speaking, one stutterer's situation and word fears can be very intense; another stutterer may show the reverse. It is the therapist's task to study each individual stutterer until she knows which *factors* are especially important in the picture he presents and then to work especially hard to weaken or strengthen these, while not forgetting the others.

We especially wish to emphasize the plural of the word *factors*. The weakness of most therapy with stutterers is that it has concentrated on only one or two of these. The psychiatrist who works to relieve anxiety, guilt, and hostility may do his job well; but the person will still stutter if his stuttering still brings penalty or frustration, or if his situation and phonetic fears have not been decreased by speech therapy. And morale alone, like love, is not enough for many stutterers. It may be for a few special ones, such as the occasional television or movie star who says he formerly stuttered—but not for most stutterers. We need a many-pronged therapy if we are to help most of our stutterers. A one-pronged therapy will help the special few who present unusual equations in which the factor hit by the prong is of major importance. It will fail with the others. There are too many factors operating in stuttering.

In the light of what we have just said, let us look at some of the ways stuttering has been treated. One of the earliest accounts goes back to ancient Greece literature, and it tells of one Battos who went to the Oracle of Delphi to find out how he could be freed of his stuttering. The Oracle gave him this prescription: "Exile yourself forever to a foreign land and never come back." We have had a few ornery cases to whom we were tempted to offer the same advice. But there is a fighting chance that Battos was helped by the Oracle's prescription. A change of environment often decreases situation fears and also permits an escape from some of the sources of conflicts in the original life situation. Or perhaps he found a Parthian maiden who loved him completely even unto the elbows, and so his self-esteem soared. Let us hope that Battos was cured, but if he was, let us understand why.

During the Middle Ages, the tongues of stutterers were burned; and even as recently as fifty years ago they were sliced surgically. Cures were reported. Once, long ago, the French government paid several hundred thousand francs for the secret stuttering cure of a Madame Leigh, who was said to have phenomenal success in treating stammerers. Her secret, when finally exposed, consisted of a small pad of cotton rolled up and held under the tongue during speech. Bizarre? Of course, but even apart from the faith healing and confidences which might have been engendered, we can see why a few stutterers might have been helped at least for a time. If your mouth and tongue were hurting or if you had to hold a pad under it, you'd have a hard time pressing that tongue hard enough to precipitate a tremor. You'd find yourself not struggling so hard. You'd find yourself expecting to have some long hard blocks and then having little ones or not having any. And so the frustration would go down, and so would the fears of words and sounds. And so would the stuttering.

About 150 years ago, a man called Columbat treated stutterers by having them say each syllable of their speech as they waved their arm or tapped on a table. This method is still in use today, even though it has had a long history of failure. But doubtless, like every other method, it has had a few successes, because, for the moment, it can reduce or eliminate most of the stuttering in most stutterers. What it does is to make all words very much alike. It reduces phonetic fears by distraction. It reduces the communicative meaningfulness of speech. It is an antiexpectancy device. Like most distractions, however, as soon as it becomes habituated, it loses its power to distract and often becomes a part of the compulsive symptomatology. There are better ways to reduce the fears of sounds and words.

Relaxation has also been used as a basic treatment for stuttering. In the late 1800s, Sandow trained his stutterers to achieve states of calm relaxation and serenity and found that much of the stuttering disappeared. (He reported some difficulty in transferring the relaxed states and the consequent fluency into situations outside his clinical facilities.) Since deep relaxation is incompatible with fear or struggle, dramatic decreases in stuttering occur in the safe situations of the therapy room; but outside, in the world of knives, it is difficult to stay relaxed enough to maintain the fluency. Nevertheless, relaxation therapy for stutterers has been used for many years all over the world.

During the last years of the nineteenth century and the first years of the twentieth, most of the treatment offered stutterers was carried out in residential centers or homes called "stammerers' institutes," usually under the direction of some former stutterer who had managed to achieve some fluency. Exorbitant fees were charged, and guaranteed promises of cure were offered in the advertisements of these institutions. The author of this text attended three of them in his youth, and he remembers wryly that the guaranteed cure at one of them was qualified by the condition that the stutterer must follow all instructions. Instruction number nine was that the stutterers must not stutter! At these institutes, group therapy was offered, the stutterers doing breathing exercises for hours, reciting isolated sounds and word drills, chanting and singing, relaxing, and speaking each syllable or each word in unison with a wide arm-swing or a finger-tap. Strong suggestion, almost hypnotic in nature, was made that if the stutterer followed the secret method, he would be completely cured. Each moment of stuttering was immediately punished and fluency was rewarded. Under this ironclad discipline and the safe protection of isolation from the real world that was provided by the institute, most of the stutterers became remarkably fluent; but the precarious fluency so attained disappeared as soon as they returned to their homes. With the advent of the new profession of speech pathology, most of these commercial institutes disappeared from the scene; but many of their methods, alas, are still in use today.

Current Methods for Treating Stuttering. At the present time we find three major types of therapy being used for stuttering: psychotherapy, techniques used to repress stuttering and to augment fluent speech, and the type of therapy advocated in this text which seeks to teach the stutterer how to stutter fluently. So far as psychotherapy is concerned, in addition to counseling and psychoanalytic procedures (which have not been shown to be particularly effective with the stutterer), we find such variants as the therapy advocated by Trojan (1965).[25] Stutterers in this treatment have sessions with the therapist where they act out and verbalize their deepest feelings for the people who have played important parts in their lives. There are also the "paradoxical intention" methods of Frankl, who has the stutterer seek out and desire the stuttering he dreads.[26] We also find the autogenic therapy of Schultz, in which an autohypnotic training including relaxation frees the stutterer from his fears and morbidity.[27] The whole field of psychotherapy is in flux, and many different psychotherapeutic approaches are currently being used with stutterers.

In the second type of approach, we also find many of the old forms of treatment being employed, though now for other reasons, but all of them seek to prevent the occurrence of stuttering. The time-beat methods in which the stutterer speaks his words or syllables in unison with finger-tapping or pulses of tone from a minature electronic metronome worn behind the ear are still being used.[28]

For example, the use of unison speech to prevent the occurrence of stuttering still continues, and a variant of this approach is called *shadowing*. Stutterers are trained to echo the speech of the therapist as simultaneously as possible. By proceeding from slow and easy materials to more spontaneous and complex, the stutterers show an immediate and marked gain in fluency.

Relaxation now appears also in the form of systematic desensitization training, the stutterer being trained in deep relaxation as he imagines himself in a series of speaking situations arranged in a hierarchic order of increasing difficulty. By repeatedly imagining each one of these in turn until the anxiety is dissipated, the stutterer is said to become free from his fears and consequently to be able to speak without stuttering. The relaxation state is supposed to reciprocally inhibit the fear and finally to extinguish it. The treatment is based upon classical conditioning. One long-term experimental study of the effects of systematic desensitization

[25] F. Trojan, "Causal Treatment of Neurotic Stuttering," *De Therapia Vocis et Loquellae*, I (1965), 265–68.

[26] V. E. Frankl, *The Doctor and the Soul* (New York: Alfred A. Knopf, Inc., 1966).

[27] W. Luthe, and J. H. Schultz, *Autogenic Therapy*, Vols. I and III (New York: Grune & Stratton, Inc., 1969).

[28] M. T. Wohl, "The Electric Metronome—An Evaluative Study," *British Journal of Disorders of Communication*, III (1968), 89–98; J. P. Brady, "Studies of the Metronome Effect on Stuttering," *Behavior Research and Therapy*, VII (1969), 197–204.

training was performed by Gray.[29] Although fifteen of his thirty subjects dropped out of the training before it was completed, the remainder did show significant reductions in anxiety and some reduction in stuttering. However, Gray concluded that "clinical observation and final disposition of the subjects suggest that in real life there was little effect of the anxiety reduction upon the frequency [of stuttering]. However there were noticeable changes informally noted in the degree of the severity of stuttering."

Operant conditioning methods are also being employed today, but most of these efforts have consisted of experimental demonstrations that a reduction in stuttering can be produced by contingently punishing moments of stuttering. Electric shocks, very loud tones, verbal disapprovals, the mandatory cessation of speaking (Time-Outs), and dosing with delayed feedback have been some of the aversive procedures used.[30]

The third major type of therapy current today (and the treatment advocated in this text is a variant thereof) is an eclectic one; but its core difference lies in its insistence that much of the abnormality of utterance shown by the stutterer consists of learned behaviors and that these can be unlearned or modified sufficiently to enable the stutterer to speak with reasonable fluency. Essentially, the stutterer is taught to stutter differently rather than to avoid stuttering, and the difference lies in the absence of struggle or inhibition or avoidance. He must learn to stutter fluently and with a minimum of interruption or struggle. Advocates of this therapy insist that the stutterer does not need to learn how to speak fluently. He already knows how to do this. What he doesn't know is how to speak disfluently. He therefore is taught to respond to his fears and experiences of speech interruption without forcing or avoidance or struggle or disguise. We repeat: he does not need to learn how to talk without stuttering. This he already knows, for most of his speech is fluently spoken. What he doesn't know is how to stutter—how to stutter fluently and without marked interruptions or struggle. This therapy is a modification therapy using the shaping of behavior, it seeks to teach the stutterer not how to speak normally but how to stutter and still be fluent. At first glance, this approach seems paradoxical, but any close examination of any stutterer will reveal that he always has some times when he stutters with a minimum of abnormality and interruption.

Moreover, this type of treatment is not solely concerned with the overt stuttering behaviors alone. It seeks also to deal with the same fea-

---

[29] B. B. Gray, *Some Effects of Anxiety Deconditioning upon Stuttering Behavior* (Monterey, Calif.: Monterey Institute for Speech and Hearing, 1968).

[30] A critical presentation of the illustrated methods used in applying operant and classical conditioning procedures to stuttering can be found in C. E. Starkweather, ed., *Conditioning Approaches in Stuttering Therapy* (Memphis, Tenn.: Speech Foundation of America, 1970).

tures that are the focus of psychotherapy—the stutterer's anxieties, guilt, and hostility and the consequences of the penalties and frustrations he has experienced. In many ways it includes an essential psychotherapeutic approach. It deals with his situation and word fears, with his morale and self-concept, with his misperceptions. We cannot confine our efforts to the stutterer's mouth alone. Many different factors are involved in the clinical picture presented by the stutterer. If we are to help him, we must deal with all of them.

A *Design for Stuttering Therapy*.   Two very important facts serve as the foundation of our own therapy for stuttering: (1) stuttering is intermittent, and (2) its specific occurrence, frequency, and severity vary systematically with the strength of certain factors which can be defined and manipulated. If we can focus our therapy on these factors so that those which make stuttering worse are weakened sufficiently and those which make for less stuttering are strengthened, the frequency and severity of stuttering will decrease, and ultimately stuttering will disappear. Therapy then is viewed as selective reinforcement and extinction. Stuttering is no mysterious curse to be eliminated by incantation or voodoo practices. Like all human behavior, it obeys certain laws.

The *Focus of Theory*.   These are the things which make stuttering worse: (1) penalty, frustration, anxiety, guilt, and hostility; (2) situation fears based on memories of past stuttering unpleasantness in similar situations; (3) word and phonetic fears based on memories of past stuttering unpleasantness on similar words and sounds. There is also a fourth factor, C, representing the communicative importance of that which is being said. Stutterers stutter more on messages and words which are especially important in communication. Stuttering, as numerous researches have shown, increases with the propositionality (communicative meaningfulness) of the material read or the thing said. There are also many things which seem to make stuttering better, but all of them appear to fit into the category of morale or ego strength and the experience of fluency.

Frequency and Severity.   The frequency and severity of stuttering usually vary with the amount of communicative stress. Most stutterers speak fluently when alone or in talking to pets or when reading in unison. A few do not. A few even stutter when they sing.

Why do we have such variations in the frequency and severity of stuttering? What causes it to appear and disappear? Why are some stutterings worse than others? We have tried to answer all these difficult questions by formulating one mathematical equation which we hope will not cause the student to bury his head beneath the covers, but instead to recognize that it will help him assemble and remember a mass of information which might otherwise be a bit indigestible. What this equation tells us is that stuttering becomes more frequent and gets more severe when:

P   Penalties are placed upon it, or past penalties are remembered,
F   Frustrations of any type are experienced or remembered,
A   Anxiety is present,
G   Guilt is felt,
H   Hostility needs to be expressed;

when:

Sf   There are situation fears due to old memories of past unpleasantness in the situation,
Wf   Certain sounds and words are feared due to old unpleasant
memories;

and when:

Cs   The speaking situation is full of communicative stress (listener-
loss, interruptions, etc.) or there are very important things to say
(propositionality).

These are the factors which make stuttering worse. They form the items
on the upper line of the equation: the dividend part.

But there are other factors which *decrease* stuttering: the morale
factor and the amount of fluency the stutterer also experiences along with
his stuttering. Some stutterers have a lot of fluent speech; others have little.
The more they have, the less likely they are to have frequent and severe
stuttering. We can represent these two factors in the divisor part of our
equation thus:

M   Morale or ego strength or self-confidence,
Fl   The amount of felt fluency.

Here then is our equation:

$$S = \frac{(PFAGH) + (Sf\,Wf) + Cs}{M + Fl}$$

This is an important equation. It explains many things about stuttering. It says that when the stutterer's morale or ego strength is high because
of achievements, success, and social acceptance, he will tend to stutter less.
If in any given communicative situation he expects or feels communicative
stress, penalties, and frustration he will stutter more. He will stutter more
if he is experiencing on anticipating anxiety, guilt, and hostility. He will
also stutter more if in scanning ahead he sees words or situations coming
which have been associated with past experiences of stuttering. Stutterers

have more trouble talking to authority figures, to people who become impatient or mock or suffer when listening to stuttering. Most stutterers are very vulnerable to listener-loss, to interruptions, to rejections, penalty, frustration, anxiety, and hostility. The pressures, then, which create more stuttering can come from without or within, from the pressures of the present, the expected agonies of the future, or the miseries of the past.

In any given speaking situation the amount of communicative stress varies. Some people are good listeners; others are bad ones. Some heckle us with constant interruptions. Some say the unfinished words for the stutterer. Some look away. Again, the message to be spoken may be difficult to express. Thinking may be confused, and so the formulation may falter. The urgency to speak very swiftly may be present. All these factors and many others put the pressure on fluency and tend to disrupt it. We include all of them under the category of communicative stress.

Our C factor also includes, as we have said, the communicative importance of the utterance. This is termed "propositionality." Stutterers often can read in unison with others without stuttering. They can blurt out whole sentences as "asides" without a bit of trouble. But when they have something important to say, something urgent that must be said quickly, they have a tough time. Even little children in the first stage of stuttering often tend to have more difficulty on certain words than others because these words carry most of the utterance's meaning. These words, therefore, carry more communicative stress. When the primary stutterer comes running home from school full of important information to communicate to his parents, his stuttering comes tumbling out in volleys; when he talks to himself or his dog, he is very fluent. There's not much propositionality in what he has to say.

As part of our general equation, we referred to morale or ego strength as a favorable factor. When stutterers are feeling confident, they don't stutter as much. The better they feel about themselves, the less they stutter. This is what one of our high-school cases wrote in his autobiography:

> All I need is self-confidence. The trouble is I haven't got much, and every time I block, I lose most of what I have. I notice that when I bring home a report card full of A's, I can talk better. For a time, a little time. When I manage to get a date with a good-looking girl and have fun, my speech almost becomes free. If I ask for a date and get turned down, I block all over the place. I finally got up nerve enough to ask for a job at a grocery after school, and got it! I felt so good from becoming partly independent and earning my own money that for two or three days I had more free speech than I've ever had. So what I need is for you to give me more self-confidence.

Unfortunately, morale is not a gift. It cannot be injected by any therapist. It is earned by acquiring more personality assets and by learning to cope with one's liabilities. Confidence comes when we do battle and succeed. It comes when we accept a challenge instead of running away from it. It gains strength when we lick our wounds after a defeat and return to the fray. It goes down when we grow morbid and bathe in self-pity. It rises when we confront ourselves, accept our limitations, and start working to fulfill our potentials despite those limitations. One of the tasks of the therapist, if he is to help the stutterer to talk more freely, is to assist him in understanding these things.

The other major favorable factor is the fluency factor (Fl). By this we mean the overall amount of real fluency the person has been having in similar speaking situations. Some stutterers seldom speak a sentence without some blocking. Others can be very fluent at times. Their sentences flow smoothly, not jerkily, when they are not stuttering. We are always alert, when examining a new stutterer, to listen not only to the stuttering but also to the smoothness of his nonstuttered speech. Those who falter, pause, hem and haw, speak by spurts, can be said to have a low amount of Fl, and their clinical problems are going to be more difficult. They will need to be taught how to make their normal as well as their abnormal speech fluent. When the morale is high and the person can be very fluent, it will take a lot of $PFAGH$ and fear and communicative stress to make him stutter.

Our task in therapy, then, is to assess the strengths of the various factors that play a significant part in the problems of each individual stutterer, and then to reduce these factors to as low a level as possible. No two stutterers will present identical equations. The treatment should be tailored to the individual needs as assessed. We have worked with stutterers who had very high morale, with others who had met few penalties. And there are some who have no word fears at all. Each stutterer presents a different diagnostic picture. This may be made clear by considering the clinical problem presented by a beginning stutterer who is markedly nonfluent, but is quite unaware of the fact.

TREATMENT OF EARLY STUTTERING

In our discussion of the development of stuttering we have seen that most children show their first marked stuttering behavior during the ages from two to six. There are a few who begin later and usually these are individuals whose stuttering originates in a primary neurosis or follows a severe illness such as encephalitis. They begin to struggle, fear, and avoid almost from the first. Most stutterers whose disorders seem to originate in the communicative pressures of speech-learning or whose histories indicate a possible constitutional etiology tend to show the excessive repetitions and prolongations of syllables and sounds and postures of early stuttering. And they appear to have very little situation or word fear. Accordingly, they present a different therapeutic problem from those of the more advanced stages. Their problem, expressed in terms of our equation, is this:

$$\frac{(PFAGH) + Cs}{M + F} = S$$

Penalty Reduction. Our task, then, is to reduce the penalties they are experiencing, not only those which parents are placing on the speech interruptions, but all penalties. They need more permissiveness and less punishment.

> One of our primary stutterers who showed the behavior of the first stage was having a very bad time with his speech. The first word of almost every utterance was spoken with repetitions or prolongations. Often the repetitions would continue for several seconds. He would say, "Ca-ca-ca-ca-ca-ca-ca-ca can I go now? His frantic parents, who had been asking him to "Stop that!" or to "Stop and begin over again!" followed our advice and ceased these admonitions. The reduction of this penalty reduced the stuttering, but too much still remained. We then discovered that they were also breaking him of the habit of sucking his thumb." As soon as we persuaded them to stop their efforts in this regard, the child stopped stuttering completely. We had reduced the *P* factor in his equation.

Reducing Frustration. Children in the first stage usually experience little frustration so far as their stuttering is concerned. A bit of it comes in during the second stage when the major reaction is the occasional expression of surprise and bewilderment, and the repetitions become faster, more irregular, and end in prolongations of a sound or posture. The child, without knowing why, is beginning at this stage to sense that speaking is hard work at times, that it isn't easy. But the major frustrations come from other sources, from the daily business of living in a world geared to the needs of others as well as to one's own needs. One of the sad things about our culture is that the age of speech-learning is made to coincide with the application of so many taboos. During the preschool years, there are so many things that a little child must learn he musn't do. The frequency of usage of the word "No!" by mothers of children of this age is probably exceeded only by that of the expression, "Oh dear!" All children of this age hear a hundred "No's" each day of their lives, and some children hear more, or feel the sharp slap of a heavy hand on their bottoms. We do not wonder that the age of three is a negativistic age; the demands for conformity are especially heavy then. All this means frustration. The child must indeed learn to behave the way our culture says he must. But he can't help feeling plenty of frustration.

In counseling our parents we must help them to understand the role of frustration in precipitating stuttering. We cannot ask them to stop being culture carriers. Their own needs for a peaceful, reasonably quiet, and orderly home life would then be frustrated. They know that each of us must learn to inhibit some of our infantile urges if we are to live in a civilized society. A child must learn to respect the needs of others. A totally ungovernable and spoiled child is an excrescence in any household. Are we then caught in a dilemma? On the one hand, to reduce the stuttering, we must reduce the frustration; on the other, if we do so, we create a continuing annoyance in the home who will provoke penalty outside the home if not within it.

The solution to the dilemma is simply to help the parents do two things: (1) *reduce* the number of the child's frustrating experiences, and (2) build up his frustration tolerance. There is no need to eliminate all frustration; we merely need to decrease it. Indeed, since life is always bound to hold many frustrations in store, it is wise to help our children learn to tolerate them.

> In counseling the mother of another of our primary stutterers, we first got her to express most of her own frustrations not only in child rearing but also in other areas. Then when the river ran dry we explained a bit about the role of frustration in stuttering, gave her a little hand counter and asked her to click it every time she used a forbidding "No!" to the boy. The first day's total was 186; the second day's 132; the third day's 71; and on the fourth day she brought back the counter, saying that Junior had stopped stuttering.

We need not and we cannot eliminate frustration; but we always can reduce it.

Increasing Frustration Tolerance.   Many an adult should learn the lesson that it is possible to increase one's tolerance for frustration. The inappropriate infantile behavior shown by our frustrated friends (never ourselves!) is evidence that somewhere along the growth line, many of us fail to learn this lesson. Perhaps it is because we have never had the teacher we needed. There are two major ways in which we can build up frustration tolerance. One is through the empathic understanding of the needs of others; the second is through desensitization or adaptation. We shall not go into the first of these save to say that children should learn that parents have rights too, and to give one illustration.

Willy was an *enfant terrible*. He had conquered his parents. He controlled them. The mother, a frantic, neurotic wisp of a woman, was very infantile herself and totally unable to cope with his nagging, his defiance, his temper tantrums. She even feared the little stuttering monster, for once he had chased her up the backstairs with a butcher knife. The father was a weak, colorless individual whose response to his miserable home life was to stay away from it as much as possible. We managed to get them to send the boy away for the summer to a camp, and for the rest of the year to an uncle's family where the laws of the Medes and the Persians and of the parents were clear and enforced. He had a bad time of it at first, but his stuttering disappeared as he learned to curb his pampered infantile urges and become a member of society. He had learned to recognize the needs of others.

The second way to build frustration tolerance involves conditioning. It follows one method for breaking a horse. First you put a cloth on the horse's back, then later a sand bag, then a saddle, then a brave little boy, and then you can jump aboard. It takes time and patience and plenty of gentling and loving along the way, but some horses are taught to accept their riders this way. Through parental counseling and observation of the child, the major frustrating factors are defined. Then they are introduced into the child's life very gradually, but persistently, and only to the degree that he can tolerate them. The consequence is that the child will adapt and gradually be able to tolerate more and more frustration.

Grant was almost four years old when volleys of stuttering appeared and went away in their usual fashion. For a week he would be very fluent; the next, he could hardly say a sentence without many repetitions. After several months of this, the repetitions began to come out irregularly and faster. Often they would end in a prolongation that rose in pitch. He did not seem to be aware of these interruptions, perhaps because he was so anxious to talk. He talked incessantly to anyone who would listen and to those like his elder brother and sister who often would not. The slightest loss of the listener's attention or any sign of the listener's impatience or any interruption seemed to precipitate a burst of stuttering. The periods of remission were shorter and further apart. He was in real danger. Occasionally he would stop and look bewildered. Talking was getting hard.

The parents fortunately were both understanding and cooperative. They loved the boy and there were no penalties to be decreased. There was little communicative stress in the picture. If anything, they had created conditions which made his communication too easy. If he began to talk, they stopped their own conversation. They asked few questions, talked slowly and simply, and gave him the floor whenever he wanted it. We could discern little evidence of emotional conflicts, anxiety, guilt or hostility. It was a wonderful home. Even the brother and sister seemed to understand, and they made things easier for Grant than most children would. The boy had simply developed an abnormal appetite for attention and for communication. He had been a bit delayed in speech and still had some errors in articulation. Perhaps, once he learned the magical power of speech, it was too good to lose. He had logorrhea. The more that appetite for speech was fed, the bigger it grew, and the less he could bear to have it frustrated.

We asked them to institute a progressive change in policy. First they were to give him their complete attention but gradually to introduce a few mild interruptions, a consciously averted glance, a slight delay in answering his questions, or in doing what he wanted. They were to do this judiciously so that the amount of his frustration would not be sufficient to precipitate stuttering. But they would put a bit of pressure on him. Then they were to return to the former policy of giving him complete attention, putting an arm around him and listening intently. Then they were to give him another dose of communicative frustration, a little larger one if possible, but again returning to the complete attention. We asked them to do this eight or nine times a day, gradually increasing the dosage of their inattention. Within a week they reported that Grant was now able to wait his turn, to accept delay in responding, to tolerate an occasional interruption. Within a month the stuttering was gone. We had reduced the large F value in his stuttering equation by increasing his ability to tolerate frustration. Frustrations other than those in speech can be handled in the same way. It is possible to build up frustration tolerance.

There is also another way of breaking a horse. You can jump on his back, drive in the spurs, and break his spirit to your will. We do not advocate this method for children, but we have known a few instances in which parents used this policy to teach their children to bear frustration. And again we have seen the stuttering disappear. But we do not advise this method. We want our children free.

Reducing Anxiety, Guilt, and Hostility.   We can reduce these reactions by reducing the penalties and frustrations which beget them. Secondly, outlets other than stuttering should be made available. Thirdly, the beginning stutterers needs extra reassurance that he is loved and accepted. We have already considered the first of these three sources; now let us discuss the second.

We find many homes where the need to express one's feelings of anxiety, guilt, and hostility is neither understood nor accepted. If a child reveals that he is afraid of big dogs, thunderstorms, going to bed, or anything else, he is subjected to ridicule and "shamed out of his silly fears." His confessions of guilt and shame evoke a slap or a smile or parental embarrassment. His expressions of hostility are punished. He soon learns to keep them to himself. But we repress these emotional acids at our peril. They want out! And they always find a way. With the stutterer, that way is often stuttering.

These taboos against emotional release can be changed for some children by parental counseling, but some parents are themselves too inhibited or emotionally involved to make the necessary changes. As Sanders says, "When parents cooperate in a counseling program with insight and determination, the outlook for the young stutterer is most favorable." [31] But there are parents who do not cooperate, who cannot accept counseling. What do we do then?

Play Therapy. We can offer the child an opportunity through play to release his forbidden feelings. We can provide him with at least one situation in which he finds a loved and loving adult who understands and accepts his feelings, who actually rewards their expression whether the child expresses them verbally or through acting-out. A quotation from the excellent book by Murphy and Fitz-Simons helps us understand what takes place in play therapy.

> One of the clinician's prime tasks is to estimate how the child is perceiving self, parents, and the world as well as how much he is distorting, misperceiving, and misinterpreting. In order to do this the clinician must provide situations and materials which will give the child the opportunities to *externalize* and project his deeper feelings. Play's therapeutic value lies in giving the child a chance to communicate some aspects of his inner world to an understanding adult, to reevaluate his perceptions and confusions; in short, to integrate. The clinician enters the child's world by allowing him to speak his own language, often a highly nonverbal, symbolic esoteric one. The child will express his needs to be aggressive; to be infantile; to suck; to mess; to do what he wants and needs to do. The child's formerly suppressed and derogated behavior will be reacted to differently by the clinician whose role is one of "new parents." The clinician submits and resubmits the child's fears, desires, hostilities, condemned wants and wishes to the child's self or conscious awareness for relearning and resocialization, for differentiation and the integration of self.[32]

We have used play therapy with many of our young stutterers and not only with those in whom we suspect a primary neurosis. Where anxieties, guilts, and hostility play an important part in the child's stuttering

[31] E. K. Sander, "Counseling Parents of Stuttering Childern," *Journal of Speech and Hearing Disorders*, XXIV (1959), 262.

[32] Albert T. Murphy and Ruth M. Fitz-Simons, *Stuttering and Personality Dynamics* (New York: The Ronald Press Company, 1960).

problem and when their expression at home is denied or prevented by the parents, play therapy is absolutely essential. Not all young stutterers need it. There are some children who show no more than a normal amount of these feelings and in whose problems other factors are more important. With the neurotic stutterer it is the treatment of choice.

Creative Dramatics.   Another method for relieving the pressures of anxiety, guilt, and hostility so that they do not contribute to the stuttering problem is that of creative dramatics. In this activity, the children, guided by an imaginative adult leader, improvise a play, take the various parts, and invent their own dialogue. Children frequently select and play parts which provide for the expression of their more intense feelings. Here is an account of an eight-year-old nonfluent child having this experience.

> He joined a creative dramatics group but took a relatively inactive part until one day when the children were playing the story of *King Midas and the Golden Touch.* Most of the children characterized King Midas as a grumpy man but not as a cruel one. Finally John said he wished to play King Midas. Suddenly the character of the king became completely different. Midas screamed at the servants, hit the table, ordered the impossible, ranted and raved and almost completely forgot the plot of the story. The children were impressed with the idea of the king, and a discussion followed. Several of the children thought that John had made King Midas too mean. Others thought maybe the previous attempts to play the king had been too mild. The children turned to John to get his opinion. "I think King Midas was a very cruel man. He's as mean as my teacher." [33]

We have found creative dramatics especially useful when much of the emotional conflict was due to sibling rivalry, fears of the local bully, or teasing by the child's playmates. In such instances, the child needs more than a permissive parent figure; he needs a permissive group. We find it very useful when play therapy fails because this particular child cannot come to have any trust in the therapist or any other adult. There are such children. There are also some children whose contact with reality is precariously slim. We do not use creative dramatics with these latter ones. Fantasy and role-playing have their dangers.

Parental Counseling.   We have referred frequently to the counseling of parents in the reduction of all of the factors that increase stuttering. Parents need education and information, but this is not all that counseling provides. They also need relief from their own anxieties, guilts, and hostilities. They need the opportunity to verbalize their own feelings in the presence of a permissive, understanding listener. They need to learn to view

[33] B. M. McIntyre and B. J. McWilliams, "Creative Dramatics in Speech Correction," *Journal of Speech and Hearing Disorders,* XXIV (1959), 277.

the stuttering child with strange eyes, objectively. Jointly with the therapist, they must explore all his problems, not just his stuttering. In so doing, they often realize their own perfectionistic strivings, their own childhood conflicts, their own present acting-out of relationships they had with their own parents long ago. There are many problems in counseling parents which produce difficulty. Some should be referred to the psychiatrist. With some, the conferences should be confined primarily to giving information. The depth of the counseling relationship should depend upon the therapist's own training and competence and on the severity of the interpersonal relationships which exist. There are Pandora's boxes no speech therapist should open.

Group Counseling. Often when the therapist can get a small group of parents together in the evening over coffee to discuss their mutual problem, the stuttering child, some real advantages are to be had. First of all, we are able to meet the fathers of these children, and often they play a most important role in the stuttering boy's difficulties. Secondly, through free discussion parents come to view their own children differently, more objectively. They get the opportunity to air and share their problems of parenthood. Each is a mirror for the other. Again the anxieties are verbalized, the guilt feelings explored, and the irritation exposed. Again the therapist plays the role of the catalyst. Group counseling can be very helpful.

Reducing the Communicative Stress. The final factor, C, in the dividend of our stuttering equation is communicative stress. All stutterers at any stage show more stuttering when they are bedeviled by the fluency-disrupting influences we now list. The beginning stutterer is especially vulnerable, and we have been able to cure more stutterers in stages one and two by reducing the fluency disruptors in the speech environment than by any other means.

How to Prevent Hesitant Speech. Hesitant speech (pauses, accessory vocalization, filibusters, abortive speech attempts) occurs as the result of two opposing forces. First, there must be a strong need to communicate; and second, this urge must be blocked by some counterpressure. Some of the common counterpressures which oppose the desire for utterance are:

1. *Inability to find or remember the appropriate words.* "I'm thinking of-of-of-of-uh that fellow who-uh—oh yes, Aaronson. That's his name." This is the adult form. In a child it might occur as: "Mummy, there's a birdy out there in the . . . in the . . . uh . . . he's . . . uh . . . he . . . he . . . he wash his bottom in the dirt." Similar sources of hesitant speech are found in bilingual conflicts, where vocabulary is deficient; in aphasia; and under emotional speech exhibition, as when children forget their "pieces."
2. *Inability to pronounce or doubt of ability to articulate.* Adult form:

"I can never say sus-stus-susiss-stuh-stuhstiss- oh, you know what I mean, figures, statistics." The child's form could be illustrated by: "Mummy, we saw two poss-poss- uh- possumusses at the zoo. Huh? Yeah, two puh-pos-sums." Tongue twisters, unfamiliar sounds or words, too fast a rate of utterance, and articulation disorders can produce these sources of speech hesitancy.

3. *Fear of the unpleasant consequences of the communication.* "Y-yes I-I-I- uh I t-took the money." "W-wi-will y- you marry m-me?" "Duh-don't s-s-spank me, Mum-mummy." Some of the conflict may be due to uncertainty as to whether the content of the communication is acceptable or not. Contradicting, confessing, asking favors, refusing requests, shocking, tentative vulgarity, fear of exposing social inadequacy, fear of social penalty in school recitations or recitals.

4. *The communication itself is unpleasant, in that it recreates an unpleasant experience.* "I cu-cu-cut my f-f-finger . . . awful bi-big hole in it." "And then he said to me, 'You're f-f-fired.' " The narration of injuries, injustices, penalties often produces speech hesitancy. Compulsory speech can also interrupt fluency.

5. *Presence, threat, or fear of interruption.* This is one of the most common of all the sources of speech hesitancy. Incomplete utterances are always frustrating, and the average speaker always tries to forestall or reject an approaching interruption. This he does by speeding up the rate, filling in the necessary pauses with repeated syllables or grunts or braying. This could be called "filibustering," since it is essentially a device to hold the floor. When speech becomes a battleground for competing egos, this desire for dominance may become tremendous. More hesitations are always shown in attempting to interrupt another's speech as well as in refusing interruption.

6. *Loss of the listener's attention.* Communication involves both speaker and listener, and when the latter's attention wanders or is shifted to other concerns, a fundamental conflict occurs. ("Should I continue talking . . . even though she isn't listening? If I do, she'll miss what I just said . . . If I don't. I won't get it said. Probably never. . . . Shall I? . . . Shan't I") The speaker often resolves this conflict by repeating or hesitating until the speech is very productive of speech hesitancy. "Mummy, I-I-I- want a . . . Mummy, I . . . M . . . Mumm . . . Mummy, I . . . I . . . I want a cookie." Disturbing noises, the loss of the listener's eye contact, and many other similar disturbances can produce this type of fluency interrupter.

We must remember that the beginning stutterer is still learning to talk. His speech is not stabilized. But the mere fact that he has some fluency, and all stutterers do, indicates that, with a little less pressure, stabilization may occur. If, through counseling the parent and often by demonstrating better practices before her in play therapy, we can just ease his burden a little, the stuttering goes away. Often we are surprised to find how quickly these children respond to the reduction of any one of the precipitating factors. This is not so true of the children whose stuttering comes from constitutional or neurotic causes however, but it is true of the large proportion of garden variety stutterers. And even the others are helped thereby.

Lowering the Standards of Fluency. Communicative stress can also come from the need to talk like others do. If the parents or other children set standards of fluency far beyond the child's ability to imitate, he is almost certain to falter. In our chapter on the development of speech we emphasized this, but here we wish to point it up again. Parents provide the models for all behavior whether they want to or not. It is not enough for parents to become better listeners; they must also provide models of fluency which are not too difficult for the child to follow. It is difficult for some parents to simplify their manner of talking to children, but most of them manage it once they understand why they should do so.

> We observed that one of the primary stutterers with whom we were working spoke in compound, complex sentences and used vocabulary which was not only that of the adult level but almost that of an English professor. We even heard him stutter on the word "innocuous," and this at six years of age. He was the only child and his parents were in their forties. They were voluble and precise in word choice. They read him to sleep each night, and the selections they chose were *good* literature. They italicized the word when they told us about it. They also played word games and lost no opportunity to teach the boy a new word.

> The counseling was difficult, but finally they came to see that they were setting exorbitant standards of speech and they asked us for suggestions. We told them to stop reading any stories to the child. We told them to make up some tales instead about very little boys. We asked them to speak in simple sentences to the child as often as they could, to stop the wordplay and teaching, and to falter a bit in their own talking. We asked them to stop talking so much. We asked them at times to play games in which they pretended that the boy was a little baby and to encourage him to talk like one. They had kept him out of school because of his stuttering, and we insisted that he be placed in the kindergarten forthwith. We continued to counsel them. In two months the stuttering was gone.

Reducing the Communicative Demands. Parents frequently report that the young child has more stuttering when he first comes back from school or from playing with the other children. They think it is because of the excitement or some baleful influence of the teacher. The better explanation often is that this is the time that parents give the child a cross-examination. "What did you do at school today?" No child remembers. He did lots of things, but he didn't memorize them. One question follows another when all he wants is a cookie and to go out to play.

Parents never seem to realize how much they question their children nor that questioning always puts the child under communicative stress. The mother gets lonely. She needs someone to talk with; and her husband, when he does get home, hides behind the paper until after dinner. She also wants to keep her close umbilical relationship with the child. She wants to know what he's thinking and feeling and doing. We can understand and sympathize, but if her needs are making her child stutter, they've got to be satisfied in other ways.

> Peter, aged five, never stuttered in school or on the playground, but he surely did so at home, especially when he talked to his mother (who illustrated the pattern outlined above). We did no counseling. Instead, with all the force and authority at our command, and enlisting her husband's aid in the matter, we insisted that from that moment she was to ask the boy *no* questions. None! Not another one for two months! She could answer his questions but she was not to demand, or wheedle any speech from him. She could talk all she wanted, but it had to be commentary, not questioning. We also got her to serve as a volunteer nurse's aid in the hospital each afternoon. The boy stopped stuttering and the father gave me a cigar (not a very good one).

Removing the Stimulus Value of the Stuttering.   A final, but very important, component of communicative stress is the unfavorable attention given to the stuttering by the parents. They call attention to the repetitive speech. They tell the child to "stop it," or to "stop stuttering." We know of no quicker way to throw a child into the third and fourth stages of stuttering than by such suggestions. They should be terminated immediately. Other parents interrupt the child when stuttering and ask him to relax or to stop and think over what he is about to say. When we tell them not to do so, they protest and say, "But it really works. If we stop him and tell him to relax or to stop stuttering he does stop stuttering. Why shouldn't we do this?" Advice again is not enough. Parents must understand how stuttering develops, how frustration and fear are born. We do point out that the child is still continuing to stutter, and is probably getting invisibly worse, that the policies they are using are frustrating in themselves, and that they are training him to fear and avoid. We help them to see that they should reduce the stimulus value of the stuttering, not make it more vivid.

Other parents do not nag their children when they hear them stuttering, but they respond to it by signals of alarm and distress, which are probably worse. They freeze in their conversational tracks. They hold their breath; they become jittery. Their faces suddenly become masks. Any little child will respond to such signals as though they were cannon shots.

When the doe suddenly grows stiff with alarm, the fawn freezes. Quite as much as when the old buck snorts! We must reduce these signals. They add too much to communicative stress.

Usually, the only way to help parents change these attitudes is by providing counseling and information. Occasionally we actually train them out of their signaling behavior by being with them as they interact with their children and helping them to respond to what the child is saying rather than to how he is saying it. But we had one set of obstinate parents who would not accept our picture of the problem and its solution. Under their constant nagging, the boy was growing worse and worse, but they still felt they should "correct him" every time he had some repetitions. Finally, in desperation, we put them into a therapy room with a group of our very severe adult stutterers and locked the door. When we let them out they were a changed couple and from that time on followed our suggestions and the child became fluent.

Building Ego Strength. We now turn to the favorable part of our equation, to those factors which reduce stuttering. These are the factors we must do our utmost to facilitate. The first of these is the M factor representing morale, ego strength, self-confidence, and security. It is difficult to define, but we know when it's low and we know when it's high. It rises and falls in all of us depending upon our success-failure ratio, but its basic ingredients are love, faith, and opportunity. Some of our stuttering children are denied all three.

One of our beginning stutterers had a father who hated him, perhaps because he wanted the babying which the mother gave only to the child. He had not desired to have children. The boy's stuttering provided the excuse he needed for the expression of his hostility. At any rate, he made no bones about his feelings. Whenever the boy tried to talk to him, the father cut him short and showed his disgust and rejection. The mother's attempt at protection only redoubled the intensity of the father's dislike. He forbade the boy to play with other children, made him stay in the house or yard "so he wouldn't get hurt," refused to let him ride a tricycle, and in every way made the boy feel he was both unpleasant and inadequate. We had no success with this child despite some heroic efforts. He is now in high school, a lonely, frightened unhappy boy, barely passing in his school work despite a high IQ. His teachers say that he has no confidence in himself. In one of our recent interviews we asked him why it was so hard for him to work on his speech. He said, "I've been brainwashed all my life. Nobody thought I could do anything, and I can't. Every time I make a half-hearted attempt I hear my father saying what I've heard a hundred times: "My God, I'll have to support you all my life." He said that whenever I stuttered bad. I think he's right.

This parent was the exception, fortunately. We have come to have a great respect for parents, once they realize their child is in danger and know what to do. Some parents have to be taught to show their love. Some have to be shown how to put aside their own anxieties and to let the child run the risks of living in a dangerous world. Better to break a leg than break a spirit! We have found the overprotective mother to be one of our major problems in this regard. The child must have opportunity even to fail. Security does not come from success alone.

How do we build up ego strength, morale, self-confidence? It is difficult to generalize. Often the therapist must accept much of the responsibility for doing the job. We ourselves have done many things. We have taught a boy to box, another to swim, another to read, another to ride one of our horses. We once took a child to a cowboy movie every week for a whole semester. Each child has his own needs.

> One little girl stutterer, the next to the youngest in a family of six girls, had failed to show any improvement in her stuttering for almost a year despite all our attempts to reduce the denominator of her own particular stuttering equation. Then one of our student therapists bought her a puppy, and she stopped stuttering. I asked the therapist, a girl, why she had bought the puppy. "It was obvious," she answered. "I have been out to Nancy's home several times, and it was clear that she had no status whatsoever. She's shy and quiet, and the other girls dominate her completely. I felt that she ought to have something she could dominate or feel superior to, someone to whom she could talk and not be interrupted, something to love. I had a puppy once and I remember."

We aren't sure that her analysis was correct, but we are sure that the stuttering disappeared. And we are certain that self-confidence, morale, and ego strength can be increased with love, faith, and opportunity.

The Fluency Factor. Fl stands for fluency in our equation, and as we have mentioned, all stutterers have a share of it, often, a remarkably large share. No child stutters all the time. Under certain conditions even the secondary stutterer is very fluent. The beginning stutterer in stages one and two can be provided with much more fluency by a few simple procedures. It is the responsibility of the therapist to see that the average amount of fluency is increased.

First of all, with the beginning stutterer, we should arrange things so that during the periods of more severe stuttering, he talks less. The converse is also true. Since early stuttering comes in waves, during the periods of excellent speech, the parents should provide him with every possible opportunity to exercise it. This simple policy has eliminated the disorder in many children.

Secondly, both in the play therapy sessions and in the home, self-talk should be encouraged. Parents should do it as they go about their ordinary activities, telling aloud what they are doing, perceiving, or feeling. In the sessions with the therapist, she should provide the same models of commentary. Few children stutter in their self-talk. It should be facilitated.

We also institute games which might be called "speech play." No attention to the stuttering of course should be involved. The child should only know that he and the therapist or parent are having verbal fun. Some of these games involve speaking in unison, or echoing, or speech accompanied by rhythmic activities, or talking very slowly and lazily. Even babylike babbling seems to help. There are hundreds of variations but the purpose of all of them is to increase the experience of fluency.

Desensitization Therapy.[34]   Any fluency under any conditions is to be sought, but fluency under conditions of communicative stress is especially to be prized. Most beginning stutterers respond favorably to a coordinated program of the type we have described, but there are some who become worse as the environmental pressures are removed, and there are many whose parents and teachers cannot be persuaded to change their unfortunate policies. What can we do with these children? Give up the case and blame the failure on the child's peculiar constitution or the parents' guilt? No, there is another alternative, if we can toughen the child, build up his tolerance to stress, and create callouses against the hecklings, rejections, or impatience. Human beings learn to adapt to extreme noise levels, to incredible heat and cold. The housefly can even eat DDT and like it. Should we not try some desensitization, just as the physician gives the shots for hayfever? Instead of lowering the fluency disrupters at home while being unable do anything about them on the school playground, should we not train our stuttering child to be able to tolerate them without breakdown? As we indicated earlier, some children lower their thresholds of speech breakdown as soon as the parents decrease their home pressures. This just makes such a child all the more helpless outside the home.

At any rate, this is what the speech therapist does. He first establishes a social relationship with the child in which the latter does not realize that he is doing any speech therapy. They may be setting up a toy railroad on the floor or participating in any other similar activity. The speech therapist then works to achieve a basal fluency level on the part of the

[34] The author owes his initial interest in this therapy and subsequent experimentation with it to George O. Egland, who first brought the concept to his attention.

child. This may in rare cases have to begin with grunts or interjections, but usually it consists of simple statements of fact, requests, observations, etc. The therapist, as he works, thinks aloud in snatches of self-talk, commenting on his activity. Soon the child will begin to do the same, and by appropriately altering the communicative conditions, and his own manner, the therapist gets the child to speak with complete fluency. In the primary stutterer, this is not too difficult. Then, once the basal fluency level has been *felt* by the child, the therapist begins gradually to inject into the situation increasing amounts of those factors which tend to precipitate repetitions and nonfluency in that particular child. He may, for instance, begin gradually to hurry him, faster and faster. *But,* and this is vitally important, the therapist stops putting on the pressure and returns to the basal fluency level as soon as he sees the first sign of *impending* nonfluency. How can he tell? Experience and training will help, but we have found usually, that just before the nonfluencies appear, the child's mobility begins to decrease—he freezes, or his general body movements become jerkier, or the tempo of his speech changes. There are other signs peculiar to each child, and a little experimentation will help the therapist know when to stop putting on the pressure just before the stuttering appears.

As soon as the therapist returns to the basal fluency level, he again begins slowly to turn up the heat, to hurry the child a little faster, to avert his gaze more often, or whatever he happens to be trying to toughen the child against. Then an interesting thing occurs. The child can take more pressure the second time than he could the first. The increment is very marked. But again, the first signs of approaching stuttering appear, and again the therapist goes down to the original basal fluency level. Most children do not seem to profit from more than four of these cycles per therapy session, since the tolerance gain decreases somewhat with each subsequent "push." It should be made clear that throughout this training, the child never does stutter, if the therapist has been skillful. What he feels, probably, is that he is being fluent under pressure. Fluency becomes associated with the feeling of being hurried. Perhaps this is why there is a remarkable transfer. The effects of this toughening to stress are not confined to the speech therapist. The child seems to be able to stay fluent even when his father keeps interrupting him. This technique, for lack of a better term, we can call "desensitization therapy." We have found it very useful.

Prognosis.   If we can locate the child soon enough and initiate the type of therapy outlined above, the chances of a favorable outcome are excellent. Children in the first two stages of the disorder usually seem to present no great difficulty if systematic treatment can be administered. For these children it seems as though all that is needed is the reduction of one or two of the factors that are precipitating the speech hesitancy so that homeostasis, self-healing, can take place. Indeed many children seem to heal themselves without treatment. We are certain that many children who start stuttering are able to overcome it without professional therapy. Therefore the prognosis is favorable.

Treatment of the Stutterer Who Has Become Aware of His Stuttering. As we have seen from our discussion of the development of the disorder, once the child begins to be frustrated by the repetitions and prolongations which interrupt his communication, the picture changes. Something new has been added to the *F* factor above the line of his stuttering equation. He is not only frustrated by having his other needs and desires blocked; now he is also frustrated by the speech itself. This is one of the major eddies in which the stutterer finds himself swirling, helpless. It too is a vicious circle or spiral. The more he struggles to release himself from the perseverative repetitions and prolongations, the more he feels frustrated, and the more he struggles. His efforts bring tensed musculatures, hard contacts, tremors, jerks, and facial contortions, all of which make speaking more difficult and unpleasant. He does not fear speaking yet, but he is having a hard time. His stuttering equation is the same, except that the frustration factor has shown a drastic increase.

$$\frac{PFAGH + Cs}{M + Fl} = S$$

The treatment of children in this stage follows much the same course as that used in the treatment of primary stuttering. We must increase the essential emotional security, remove the environmental pressures that tend to disrupt speech, and increase the amount of fluent speech which he experiences. Every effort should be made to prevent traumatic experiences with other children or adults who might tend to penalize or label the disorders. By creating a permissive environment in which the nonfluency has little unpleasantness, much can be done to help the child regain his former automaticity of repetition. The wise parent will find ways of distracting the child so that the struggling will not be remembered with any vividness. Some parents have increased their own nonfluency, reacting to it with casualness and noncommittal acceptance. One of them used to pretend to stutter a little now and then, commenting, "I sure got tangled up on that, didn't I? What I meant to say was . . ." It is also wise to provide plenty of opportunity for release psychotherapy, for ventilation of the frustration. Let them show their anger. Help them discharge it.

If teasing has reared its ugly head and the child does come home crying or unpleasantly puzzled by the rejecting behavior of his playmates, the situation should be faced rather than avoided. Here is a mother's report:

Jack came home today at recess. He was crying and upset because some of the other kindergarten children had called him "stutter-box." And they had mocked him and laughed at him. He asked me what was a stutter-box and for a moment I was completely panicky, though I hope I hid the feelings from him. I comforted him, and then told him that everybody, including big people, sometimes got tangled up in their mouths when they tried to talk too fast or were mixed up about what they wanted to say. Stutter-box was just a way of kidding another person about getting tangled up in talking. I told him to listen for the same thing in the other kids and to tease them back. Later on that day he caught me once and called me a stutter-box. We laughed over it, and I think he's forgotten all about it today. I hope I did right. I just didn't know what to do.

The desensitization therapy used with the third-stage stutterer varies in one respect from that used in the first two stages. We do not use complete fluency as our basal level from which we start and to which we return after gradually increasing the stress. Instead, it is wiser to use the first appearance of tension in the repetitions or postural fixations as the cue to return to the basal level. As in primary stuttering, we try to harden the case to the factors that precipitate his nonfluency, but in this third stage of stuttering we keep putting on the stress (the interruptions, impatience, hurry, etc.), even though the repetitions begin to appear. But we stop short and return to our basal fluency level just before the tension, forcing, or tremors show themselves. By this technique, it is possible to bring the child back to a condition where there may be many of the primary symptoms, but little or no struggle reactions.

Direct Therapy. Depending upon how far the child has entered this stage of frustration and struggle, there comes a moment when direct confrontation of the stuttering is necessary. There comes a time when the child needs some adult to show him that he need not struggle, that it is better to let his speech bounce and prolong easily, that this way "the words come out faster and easier."

This new direct attack on the problem should be done by the professional therapist but we have found it wise to do it in the presence of the parents so that they can feel the objective attitude employed and observe what we do. Here is a glimpse from the transcript of one such session:

Therapist: I understand that you've been having a lot of trouble talking lately, Peter.

Peter: Yea, I, I, I, I've been sssssss . . . stutt . . . stuttering." (*The boy squeezed his eyes shut and fast tremors appeared on his tightly closed lips. The word finally emerged after a surge of tension and a head jerk.*) "I've been stuttering bad."

Therapist: So I see. Let's try to help you. I know what you're doing wrong. You're fighting yourself. You're pushing too hard. Let me show you how you just stuttered and then show you how to do it easy. (*Therapist demonstrates.*)

Peter: Oh!

Therapist: Now I'm going to ask you a question, and if you stutter while answering it, I'll join you but show you how to let it come out easy. OK? All right, how close is the nearest drugstore to your house?

Peter: It's over on the next b . . . b . . . bbbbbbblock. (*While the boy is struggling, the therapist first duplicates what he is doing, and then slowly slides out of the fixation without tension. The child hears him, opens his eyes to watch him, and an expression of surprise is seen on the child's face.*)

Therapist: Yea, I told you I was going to stutter right along with you, but you'll have to watch me if you're to learn how to let the words come out easy. Let's try another. If I went through the front door of your house, how would I find your room?

Peter: YYYYYYYYYYou'd . . . (*The child joined the therapist in his grin.*) Yyyou'd have to ggggggo upstairs.

Therapist: That second time you didn't push it so hard, did you. Good. You went like this . . . (*Therapist demonstrates.*) Look, you've got to learn how to stutter my way, nice and easy, either like th-th-th-this or like th . . . is. (*Therapist prolongs the sound easily and without effort.*) Now let's play a speech game of follow the leader. You be my echo and say just what I say and stutter just like I do. Sometimes I'll stutter your way and sometimes my way, the better way, the way you've got to learn to do it.

The session continued along this line and, before the end of the half-hour, Peter was beginning to cease his struggling. It took four more meetings before he really learned how to stutter easily, but the parents reported a marked reduction not only in the severity but in frequency as well. We saw him again after four months and the only stuttering behavior he showed was that of the first stage. Within a year it was gone. Children learn quickly and forget their troubles quickly.

The Conspiracy of Silence. Many parents have been told so often that they should always ignore the stuttering that they continue to do so even when it sticks out like a second nose. This is very unwise. When the child is struggling with his stuttering, when he is obviously reacting to it, no good is obtained by pretending that it doesn't exist. There is a time for ignoring it, for distracting the child's attention from it, but there also comes a time when we must confront it and share the child's problem with him. Otherwise, he will feel that his behavior is shameful, unspeakably evil. He will feel that his parents cannot bear even to mention it. This is the road to fear and avoidance. It is a dangerous road to travel alone and in the dark.

Treatment of the Confirmed Stutterer. The stutterer who shows the avoidance behavior characteristic of the final stage of stuttering presents the most difficult therapeutic problem. Something new has been added—fear. The equation is now complete:

$$S = \frac{(PFAGH) + Cs + (Sf \times Wf)}{M + Fl}$$

Situation fears times word fears (and we think they multiply rather than add) create a most potent influence in determining stuttering frequency and severity. Often this influence of fear overshadows in importance all the other factors. Certainly it makes for more penalty, creates more frustration in communication because of the avoidance, and adds a constant supply of anxiety, guilt, and hate. We now cannot content ourselves with reducing *PFAGH* and communicative stress, building morale, and providing more experiences in fluency. We must do these things, but we must do more: we must now find ways of reducing the fears of speaking situations, the fears of words and sounds. Stuttering now has become its own cause. It is self-reinforcing. Somehow we must get the person out of the whirlpool.

Current Methods. There are presently three major ways of treating these confirmed stutterers being employed in this country. One is through psychotherapy alone. We are not impressed with the results of this method. A few are healed, usually those whose stuttering is fairly mild or of neurotic origin. Psychotherapy certainly can reduce anxiety, guilt, and hostility; but in the stutterer who has spent some time in the fourth stage of the disorder, the situation and word fears together with the habituated struggle reactions cannot be ignored. These also need therapy.

The second major method for treating this advanced form of stuttering does attempt to eliminate the fear and struggle component, but it does so largely by suggestion and distraction. This school of speech therapy, numbering among its adherents many of the older workers in the field, attempts to teach the stutterer methods for avoiding or preventing fear and occurrence of stuttering blocks. It aims to eliminate the emotional factors which precipitate the symptoms. The stutterer is urged to believe in the theory advanced by the clinician, and nothing is left undone to convince him he can be cured. Strong clinical suggestions and even hypnosis are used to strengthen his confidence in the remedial techniques. Routine breathing and vocalization exercises and rituals are employed. Through the use of distractions of all kinds, the fear of stuttering is kept from consciousness. Gestures, head movements, and other forms of muscular reinforcement are used as starters. Strange methods of vocalization—preceding all consonants by a vowel, sing-song speech, the "octave twist (in which the stutterer is taught to shift the pitch of his voice an octave when he feels blocked)," stereotyped rhythms of stress or phrasing, slurring of the consonants, and many other similar devices—are used to keep the fear from becoming potent enough to precipitate stuttering. Every effort is made to get the stutterer to forget his fears and symptoms. He is urged to consider himself a normal speaker. By the use of speech situations and types of communication arranged according to graduated levels of difficulty, his confidence is nursed along until it becomes sufficient to enable him to speak without fear or stuttering at each successive level. Group techniques help to decrease the fear and increase the suggestion.

In most cases, this type of treatment produces immediate release from fear and stuttering. The stutterer believes that at last a miracle has happened. Hesitantly he applies the formula and lo! it seems to work. His confidence grows by leaps and bounds, and, as it does, his fears decrease. He writes his clinician a glowing letter of praise and thankfulness and departs for his home. Occasionally, his new speech fluency continues for the rest of his life. Whenever fears arise, and they are inevitable, he applies the formulas given to him by the speech correctionist. If the environmental pressures are not too great, and novelty, suggestion, and faith are still effective, the formulas successfully dispel the fear. He realizes that he can still speak without stuttering.

Unfortunately, like most of the devices the stutterers themselves have invented, the formula devices soon become habitual and relatively unconscious. When this happens, they no longer are able to take the place of fear in the stutterer's mind, and relapse usually occurs. Giving the stutterer a period of free speech does not solve his problem if, and when, fear returns. Nevertheless, in the safe haven of the speech clinic, where belief and novelty are important factors and both group and clinical suggestions are everywhere, the stutterer finds great relief. Under such conditions, few stutterers experience much trouble; but unfortunately, such conditions do not exist in ordinary life. When the stutterer returns to his home or former environment, or meets situations that remind him of past failures, there is no one around to tell him that his fears and blocks are mere bugaboos which will disappear if he follows the formula. Life is not made up of easy speech situations or optimal conditions for communication. He finds that he cannot remain relaxed when he applies for a position. He finds it impossible to remain permanently unemotional. The self-confidence so carefully and painstakingly nurtured by the speech therapist collapses like a house of cards. The formula suddenly seems to have lost its charm. Faith crumbles. The stuttering returns in all its viciousness, often with greater frequency and severity than before. The stutterer attempts to relax, but fear and panic prevent relaxation. He starts his arm-swing, or "octave twist," or whatnot, and finds that suddenly it does not keep out the blocks. After repeated failure, he finally gives up and resumes his hunt for a new miracle worker to cast out his "stuttering devil." Meanwhile, the speech therapist has new stutterers to whom the formula may be taught.

Relaxation. Another basic technique used in helping the person not to stutter is that of relaxation. For many years it served as the basis of all therapy with stutterers. They were asked to relax completely, on the cot and off. They were told to put themselves to rest, that all was well on the blue horizon, that no thunderclouds were visible. Powerful suggestion, even including hypnosis, was used. When a state of relaxation was obtained, the case was then asked to speak, quietly and serenely, the carefully graded sounds and sentences of his therapist. Usually no stuttering appeared when the person followed these directions and was safe in the harbor of his therapist's arms or voice. It was almost as easy as speaking alone. There were no tensions to form the substructure of tremors; no sudden ballistic movements were permitted. There was no stress—often no real communication. But it is hard to be a rag doll in a steel world, as Martin Palmer once said. To be serenely relaxed under a descending sword or piledriver is not a natural response. Life for the stutterer is full of threats, old and new. To ask him to be relaxed is to ask him not to fear. Sure, he can do it when he is safe, but not otherwise. Some few stutterers have been cured this way. Through relaxation many of them have had a bit of temporary relief and hope, but most of them have been left still stuttering and with added guilt feelings because they do not relax as they've been told they should. It's a nice treatment—for the therapist.

The third method is now perhaps the most widely used, although the way it is administered often differs with clinics and therapists. First of all, it is devoted to a total attack on all the factors that increase stuttering. It provides a nonpunitive situation in which stuttering is sought and encouraged. The exhibition and confrontation of stuttering are rewarded so that it can be studied and explored and varied. When possible, other penalties being suffered by the stutterer are reduced by environmental manipulation. The P factor is therefore treated. Frustration (the F factor) is also reduced by this permissiveness about stuttering, and at the same time definite steps are taken to build up the stutterer's frustration tolerance. Anxiety, guilt, and hostility (A, G, H) are not forgotten. Through group sharing of experiences, through acting-out the conflicts during the speech assignments, or by professional counseling or other forms of psychotherapy when indicated, these factors are also reduced. Communicative stress (the Cs factor) is not, as in the earlier stages, primarily treated by reducing the stress and creating especially favorable speaking situations. Instead, the stutterer is deliberately subjected to judiciously chosen speaking situations in which stress is present, and he is taught to resist this stress. The M factor (morale) is augmented in many ways: through the close support of a sharing therapist, through the creation of new assets and the elimination of old liabilities, but especially by means of the sense of achievement procured by the successful performance of speech assignments and the conquest of fears. Through various means, later to be described, the stutterer is made aware of the amount of fluency (the *Fl* factor) that, despite his stuttering, he always possesses, and especially of the fact that one can stutter and still be fluent. To sum it up, this total approach tackles each of the features of the disorder, not just a few of them.

In the preceding paragraph we have shown how this type of therapy treats the *PFAGH* and *Cs* and *M* and *Fl* factors. But it is in the way this therapy attempts to reduce the situation and word and phonetic fears (the *Sf* and *Wf* factors) that it seems to be unique. It stresses the welcoming of stuttering as behavior to be confronted, analyzed, and manipulated or controlled. It works hard to eliminate all forms of avoidance, since avoidance increases fear. It also attempts to associate more fluent forms of stuttering with the situational and word cues that formerly produced avoidance or struggle. It teaches the stutterer that he can stutter fluently. The expected unpleasantness is reduced and with it the fears.

It is obvious that the author of the text is an advocate of this methodology, perhaps because, as a stutterer himself and as a speech therapist, he has experienced the inadequacies and restricted scope of the other methods. This brief summary of the purposes of this particular variety of stuttering therapy was intended to point up the contrast between it and the other two. Now let us outline the sequence of therapy and tell what we do.

The Sequence of Therapy. Let us coin another acronym to put the matter succinctly: *MIDVAS*. The separate letters of this word refer to the main phases of our therapy for the secondary stutterer, and they follow the order of the letters of the word. *M* is for motivation; *I* is for identification; *D* for desensitization; *V* for variation; *A* for approximation; and *S* for stabilization. This is the sequence of our therapy. We structure our therapy plan so that each new phase has a special emphasis, but all preceding goals are continued. New experiences are added but the old are reviewed. It is cumulative therapy. For convenience of exposition, we shall describe the treatment as though it were being administered to severe adult stutterers. Modifications must of course be made for young children or for the very mild stutterer, as well as for the special needs of any given individual. All stutterers present special problems. All need special treatment, but there still are general principles and practices which help all of them.

Motivation. One who has not worked much with secondary stutterers would expect to have little trouble motivating them to do the things necessary to find relief. Certainly, the interruption to communication, the social implications and deprivations, and the struggling and the fear are unpleasant. Why then do we find so much resistance? For we certainly do. We think there are two answers. First, it is always difficult to confront one's abnormality, to expose it enough to modify it, and this resistance is found in healing all emotional ills. Indeed, unless resistance occurs in psychotherapy, we can be pretty sure that any apparent insight and improvement in adjustment is superficial and temporary. Secondly, the fact of the stutterer's fluency when alone or in nonstressful situations makes him feel that no major overhaul is needed. But deep in his bones he knows he has a tough job to do, that the seizurelike behavior and the panic of his fears are not going to yield to any waving of a savior's hands; yet it is only human to hope for easy miracles. We keep in our desk a little bottle full of pink aspirin with a label reading: "One of these will cure stuttering forever." In an early session, we always hand a new stutterer the bottle. He always grins and hands it back. We have never had one so much as open it in thirty years. They know.

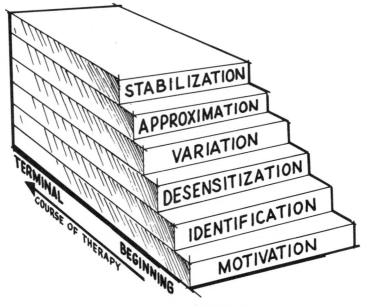

Figure 28: *MIDVAS*

The Role of the Therapist in Motivation. When the secondary stutterer first comes for therapy, he speaks with great difficulty usually; and we have found it wise to begin by revealing our own role and competence. We don't tell him how good we are; we let him find that out. But we do define our role, not as a teacher or preacher or medicine man, but as a guide and companion on a joint quest. We do this in the initial interview, explaining why we ask the questions we do, and sharing with him the implications of his answers. When he stutters, we provide a running commentary of our own objective evaluations of his behavior. When he avoids, or postpones a speech attempt on a feared word, or uses some trick to start his utterance or disguise the stuttering which occurs, we recognize and identify what he has done with complete acceptance. This always seems to surprise the stutterer. He always seems to feel that his little devices for avoiding or escaping from his difficulty are his own personal secret. And he is always surprised at the acceptance. The only listener responses he has remembered are those of rejection or embarrassment or pity. Suddenly he finds not only a permissive listener but one who understands. This is one of the crucial experiences in all successful therapy. Often, at this point, he will begin to stutter very severely as if to test the genuineness of the therapist's acceptance, and again he is surprised to find that the behavior is welcomed, rewarded.

Another crucial experience which the stutterer should have as soon as possible is that of observing his therapist actually *sharing* his abnormality. Here is the transcript of one such experience:

Therapist: You had a pretty long and complicated block on that word "people." Let's see if I can duplicate it. First of all you squeezed, then protruded your lips like this. Then I think you gave a quick little gasp like this . . . and then. . . . No, I don't have it right. Let me have another bad one so I can learn what you do.

Subject: Pppeople. That time it came out easy.

Therapist: Yes it did, but I wish you could show me a more severe one, the kind that make you panic, as you said a moment ago. I've got to feel it in my own mouth to know what you do so I can understand what the problem is. You've got to teach me.

Subject: Yyyyou mmmmean you want me, you want me, you want me to teach you to stttttt . . . stttttttttutter like I do?

Therapist: To know how you feel, to know what you do, I've got to do it too. And not just here but in real speaking situations. As soon as I've learned how you do it, I'll make a phone call and try it out, and you can tell me how close I am, and if my feelings are similar to yours.

Subject: Holy C-C-Cow!

We do not only repeat the stutterer's behavior; we also share it as it is happening. By pantomiming what he is doing as he is doing it, we become a human mirror for him. When he first experiences this, old memories of the mockery of playmates long ago flood back and suspiciousness is aroused, then allayed as he finds that the therapist is actually trying to understand and share his burden of abnormality. This interaction not only helps to produce a close relationship of the stutterer with the therapist, but it also partially extinguishes some of the persisting evil effects of old traumatic wounds.

Another important experience occurs when the therapist reveals that he is interested and desires to share not only the outward behavior of the stutterer but also to understand his inner feelings. We find it wise to begin with the feelings created by the immediate moment of stuttering. A few stutterers are able, with skillful counseling, to express these feelings, but most are not. The stuttering itself interferes with expression. As Fenichel put the matter in a nutshell, when speech, the healing tool of psychotherapy, is itself infected the task of the therapist is hard. We have therefore found it wise to verbalize the patient's feelings for him. We do this tentatively and ask for corrections and additions. Here is a portion of the transcript of a session in which this took place:

> *Therapist:* When you were stuck that time, what were your feelings?
> *Subject:* I don't know. All, all mmmmmmmmmmmixed up, I gggg-guess.
> *Therapist:* You probably felt helpless . . . sort of as though your mouth had frozen shut. . . .
> *Subject:* And, and and I cccccouldn't open it. Yeah.
> *Therapist:* You couldn't open it. It was almost as though you had lost the ability to move a part of yourself when you wanted to. . . . Sure must be frustrating. . . .
> *Subject:* Sssure is. BBBBBurns me up. I, I, I, jjjust hate mmmmm . . . Oh, skip it . . . I don't know.
> *Therapist (accepting ly):* It almost makes you hate yourself when you get stuck like that.
> *Subject:* Yeah, dih-dih-disgusted with mmmmmyself and everything else. . . .
> *Therapist:* Some stutterers even find themselves hating the person they are talking to.
> *Subject:* Yyyyea. I, I, I, I, I, wwwwwas huh-huh-huh-hating yyyyyy-yyyyyou just then.
> *Therapist:* Uh huh. I know.
> *Subject (blurting it out):* How, howcome you know all these th-things?

If these three crucial experiences, which will be repeated many times in many different forms, are scrutinized, it is apparent that we are already at work on the stuttering equation. The case finds for the first time that stuttering is not being penalized, but encouraged. Frustration declines a bit as he discovers that his therapist is in no hurry, that this ear is always open no matter how long the blockings last. He learns that here he can pour out a bit of anxiety, guilt, and hostility with impunity. In the therapy situation, communicative stress is reduced. It is easier to talk here. Moreover, since stuttering is actually sought and encouraged, the fears are reduced. We do not fear that which is rewarded. Finally, and perhaps most important of all, there comes an increase in morale as the stutterer finds that he is not alone, that someone who seems to understand his problem has faith that he can solve it. Moreover, burdens which are shared are thereby divided. The load lightens. All of these changes reflect themselves in increased motivation. The M in the equation can also stand for motivation.

Goal Orientation. But the therapist is not only an understanding companion sharing part of the load; the stutterer soon comes to feel that this person is also a competent guide. At least he seems to know one way out of the swamp. Let us outline how we help him to come to this conclusion.

First of all, we try to provide some person whom he can see or hear who has been able to conquer his stuttering problem. Usually we have several around who are determined, despite our usual discouragement, to become speech therapists. We also have the tales of many others on tape, tales that often exaggerate a bit the difficulties encountered, and we must use them with care so that the new sprout of hope will not be withered by the frigid windiness of their exaggerated accounts of what they had to do. We use films for the same purpose.[35]

Next we try to help the stutterer realize that he possesses in his own present speech both a certain amount of fluency and also, what is more important, a certain amount of stuttering that does not interrupt communication unduly or show much abnormality. This latter item is of utmost importance. All stutterers have some moments of stuttering which are unforced and unaccompanied by struggle or avoidance. We point these out when they occur and often make a tape in which many samples of these fluent, normal stutterings are combined. We ask the stutterer to listen to this tape frequently. Also in our pantomimic sharing of his stuttering, we often repeat again and again these fluent stutterings so that he can see them, and we ask him to repeat them also. We point up this easy, fluent sort of stuttering as a goal object. Even a rat runs a difficult maze better when he has a taste or smell of the cheese to be found at the end of that maze.

At this point the stutterer often objects.

> *Subject:* Yyyyou mean, you mmmmmmmmean that it's possible to stutter easy like that even when you're scared green?

[35] One which we have found useful in this regard is "Great Clinicians: Stuttering," which can be procured on rental from the audio-visual department of the University of Wisconsin.

Therapist: You feel it isn't possible. (*Nods acceptance of the feeling.*)
Subject: Oh nnnnnnot when you're really petrified, nnnot wheh, when
you can see th . . . em c-c-c-coming and the fffffffffffear builds up.
Therapist: Real hard fears are bound to throw you into long hard
blocks. . . .
Subject: Yeah, but mmmmmaybe, maybe not. Maybe it is ppppppos-
sible to let them kind of leak out, hey? MMMMaybe I c-c-could
llllllearn. . . . (*He shakes his head.*)
Therapist: But you have your doubts. . . .
Subject: SSSSStill those other gggguh-guys say they can stutt . . .
stutter. . . . Hey, I'm doing it right now. I just had an easy bbb-
block on sssss, on ssssssstut. . . . Why can't I say it now? On ssssss-
stutter. I, I, I, dddddid have one, dddddidn't I?
Therapist: Sounded like it.
Subject: And, and, and mmmaybe the fffffears wwwwwwwon't al, al, al,
al, always be so strong. Even already I dddddon't seem to bbbbe
quite ssssssssssso sceh, scared. YYYou know it's true. I, I, I, I dddddo
have dddddifffferent kkkinds of bbbbblocks.

At some such moment it is possible to help the stutterer to have another very important experience: the realization that it is possible to stutter
in many different ways and that some ways may be better than others. We
make it possible for him to observe and duplicate the kinds of stuttering
shown by other stutterers. We also ask him to experiment a bit in modifying his own.

Therapist: I notice that usually on a word beginning with *b* or *p* you
squeeze your lips tightly and then open them and suck in a little air
just before the release comes—like this. . . . (*Therapist demonstrates.*)
Subject: YYYYeah, and it, it, it, it mmmmakes a ssssssssssssssssucking
sound I don't like.
Therapist: You hate that sucking noise.
Subject: Yeah. (*It is evident that he is not going to pursue the subject
further.*)
Therapist: Then let's see if you stutter on words like that without
sucking.
Subject: Huh?
Therapist: Let's see if you can say these names in the phone directory
beginning with *P* and try to keep the sucking noises out.
Subject (*doubtfully*): OK. PPPP(*suck*)Partridge; PPPPPP(*suck*)Par-
sons . . . I can't.
Therapist: OK (*acceptingly*).
Subject: LLLLLLet me rrrrreally try th . . . is tttttttime . . . PPP-
Puhpuhparparpartridge. Hey! I did it! What do you know! Yyyyou
mean I, I, I, I don't have to ssssssuck?
Therapist: Looks like it.

This is another of the crucial experiences which are the mile markers on the road to freedom. There are many of them.

Mapping the Route to the Goal. It is also necessary that a clear picture of the course of therapy be given to the stutterer. He needs some kind of a map before he becomes willing to undertake a journey, even though he now knows he has a guide. We have found it useful to give him some understanding of *MIDVAS* and also of the stuttering equation. This first phase of therapy requires the imparting of information. The stutterer is usually as ignorant of the nature of his disorder as he is of the behavior he uses so compulsively. He needs to know something of the causes of stuttering and the way it develops, and we also help him to find information about the way stuttering has been treated in the past as well as how it is being treated today by other therapists. We do not believe in blind therapy. We want him to know where he's going, where he is, and what he has to do. We find that we get a better motivated case this way.

The Second Phase of Therapy: Identification

As soon as possible we move directly into the second phase of our therapy, in which the basic goal is the identification and evaluation of the various factors in the case's *personal* stuttering equation. There is no emphasis on trying to speak more fluently. Just the converse. The stutterer is to seek out stuttering experiences and to analyze the behavior and identify the forces which created it. This is the period of self-study, of self-exploration. (Note that this goal-structuring increases the approach and decreases the avoidance vectors in the approach-avoidance conflicts.) The objective observation of the stuttering behavior gets down to what the semanticists might call "first-order facts." The more the stutterer stutters, the more opportunity he has to make his observations. The therapist shares and rewards these discoveries. He also provides structured experiences which will make them possible.

Speech Assignments. One of the unique features of this type of therapy is the use of the speech assignment. In addition to the stutterer's own attempts in self-therapy, certain required activities and experiences are devised by the therapist to provide guidelines and models for what the case should be doing himself. Some stutterers need few of these; others need many; but the emphasis is always on self-therapy. The devising of self-assignments is constantly and vividly rewarded. Usually, the therapist-formulated speech assignments are given more frequently in the early phases of therapy, and especially during the phase of identification. Reporting the experiences *and feelings* evoked by these experiences is a very necessary part of the clinical routine. This may be done orally either in private sessions with the therapist or in group sessions with other stutterers, or the reports may be written in certain instances. Often we use both oral and written reports. The mere act of preparing and handing in reports of self- and therapist-assigned experiences gives a sense of achievement which has profound and cumulative effects upon the M factor in the equation. Moreover, these assignments often provoke the resistance and testings of the relationship between stutterer and therapist, that when worked through, create new insights and energies for healing. They make it possible for the therapist to share significant moments in the stutterer's life; they reveal the basic feelings which can then be accepted and reflected upon. They help the stutterer to know where he is and how much he is doing and how much he still must do. They provide an objective account of the course of therapy. We have found them very useful.

Typical Assignments in Identification. Since this is a general and introductory text in speech correction and not a manual for stuttering therapy, we can do no more than provide one or two typical assignments for each of the subgoals involved. There are hundreds of other possible assignments which might be more appropriate for a particular case. The stutterers themselves often invent better ones than we can design. Since the basic goal of this phase of the therapy is the identification of the various factors in the stutterer's personal equation, the illustrative assignments will be organized about these factors. Often, in a single day's work, the stutterer will perform one of the therapist's assignments for each of the factors, and also a self-invented one of his own for each of them. There are also times when he may do nothing. He gets the therapist's warm approval for the first of these responses, and the other is accepted as part of the difficulty. However, if the case proves entirely unwilling to work, therapy is terminated. Even a psychoanalyst has to get them on the couch now and then.

Penalties. Many secondary stutterers have become a bit paranoid about the reactions of listeners to their stuttering. Even when no overt rejection is evidenced, they think the listener is merely covering up a punitive or embarrassed reaction. It is vitally necessary that they do some reality testing. Some assignments which could begin this testing might run like this:

> Keep track of the number of listeners who frown or show objective signs of impatience when you stutter. What proportion do not? Get a sample of ten strangers with whom you stuttered obviously to determine the proportion.
>
> How many store clerks did you talk to before you found one who showed signs of mirth or mocking when you stuttered? Try a minimum of five.
>
> If possible, ask one of your friends how he really feels when you stutter to him. Ask him to tell you the truth. Report what he said and whether you think he was honest.

Here is one stutterer's own self-assignment report:

> I've been wondering maybe I've been blowing this fear business all up.
> Maybe most people don't really give a damn whether I stutter or
> not. Maybe they figure it's my problem, not theirs and they let it go
> like that. Then I got to thinking how many people can I remember
> who really did laugh in my face when I stuttered and you know I
> couldn't remember a single one except Wilbur Ketchum when I was
> a kid and he was goofy anyway and laughed all the time. So I got to
> thinking and thought I'd try something out. I called on the phone a
> whole mess of people and asked them things like "Is Wilbur home"
> or "May I speak to Jane, please" and I stuttered plenty but I cocked
> my ear to see if I could hear any laughing or giggling. I just got one
> who did. It was a little girl who answered the phone. All the rest just
> waited till I got it out. I was sure surprised. Maybe I have been exag-
> gerating.

And here is another:

> Had a lulu of a penalty today. It threw me. Was talking to a stranger,
> a man about sixty, and asked him how to get to the bank. He got
> mad when I stuttered. He said, "If you can't talk any better than
> that don't ask questions." And turned away. Felt like quitting right
> there. Made me feel dirty mouth. But I said to myself why does he act
> like this? What kind of a guy is this? So I follow him around and
> listen. He gets some tobacco in a store and he raises hell with the
> clerk for not having his kind. Then he goes to another place and gets
> his tobacco but growls at that clerk. I tailed him into Gilmore's, and
> there he was giving some other clerk hell for something. So I guess I
> got a bad one and it wasn't just my stuttering. Felt pretty good after.

These assignments happen to revolve about the speech disorder itself,
but we wish to make clear that we explore all penalties, not just those
evoked by stuttering. Punishment of any kind seems to add an increment
of stuttering. During this phase of treatment the case tries to locate and
assess the importance of all penalties, present and past. He becomes aware
of sources of rejection other than his stuttering. One girl changed her
hairdo and bought new clothes and a red hat instead of the mousy-looking
apparel she had been wearing. A boy learned how to dance when he found
he could get dates easier for such affairs than for the movies. As a result
of some vivid experiences, one man began to see that he was getting more
rejection for his aggressive sarcastic reactions to other speakers than for
the fairly mild stuttering which he exhibited. And he also found that his
stuttering began to decrease. One of our college students wrote an essay
on "My History of Penalty" and won a prize for the composition. Often,
in group sessions, the memories of past penalties are ventilated, and again

not just those concerning stuttering. In this phase of therapy, we make no attempts to eliminate the behavior that provokes the penalty but merely to explore and to define it, but often the stutterer starts making some changes anyway. The emphasis at this phase of therapy is merely to *iden-tify* those penalties which contribute to stuttering.

Frustration. In exploring this factor the stutterer compiles an account of the frustrations characteristic of his present situation and also a history of those of the past. He also thereby becomes aware of basic drives and needs other than to speak fluently. Many stutterers become so focused on stuttering that other major problems are completely disregarded, even though they contribute to the disorder and may be more easily rectified. In the identification phase of therapy, the whole target, not just the bull's-eye of stuttering, comes into view. Here are a few typical assignments:

> Keep a pad and pencil with you all morning and write down *every* time you feel frustrated, not just those times when you stutter. Try to report why you felt this way and what the frustrating situation was.
>
> Frustrate your roommate three times and report how you did it. Then ask him to frustrate you as often as he can for an entire day and report how he did it.
>
> In speaking to some friend, keep stuttering on a word until he says it for you or finishes your sentence. Do this a minimum of three times. Report your feelings.
>
> In what ways were you especially frustrated as a child? What were your parents' major frustrations? Prepare a written and comprehensive answer to these questions.

Here is the report of a self-initiated assignment in exploring the frustration factor.

> My roommate in our girls' dormitory has a nasty little habit that's been driving me to distraction. She sniffs. She sniffs when she's studying. When it's quiet all I can hear is that sniff, sniff, and I almost go wild. It's a tic or something. I used the radio for a while to cover it up, but she says she can't study with it going. I asked her if she couldn't stop it and she said no, that if it didn't bother her why did it have to bother me. I told her it still did and she said that's too bad. Lately I've been doing all my studying at the library, but that's pretty inconvenient. Well, I've been thinking about frustration and how it may affect my stuttering, and I know her sniffing makes me jittery so I said to myself, "All right, let's see if you can learn to bear it." Ruth's a very nice girl in other ways and we have lots of fun together. So I said to myself, "Let's measure how many sniffs you can count before you get nervous, and then you can give her one stutter for every five

sniffs." That made me grin to myself. Well, I stuttered eleven times to her before we went to bed, ten for her sniffs and one for myself. It actually took fifty sniffs and three hours of studying before I couldn't stand it any longer. I guess I can get used to it if I can only use a little psychology on myself.

Anxiety, Guilt, and Hostility. For some stutterers only professional counseling can help to ease the pressures of these emotions. There are therapists who are qualified to do such counseling. Other therapists cannot and should not do it, and the patient must seek help elsewhere. Professional psychotherapy for the stutterer whose disorder is primarily neurotic in nature is a must. But most stutterers, in our opinion, do not fall in this category. Yet they all have some anxieties and guilts and hostilities which need ventilation and release. Fortunately, the speech assignments devoted to other factors usually bring about the expression of many of these feelings that the therapist must permissively accept and reflect. Usually in this early phase of therapy we do not use many direct assignments in exploring these factors, but some illustrations may be given.

Interview some friend and try to discover what anxieties he possesses. Report which ones you also have.

Here is a list of behaviors (list is provided) which create feelings of guilt in children. Which of these do you remember experiencing?

Keep stuttering to strangers until you have a clear experience of hostility. Describe this as vividly as you can.

For what things other than stuttering do you tend to punish yourself? Watch yourself all this day and see what you might discover.

Communicative Stress. Here we confront the stuttering directly. In this phase of treatment, the case explores and identifies the types of communicative stress to which he is most vulnerable. Again he is *seeking* speaking experiences instead of avoiding them, which is healthy in itself and a reversal of old practices. Here are some typical assignments.

Which of these two audience reactions seems to produce more stutterings: (1) interruption by having the listener finish what you are trying to say or (2) having him look away when you're stuttering? Collect two experiences of each kind and report.

Read a passage aloud to some other stutterer very swiftly; then another of equal length at a normal rate; then another at a normal rate; and finally a fourth at a fast rate. Using hand counter, have him count how many blocks you have under fast and ordinary speaking rates, averaging the two trials for each. How much of a factor is speed in producing more stuttering? Report your findings.

Tell a joke to some friend. Do you have more stuttering on the words that carry the key meaning, or on the punch lines? Why?

Analyze four speaking situations which produced different amounts of stuttering and attempt to identify the kinds of communicative stress present in each.

Read aloud the names on one page of the telephone directory to some other person and have him indicate which ones you stuttered on most severely. Were some of these strange unfamiliar combinations of sounds such as occur in foreign names?

What kinds of attitudes shown by your parents when you were trying to talk to them seemed to produce the most stuttering when you were a child?

Collect an experience of each of these types: Interrupt another person when he is talking. Ask a favor. Repeat in other words what some-one has just said. Arrange these, if possible, according to a progression of decreasing stress. Talk aloud to yourself when alone, answering the phone, and making a phone call.

Situation Fears. In exploring these, the stutterer should not only identify those of the present and the past but also attempt to assess their intensity. He should also try to discover what he specifically dreads. Many very important insights come from this sort of investigation. He may even find that he doesn't know what he is afraid of. The stutterer should also study the relationship between situation fears and the amount of actual stuttering that does occur. He may find that the correlation is not as high as he thinks it is. We find that experiences of this sort are very salutary because they weaken the *fear of fear*. Often these people seem to be more afraid of the fear than of the stuttering itself. By seeking out what is dreaded, by exposing and analyzing it, the evil subsides a bit.

Some typical assignments are as follows:

Before you enter five different speaking situations, predict on this five-step scale how severely you will stutter. Then, after you have left the situation, record how badly you actually did stutter.

What three speaking situations in your whole life do you remember as being the worst? Why were they the worst?

Apply for a job at some restaurant. On your way down town, try to identify and remember the kind of thinking you were doing and what you were especially dreading. Report this in writing.

Word Fears. This factor, as we have said, includes not only fears of specific words but also the phonetic fears of sounds. It might be objected that by focusing the stutterer's attention on them, we only make them that much worse. All we can say in this regard is that any increment of this sort is negligible. They already have their full strength based upon a thousand memories. Stutterers also fear these phonetic fears; they attempt to distract themselves from them, to repress them, to escape from them. We have found it healing to look them plumb in the face.

Here are some typical assignments:

When a stutterer reads and rereads a given passage, the number of stutterings decreases through adaptation. Usually those words on which stuttering persists longest are the most feared. Therefore, to discover them, read a given passage four times and have someone else underline all words on which you stutter each time. Then take the fourth reading's underlined words and try to tell why they resisted adaptation.

Underline all the words of a reading passage on which you expect to stutter, and then read it aloud to some other person. Have him underline all words on which you actually do stutter. What percentage of correct prediction did you show?

Take two of the sounds which you feel are your "Jonah sounds," those most feared, and prepare a reading passage which is full of them. For example, if you usually fear *s* words and *m* words, prepare a passage which has many sentences such as this one: "Many snakes must search such marshes as may be seen by the seashore." Read this aloud to some other person and have him underline all words on which you stutter. Compute the percentage of *s* words and *m* words on which you actually stutter.

Before you make a phone call, prewrite what you plan to say. Underline all feared words and predict the severity of stuttering on each. Use a five-step scale of severity. After you have finished, score each underlined word in terms of how severely you did actually stutter on it.

What kind of rehearsals do you use when fearing a specific word? Investigate and report on five of these.

The **M** *Factor.* We also feel it very important for the stutterer to study his own variable feelings of self-worth. As we have said, stutterers are focused so much on their stuttering that they fail to see their other difficulties. In much the same fashion, they are also unable to evaluate with any objectivity the other assets they possess. In this phase of the treatment they learn objectivity, and it is important that they apply it to the favorable factors as well as to the unfavorable ones. While much of the increase in ego strength comes from the sense of achievement gained by working on their stuttering and from the identification with a strong therapist, nevertheless we find that certain assignments can have a real effect. Here are some samples.

Prepare a list of all your personality assets and liabilities. Shyly we suggest that you include stuttering among the latter.

Write up an account of all the things for which you have received approval from others.

Keep a mood chart in which you assess your feelings of morale four times a day: after breakfast, lunch, and dinner and before you go to bed. Make a graph of your mood swings for an entire week of a five-step scale with these values arranged on lines from top to bottom: (1) Whoops! (2) Feeling good. (3) Uncertain. Don't know. (4) Depressed. (5) Mighty, mighty lowdown.

Who are the people who have evidenced some faith in you? Why do you suppose they evidenced this faith?

The Fl Factor. Only the stuttering seems to have stimulus value for the stutterer, never the quite evident amount of fluency he also possesses. Again we must help him assess the real state of affairs. At this stage he has become morbidly conscious only of his abnormality, not of his normality. Also, most secondary stutterers have an exaggerated concept of what constitutes normal fluency. They do not realize that normal speakers are also nonfluent, at times of stress very nonfluent. This area must also be investigated.

Here is a tape recording of one of ex-President Eisenhower's press conferences. Record how many hesitancies he demonstrates.

On what percentage of words do you stutter? Make tape recordings of yourself (1) reading to another person, (2) explaining something to a friend, and (3) making phone calls. Count the words spoken and the stutterings, and find out how fluent you are in each.

Listen to the conversations of other people, and be able to show us all the different kinds of nonfluencies they demonstrated.

In this section describing the *identification* phase of therapy we have tried to show how we help the stutterer recognize the scope of his problem as expressed in terms of the various factors that make his stuttering better or worse. We would like to reemphasize here that this exploratory phase by itself often produces immediate decreases both in the amount of stuttering and in the intensity of the fear and avoidance. As in motivation, identification experiences will continue throughout therapy. We find, however, that we have more success when we stress it early in the treatment.

DESENSITIZATION PHASE OF TREATMENT

The third major phase in the treatment of secondary stuttering we have termed "desensitization" because our major goal in this part of the therapy is to toughen our case to those factors which normally increase the frequency and the severity of his stuttering. It should be pointed out at once, however, that the methods used are not the same as those used in desensitizing the stutterer in stages one and two. We now work directly, rather than indirectly. We neither use basal fluency levels, nor introduce the stress without the case's knowledge that we are doing so. Instead, we enlist his cooperation and provide him with challenges. His task now is consciously to learn to endure the stresses which formerly threw him into inadequate and abnormal behavior. He seeks them deliberately; and the therapist, with the case's cooperation, deliberately provides them. His goal is to remain integrated despite forces which tend to cause disintegration. His task is to decrease his hypersensitivity, in short, to toughen himself.

Human beings are wondrously adaptable. They can exist in the Arctic Zone and on the equator. They can even live in big cities. They can endure anything once they put their minds to it. Rats can be trained to bear electric shocks of great intensity with proper schedules of reinforcement. Surely, we can hope that our stutterers can improve in their ability to resist and endure the stresses they must encounter. In this phase, we are raising the thresholds of breakdown. It is very necessary that the stutterer understand why this is being done. But there are immediate rewards from desensitization. He will soon learn that as he becomes more hardened, he stutters less and suffers less. As he becomes tougher, he finds that penalties do not throw him so quickly; that frustration has a less evil effect; that he can tolerate more anxiety, guilt, and hostility than he could before; that communicative disruption and fear do not precipitate stuttering as frequently as once they did. And the morale factor rises, as any soldier knows, once he has learned what he can endure.

It is obvious that the administration of this phase of therapy takes some skill and empathy on the therapist's part. By now he should have gained a clear picture of his case's sensitivities and the energies the latter might marshal to modify them. He must not overload. Indeed, often the therapist must keep the case from overloading himself. But there must always be present the faith that comes from realizing the enormous potentials that all humans seem to possess, and the support which only a loved and respected therapist can give. Evidence must be provided that the therapist can also share these experiences, can also bear the stress, can also suffer but endure. Often he must become the receptacle for the hostile attacks that result from the hurt the stutterer experiences when he tries and fails. But the therapist knows that if he can accept these, the stutterer can try again. And he knows, as does Britain, that you can lose a hundred battles and still win a war.

Again, assignments are given which provide opportunities for desensitization to occur. Again, the stutterer is prevailed upon to construct his own assignments and to bring to the therapist for sharing and analysis the trophies and the failures which result. Group therapy provides an excellent situation for sharing these accounts, and the stutterers vie with each other and support each other. For example, we have found, in such a group, that if one girl shows she can make progress, all the males have to do more. Also, as they often do assignments together, a sense of comradeship is established which relieves the feeling of isolation so many stutterers know so well.

Usually, we begin fairly gradually to introduce the stress challenges, and the therapist sets models for the case to follow. We have found it wise to enter a store or similar speaking situation and to fake a very long stuttering block in the presence of the stutterer or stutterers. And we show we are not upset, that we remember exactly what the clerk did and how he reacted. We also verbalize our own feelings honestly. And then we do it again. We have found this often to be another crucial experience in the stutterer's life. The fact that another human being, a normal speaker perhaps, would be able to undergo such an experience and remain well-integrated and relatively unperturbed, seems to impress the stutterer greatly. After a few of these demonstrations, he is willing to try himself. We now list just a few illustrative assignments and experiences.

Penalty.

Keep making phone calls and fake one long repetitive block until one listener hangs up on you. Time the faked stuttering with a stopwatch, and report how many people you called before one did hang up.

Ask one of the other stutterers to yell at you "Stop that damned stuttering!" every time you do so as you read a paper aloud.

Ask one of your friends to laugh at you every time you stutter in a conversation. Explain that you are trying to be able to resist going to pieces when such reactions occur.

Keep your collar buttoned, but do not wear a tie all morning. Report all actual and suspected penalties.

Irritate some other person until he attacks you. Then explain why you did it.

Frustration.

Prewrite everything you say before you say it for an entire morning. Report your feelings of frustration but try to hold to the assignment despite the desire to talk without the annoyance of putting it down.

Do not smoke at all today.

During the noon hour, before you say the first sentence of any conversation, tap your toe once for each word within it.

Do some cumulative reading aloud. Read the first word; then the first and second; then the first, second, and third; and so on.

Have real or faked stuttering on every word of (1) a reading passage, (2) a conversation, and (3) in asking a stranger to direct you to the nearest movie theater.

Anxiety, Guilt, and Hostility.

Deliberately stutter to one person in a mildly hostile fashion, and then to another in a very hostile fashion. Smear him with a little of it, then with a lot of it. Report his reactions and your feelings.

Verbalize some of your worries about the future to five different listeners, one at a time. Say the same things each time. Report your feelings.

After each of five faked stuttering blocks, stop and say this to your listener, "I'm sorry I stuttered so hard. I'm sorry I took so much of your time." Report your feelings.

Using a hand counter, click it every time you feel ashamed during your conversations at meal times. Do this for three days in a row and see if the number doesn't decrease.

Communicative Stress.

Find someone who habitually interrupts your attempts to speak or finishes the words for you on which you are stuttering. Every time he does either, go back to the beginning of your sentence and repeat the whole thing. Report what happened.

Ask your roommate to heckle you as you explain something. Try to keep from hurrying or getting upset. And do not stop moving forward even though you stutter. Do not stop or repeat. Have him heckle only a little at first, then turn on the heat.

Interrupt another person three times in one conversation but do not hurry when you do so. Wait till he stops to take a breath but then interrupt him. Report your feelings.

Find one listener who seems to stop listening or who always says "What?" or "What did you say?" Keep talking to him till he has done this five times.

Situation Fears.

Make twenty-five phone calls before you go to bed tonight.

Stop at every residence in one block; go to the door and ask if someone with your own name lives there. Stutter at least once, real or faked stuttering, at each house.

Smile and say hello to every girl you meet on your way to school.

Remembering one of the worst speaking situations you've ever had in the past, try to invent another which has some resemblance to it, and enter it.

Apply for a job at every store in one block downtown.

Ask a policeman how to get to the railroad station.

Word Fears.

Prepare a reading passage containing your most feared words, and make a tape recording of four readings of this material to the same listener.

In speaking to a friend, repeat each stuttered word either until you no longer stutter on it, or until you have tried it ten times.

Make a list of five of your most feared words and deliberately introduce them into conversations. Write each word on a small slip of paper and hold each of these in your hand until it has been used.

Prepare prewritten phone calls in which you load what you have to say with words beginning with your feared sounds. Example: "Sammy Smith speaking, is my sister Sue staying with Sandra this evening?" Keep calling till you've got it all out and without going haywire.

Purposely fake repetitions of the first feared sounds of words until you find yourself calm, then say the word. Collect ten of these.

Hold the silent posture of the feared sound of a word until you have tapped your toe five times. Collect another for ten toe-taps, and, if you can bear it, another for twenty toe-taps. Be sure to count the toe-taps.

In making a phone call, time your deliberate prolongation of the first sound of one feared word for two seconds. Then do it again to another listener for three seconds; and if possible, to another for four seconds. Don't count any who hang up.

Let us repeat that these are merely illustrative speech assignments, any one of which might be entirely inappropriate for certain stutterers. Moreover, we have not indicated—and cannot indicate—the wide variety of assignments possible under each heading. Each therapist and each stutterer must invent his own. We have found it wise to keep the busywork at a minimum, to ask for as little performance as possible and yet enough to produce some impact. Assignments must be so structured that an objective report can be produced. They must provide enough stress to permit desensitization to occur. For any given case, their difficulty must be so tailored that more success than failure ensues, but failure is not to be avoided entirely. Indeed, in the sharing period with the therapist and other stutterers, often the failures when expressed and accepted do more good than even the successes. But there must be therapist approval and reward for meeting these challenges. And constantly we must emphasize the basic purpose these desensitization experiences are designed to fulfill: the building of a thicker hide on the stutterer's sensitive soul.

THE VARIATION PHASE OF TREATMENT

It is not enough to motivate, to identify, and desensitize, although these bring reductions in the frequency and severity of stuttering. In this new phase of therapy we begin to change, to modify the reactions to the factors that determine stuttering. Our purpose is to break up the stereotypy of the stutterer's responses, to attach new responses to the old cues. Much of the strength of habitual compulsive reactions lies in their stereotypy, in the consistency of their patterning. Varying them weakens them. Until new responses are made available, the stutterer has no choice except to yield to the old ones. We must help him to know that he has this choice. We cannot persuade him through intellectual argument. Only by behaving differently can he know that it is possible to behave differently.

This variation phase of treatment is usually short in duration because it passes directly into the next one of approximation, in which we seek to help the stutterer learn not just *new* responses to old pressures, but *good* responses. By "good" we mean only that new responses can be learned which will facilitate fluency rather than reduce it. There are always better ways of responding to penalty, frustration, word fear, and all the other evil factors than those the stutterer has habituated to compulsive automaticity. We must help him learn new responses which do not continually reinforce his stuttering as his old responses do. But before these new ways of behaving can be learned, the old ways must be weakened. Variation must precede approximation. The stutterer must realize that he has a choice of responses before he can pick out and master a better one.

Again we seek to provide for the stutterer experiences in which this learning may occur and to motivate him to seek such experiences himself. Let us reverse our usual sequence of presentation and begin with the factor of word fear.

Varying the Reactions to Word Fear.

Read a passage omitting all words on which you anticipate any stuttering.

On every other word on which you stutter, be sure to stutter repetitively but slowly on the first syllable. Do this to three listeners.

Underline the feared words in a reading passage and substitute (or add) a tremor in your right leg for each one that you find in your lips or tongue.

In a phone call, when you find yourself using such stallers as *a* . . . *a* . . . *a* . . . , vary them so that you also use *um, uh, ub, oops,* and *Ozymandias*. Your job is to vary the way you usually postpone.

During three moments of stuttering attempt to shift the focus of the tension from where it usually resides to some other parts of your body. Report what you did.

Instead of gasping as an interrupter of your tremors, try blowing out a puff of air on four of your stuttering blocks.

Since you usually lower your head whenever you stutter, watch yourself in a mirror with an observer, and raise it instead.

Instead of shutting both eyes as you usually do when stuttering, try shutting only one. Work before a mirror until you get ten successes.

Varying the Reactions to Situation Fears.

You have said that when you enter a phone booth to make a call, you hurry too much and go all to pieces. Today, enter five phone booths, stay in each for two minutes before you call me. When I answer, just make noises and hang up. Report your feelings.

You report that when you must do an errand, you rehearse over and over again what you plan to say, picking out easy words and revising sentences. Today, do three such errands with a friend but you are to say only what he tells you and to say it exactly as he does. He is not to tell you what to say until the last minute. Report your experiences.

Ordinarily you walk around the block several times before entering a store to ask for something. Today, ask questions in three stores, but stand absolutely still looking in the display window for as long as it would take you to walk around that block. Then go in and ask for it. Report your introspections.

In your trigonometry class today, sit in the front row for a change. Get there in time so you can.

Varying the Reactions to Communicative Stress.

Get a companion and hunt for the noisiest places you can find. Try not to speak more loudly to your friend but speak more slowly and distinctly.

Ask some acquaintance to do you a favor you know he will not grant. Do not apologize or appear uncertain. Just ask him.

Criticize your roommate for some of the behavior you do not like and return to it until he gets angry. Speak very slowly as you do so.

When one of your listeners looks away while you stutter, speak more loudly or do something different so he will look at you.

Varying the Reactions to Anxiety, Guilt, and Hostility.

You say you find yourself worrying vaguely about everything and find it hard to get to sleep. Tonight, assign yourself to worry on purpose and do so aloud in self-talk just before you hop into bed. Worry aloud about everything you can possibly think of.

You've reported that when you've felt ashamed about something you did or didn't do, you found yourself biting your fingernails to the quick. Keep a pocketful of peanuts and remember to bite one of them (only one) instead whenever you start to nibble a fingernail or find yourself feeling guilty or ashamed.

You've reported how frequently you keep reviewing your wrongs and hates. This evening before you go to bed, write out as many of them as you can on toilet tissue, read them again, then flush them down the drain.

At the beginning of each hour, by your watch, verbalize to yourself a statement of one anxiety, one guilt, and one hostility. Try not to repeat yourself. Do this for each hour of the afternoon.

Varying the Reactions to Frustration and Penalty.

Every time you feel frustrated this evening, smile and continue to smile until the frustration has subsided.

Whenever a listener interrupts you or finishes a word on which you are stuttering, say to him, "Don't interrupt me. I've got a hard enough time talking anyway."

Collect three instances in which a moment of stuttering causes you feelings of frustration or evokes listener penalty and in which you repeated the same word over and over again at least three times.

You say your stuttering often produces smiles on the faces of your listeners. Suddenly ask one of them why he's smiling.

As we write this chapter we are constantly aware of the inadequacy of our presentation of such assignments in reflecting what actually occurs in therapy. These assignments by themselves have no value. Only when shared with the therapist and when feelings are expressed and when rewards are appropriately timed, do the experiences they evoke have potency in modifying the attitudes and outward behavior of the stutterer. It would be easier and perhaps safer to resort to statements of vague general principles, but students seem to profit more from specific examples. So be it!

The Approximation Phase of Therapy

Once the stutterer has learned that his habitual reactions to the factors which make stuttering worse can be varied, we try to help him learn *new responses which will diminish that stuttering*. We now seek not just different responses but the best responses, those which tend to extinguish stuttering rather than reinforce it. Why do we call this phase the approximation phase? Because we feel that new responses are acquired, not by sudden exchange, but by gradual modification. You just don't stop stuttering severely and suddenly begin to stutter easily. Again, it's like learning to target-shoot. You shoot and miss; then you change a bit of your behavior and shoot again. Your attempts result in a coming closer, in an approximation to the behavior needed to hit the bull's-eye consistently. By approximation we mean the progressive modification of behavior toward a goal response. It is operant conditioning.

The basic goal then of this phase of therapy is to learn how to stutter and to respond to stress in such a fashion that the disorder will not be reinforced. The therapist's responsibility is to see that rewards are felt whenever the stutterer moves closer to this goal. Approval is contingent upon progress, not merely upon performance. Happily, the relief from communicative abnormality seems to follow the same course, and provides even more powerful reinforcement. The goal is getting nearer now.

In our discussion of this phase of therapy, we will confine ourselves to the exposition of what we do with the fears and experiences of stuttering itself. It must be remembered, however, that the characteristic responses to penalty, frustration, and all the other disturbing factors must also be modified in the direction of nonreinforcement of the stuttering. There are better responses to penalty, to communicative stress, than those the stutterer first brings to us; and these he can also learn by progressive approximation. However, here we will concentrate on the stuttering behavior.

Stuttering in Unison. One of the best ways we have discovered to help the stutterer learn an easier, nonreinforcing kind of stuttering is to do it with him. He watches us and hears us as we join him in his stuttering, duplicating the first of his behavior, but then we ease out of the tremors, cease the struggling, and smoothly finish the word. Often at first, the contrast between his continued struggles and our smooth utterance tends to shock him, but gradually he begins to follow our lead and to stutter as we do. He finds us sharing his initial behavior but then diverging. We make the changes gradually, at first setting models of minor changes which he may be able to follow, and rewarding them when they appear. Once he can make these minor changes (e.g., stuttering with his eyes open rather than closed), he gets no more approval until a further change occurs (e.g., lips are loosened from their tensed closure), and so on. We move only as far as the case is ready and able to go in any given session. It is vitally necessary that this training be done under some stress, stress that can be felt but not stress that overwhelms. To sum it up, we share and show him how to shift, how to change his responses. Verbalization of feelings is always encouraged, and this phase of therapy often produces some new storms. But the mere fact of the sharing, the fact of the therapist's faith, the fact of his patient acceptance of failure as a necessary part of learning—all these create a favorable climate for change and growth.

Cancellation.[36] As soon as any change in the stuttering behavior has been learned, the stutterer is encouraged to use it in cancellation. By this term we mean that the stutterer stops as soon as a stuttered word has finally been uttered; pauses; and then says it again, this time using the modification he has learned in unison stuttering with his therapist. He still stutters this second time, faking, if he must, a duplication of the same stuttering he has just experienced; but now he modifies it in accordance with the new behavior he has learned. Then he finishes his sentence. Communication stops once he stutters, and it continues only after he has used a better stuttering response. This also is powerfully reinforcing.

Pull-outs. This awkward term, stemming from the stutterers' own language usage, refers to the moment of stuttering itself and what the stutterer does to escape from his oscillations or fixations. Evil pull-outs are the jerks, the sudden exhaling of all available air. These only increase the penalty and all other factors that make for more stuttering in the future. There are better ways of terminating these fixations and oscillations, and once these new ways have been learned in unison speaking with the therapist, and practiced frequently in cancellations in all types of speaking situations, the stutterer should begin to incorporate them within the original moment of stuttering itself. Any change for the better should be incorporated as often as the stutterer can manage it. Thus the new behavior moves forward in time, from the period just following the stuttering into the moment of stuttering itself.

Preparatory Sets. Our next step is to move it even further forward, into the period of anticipation, into what has been called the "prespasm period." Usually, in response to word or phonetic fears, the stutterer actually makes little covert rehearsals of the stuttering abnormality he expects. These preparatory sets to stutter often determine the kind and length of abnormality which result. Therefore, once the stutterer has

[36] An illustration of a complete operant conditioning program for getting the stutterer to use cancellation, pull-outs, and preparatory sets will be found in Speech Foundation of America, *Conditioning In Stuttering Therapy* (Memphis, Tenn.: Fraser, 1970).

shown that he can incorporate the new change not only in cancellation but also during the actual stuttering behavior, he is now challenged to incorporate it within his anticipatory rehearsals, to plan to stutter this new way. Often we help him by rehearsing for him and by getting him to duplicate our model before he attempts the word he has indicated he will stutter upon. Again, we reward the successes and disregard the failures. Again, we reward progressive change.

As each new modification of stuttering is learned and starts up the series of experiences in cancellation, pull-outs, and preparatory sets, new modifications are being born, either with the help of the therapist through unison stuttering or through self-discoveries. With each new change comes a decrease in the severity and often in the frequency of stuttering as well. Fears of words, then of situations, lose their intensity. The stutterer's self-confidence begins to grow with each new achievement. The fluency factor grows larger. He becomes able to tolerate more communicative stress. It is also interesting to watch how he applies the same therapeutic principles to his other inadequate behaviors. He begins to modify his old inadequate reactions to penalty and frustration; and the ways he handles his anxieties, guilts, and hostilities improve. Progress comes swiftly on all fronts. Instead of avoiding stuttering experiences, he hunts for them so he can try out his new skills. Avoidance declines.

Perhaps some glimpses of the actual interaction between therapist and case would be helpful here, although it is impossible to indicate the changes in behavior which occur. The student will have to use some imagination.

> This stutterer, when he attempted a feared *p* or *b* or *m* word, characteristically assumed a wide-open-mouthed posture, invested it with a strong tremor, then attempted to release himself from it by a sudden movement in which the head went up but the jaw went down. The final utterance of the word always emerged from one of these jerks. Often he would have to use two or three of the latter before release occurred; and if one failed, he then returned instantly to the tremorous highly tensed open-mouth posturing.
>
> *Therapist:* Today, let's see if we can't learn to stutter a bit more easily than you've been doing it on that feared *p* sound of yours.
> *Subject:* GGGGGGGood. I'm rrrrready.
> *Therapist:* On these cards I have written some *p* words that you have often stuttered on, and I'm hoping that you'll stutter on a few of them at least.
> *Subject (opens mouth and has his characteristic abnormality):* . . . (*jerk*) Probably!
> *Therapist:* Well, I won't need the card, I guess. I'll ask you a question now, and if you stutter on the answer, I'll join you, do just what you

do at first, but then do something differently too. Try to follow my lead. Here's the question: Do you think you'll have some stuttering on these words?

Subject: (*Open mouth in same tremorous posture, which the therapist duplicates almost exactly; but therapist slowly closes mouth while continuing the tremor so that finally the tremor is occurring on the lips alone. The stutterer also closes his lips as he watches and follows the model; but just before he says the word "Probably" his mouth again opens suddenly, and the head-and-jaw jerk of release precede its utterance. The therapist's utterance finally emerges from the closed-lip position, so the two performances, at first fairly identical, later diverge.*)

Therapist: Good. You made some change. Not enough, but at least you managed to produce the only posture that the first sound of "probably" can use. Here's what you did . . . (*demonstrates*), and here's what you always have done in the past . . . (*demonstrates*), so you can see that you made some change for the better. Nobody can say "probably" with his mouth as far open as your Grand Canyon of the Colorado. Now show me both ways. Show me, by faking if you must, how you usually stutter on the word, and then how you just changed it a bit.

Subject (*demonstrates old way*): . . . (*jerk*) Probably. . . . Hey, that . . . (*jerk*) bbecame real! (*Therapist grins, and the stutterer then demonstrates the changed stuttering pattern.*)

Therapist: Pretty good! Now let's try some of these *p* words, and be sure to get your mouth closed and hold it closed a bit before you jerk it out. Remember I'll be joining you every so often . . . not always.

They work on eight different *p* words this way. The therapist gives approval intermittently but only for lip closure during the stuttering. Then he says:

Therapist: Now let's hear about that job you have with the *Gazette*. Forget about doing anything about any other stutterings, but if you have one of your old unchanged blocks on a *p* word, stop immediately, pause until I give you the signal, and then cancel it by stuttering again on the word but in the changed way.

Subject: OK. Well, I, I, I dddddelivered ffffffffforty . . . (*jerk*) papers. . . . (*Therapist signals and case stops. Therapist pantomimes changed stuttering pattern, then nods, and case cancels in the new way*) . . . ppppp . . . (*jerk*) papers. How's that?

Therapist: Attaboy. Good. Let's do some more cancelling. Tell me some more about your deliveries. (*The stutterer begins but forgets to cancel on the first p word.*)

Subject: Oooops, I fffforgot.

Therapist: It's hard to remember when you're interested in what you're saying. (*The stutterer gets some more cancellations, and then he uses his new change in the first attempt on another p word.*)

Subject (*surprised*): Hey, I used it in the mmmmmmmmmiddle.
Therapist: Good. Good! How about trying to get some more of those
in the middle of your stutterings? Look, here's how you did it. . . .
(*Therapist demonstrates.*) You don't *have* to keep your mouth open
when you try to say a *p* word.

They collect several more experiences, some successful, which the
therapist rewards, and some failures, which he ignores. Several times
the case failed but then cancelled. This was reflected and rewarded.
Once, he successfully rehearsed it before succeeding.

Therapist: How do you feel about this experimenting?
Subject: MMMMMan! It's ffffffffffascinating. I, I, I, I think I'm
ggggggetting the idea. MMMMaybe I can do it easier, hey?
Therapist: Want to try changing it a bit further?
Subject: Sure.
Therapist: OK. Now, let's see if you can stop jerking just before the
word comes out. Look, here's what you do (*demonstrates*). . . .
Can you also do this? . . . (*Demonstrates the elimination of the
jerk release and shows how the utterance could come directly from
the tremorous lip posture.*)
They then work on this new change in the same way. Now the therapist only rewards the new changes. The session ends in some fairly
potent expression and reflection of feelings revolving about the stutterer's fear of hoping too much and his many doubts about the future.

We cannot end this section on approximation without reminding the
student that most of the progress made must be due to the stutterer's
solo efforts. Many speech assignments are devised to provide the necessary
opportunities for progressively modifying the stuttering behavior under
stress. But this is how we begin.

Stabilization. The final phase of stuttering therapy we have called
stabilization. For lack of a clear-cut program of this sort, many stutterers
have experienced frequent relapses and despair. It is not enough to bring
the stutterer to the point where he is fluent, where he can speak with little
struggle or fear. We must stabilize his new behavior, his new resistance to
stress, his new integration. Anxiety-conditioned responses are very difficult
to extinguish entirely. New adjustments must be made, new responsibilities
undertaken now that the stuttering excuse is no longer valid. Terminal
therapy must be done carefully. It must be done well. We always keep in
fairly close touch with our secondary stutterers for two years after formal
therapy is terminated. Many of them occasionally avail themselves of our
counsel for many years, often on matters other than stuttering.

Often stuttering seems to go out the same door it entered. More of
the easy and unconscious repetitions and prolongations appear; periods of
fairly frequent small stutterings alternate with periods of very good fluency.

Sudden bursts of fear and even avoidance occur. Under moments of extreme stress an occasional severe blocking may be evident. It is important that the stutterer understand this and accept it as part of his problem. Often the therapist must be available for the verbalization of these traumatic episodes and receive the confession of avoidance and compulsive behaviors with accepting reassurance and remedial measures. However, it is possible to prevent much of this stress by an organized program of terminal therapy.

Fluency. Even when the stuttering disappears, there remain gaps in the flow of speech where the stuttering formerly occurred. These people have had so little experience in smooth-flowing speech that some training is needed to provide it. One of the best ways we have found to do this is through echo speech or shadowing, in which the stutterer, while watching TV or observing some fluent speaker, follows in pantomime the speech that is being produced, saying it silently as it is being spoken aloud. Often we train the stutterer to repeat whole sentences exactly as the speaker spoke them. We also ask him to cancel whole sentences of his own in which gaps or hesitancies appeared so that they can be made to flow more smoothly. We persuade him to do much self-talk when alone. We emphasize display speech of all types so that he can get the feel of fluency. At the same time we also show him that even excellent speakers have some nonfluencies and that these are different from the residual breaks which come from a long history of broken speech.

Faking. We also train our stutterers to fake easy repetitive or prolonged stutterings, to put these into their fluent speech casually in certain situations every day. We ask them, too, to demonstrate an occasional faking of a short block of the old variety and then to follow it with a cancellation. Occasionally it is wise to fake a pull-out or some of the modifications of postures and tremors so that these basic skills may remain fresh for use in emergencies. Most stutterers dislike doing these things, and they will not do them unless the activities form a basic part of the stabilization phase of treatment.

Assessment. The practice of taking an honest daily inventory must be encouraged. In this phase of treatment, we help the stutterer to learn to survey his own personal stuttering equation, to assess the variations in strength of the various factors, and to be honest in his evaluations. Here the accepting attitudes of an understanding therapist are most essential. He hears the confession and turns it into an inventory, for these are not sins but the natural residues of a severe disorder of communication.

Resistance Therapy. In this final phase of active therapy, we work especially hard to help the stutterer learn to maintain his new methods of fluent stuttering and fluent speaking in the face of pressures of all kinds. When he first comes to us, the stutterer has but two choices: to stutter on the feared words or to avoid them. We now have given him a third choice, the ability to stutter in a relatively fluent and unabnormal fashion. It is necessary not only to stabilize his new behavior of this third choice under conditions of stress but also to give him a fourth choice—to resist stuttering.

In helping the stutterer to resist communicative stresses of all kinds and yet maintain his new ways of short, easy stuttering, we (both stutterer and therapist) deliberately create conditions in which the pressures to stutter in the old way are strong, and then the stutterer does his utmost to resist them. We seek out and enter the feared situations of the past; we look for more and more difficult situations. By programming this stress so that the stutterer is largely (not always) able to beat it and yet can stutter easily when he does stutter, we enable him to strengthen the new behavioral responses to the old cues, to the old stresses which once set off the old abnormal responses of avoidance and struggle. This stress strengthening is even good for concrete beams; it is good for stutterers in the terminal stages of therapy.

But there is another form of resistance therapy which goes further and which holds the promise of curing stutterers and not merely making them fluent. It provides the fourth choice we mentioned earlier. Stutterers have long known a curious experience, namely, that occasionally they are able to summon up their powers and just refuse to stutter. It sounds unbelievable, but most stutterers will so testify; and often this occurs under conditions of great stress. They do not know what happens, nor do we. However, we have found that in the terminal stages of therapy, when avoidance has been pretty well eliminated, and when, if difficulty does come, it can be handled without great distress, we can train the case to resist his urge to stutter. Let us illustrate.

A simple procedure is to have the stutterer read in unison with the therapist. Under these conditions he will be very fluent. He is also very fluent in automatic echoing or shadowing. But then the therapist deliberately introduces some stuttering into his own speech and challenges the stutterer to resist him, in other words, to continue to speak the words as fluently as when the therapist was using fluent speech.

This is a strange and a new challenge. It is possible to resist the therapist's behavioral suggestion that he must stutter! There is no avoidance of feared situations, words, or sounds here. There *is* the resistance to suggestion, a resistance which stutterers need badly. Why should they always yield? By judiciously using the principles of desensitization therapy and introducing just enough stuttering in the model so that the case wins more often than he loses, it is possible to teach him to battle rather than succumb. There's no virtue in stuttering if you can resist the influences which tell you that you must. In this technique there is no avoidance, no running away. The challenge is proffered and accepted. No postponement, starting tricks, or other devices are permitted. The stutterer is simply to say the word if he can without stuttering, at a moment when the therapist is trying to make him have some stuttering. Once the principles of this resistance therapy have been mastered, the stutterer, through speech assignments and self-therapy, continues to battle the suggestion that if he has fear, he must stutter. Other ways of resisting stuttering involve the monitoring of speech by proprioceptive feedback and the use of masking noise or the echo device called the delayed auditory feedback apparatus. Descriptions of these will be found in references 8, 20, and 54 at the end of this chapter.

Treatment of the Young Secondary Stutterer.   In order to spell out exactly how we treat the secondary stutterer, we have described our therapy as it would be administered to a person who is relatively adult. With slight modifications—especially those in which the therapy is done with the therapist in the safety of the speech room—the suggestions made are useful with the person of high-school age. But there are secondary stutterers in the elementary school. Indeed, we have had to treat children as young as three and four years who showed all the overt and covert behavior characteristics of the fourth and terminal stage of the disorder. Most of them begin to come to the speech therapist later, when they are at least in school and in the third grade or above. How do we treat these children?

The general pattern of treatment is the same. It also follows MIDVAS. We begin by identifying with the child during his stuttering, sharing it, helping him confront it without shame. We teach him to watch it, feel it, try to change it so that when he does stutter he does not avoid or struggle. We give him models and have him imitate us directly as we show him how to ease out of his tremors, his hard contacts, his hypertensed mouth postures. "Watch me," we say. "Look! Here's how you stuttered just now. Now see how I can start the way you do but ease out of it . . . like this. Try it again." Fortunately, in these younger children, the disorder is as yet not too deeply rooted. They unlearn more easily. Once they put their trust and love in you, they will follow your demonstrations and directions most willingly. We almost always use play therapy along with the speech work to relieve the pressures of PFAGH. We provide situations in which there is little communicative stress. We do desensitization therapy often, as though the child were still in the earlier stages. We give him many experiences in being completely fluent through the use of echoing, unison speaking, rhythmic talking, and relaxation. We do our utmost to build his ego strength in every possible way. We use no speech assignments but, through parental counseling and home and school visits, we gradually incorporate his new ways of talking into his entire living space. We can help these children.

REFERENCES

Articles

1. Andrews, G. and Harris, M. *The Syndrome of Stuttering.* London: William Heine, Limited, 1964.
Read the chapter on syllable-timed speech and summarize.
2. Berlin, S. and Berlin, C. "Acceptability of Stuttering Control Patterns." *Journal of Speech and Hearing Disorders,* XXIX (1964), 436–41.
What were the different kinds of stuttering patterns used, and which was preferred by listeners?
3. Cooper, E. B. "A Therapy Process for the Adult Stutterer." *Journal of Speech and Hearing Disorders,* XXXIII (1968), 246–60.
Outline this therapeutic approach.
4. Douglass, E. and Quarrington, B. "Differentiation of Interiorized and Exteriorized Secondary Stuttering." *Journal of Speech and Hearing Disorders,* XVII (1952), 377–85.
What are the differences between these two "types" of stuttering?
5. Egland, G. O. *Speech and Language Problems.* Englewood Cliffs, N.J.: Prentice-Hall, Inc., 1970.
Read pp. 233–42 and list the major suggestions for treating a beginning stutterer.
6. Emerick, L. L. "Bibliotherapy for Stutterers: Four Case Histories." *Quarterly Journal of Speech,* LII (1966), 74–79.
Who were the famous stutterers described in this article, and what were their stuttering problems?
7. Glasner, P. J. "A Holistic Approach to the Problem of Stuttering in the Young Child." In D. A. Barbara, ed., *Psychological and Psychiatric Aspects of Speech and Hearing.* Springfield, Ill.: Charles C Thomas, Publisher, 1962.
What is the author's view of the nature of this early stuttering, and how it should be treated?
8. Gruber, L. "Sensory Feedback and Stuttering." *Journal of Speech and Hearing Disorders,* XXX (1965), 373–80.
What is the author's argument concerning the role of feedback in stuttering?
9. Hejna, R. F. *Interview with a Stutterer.* Danville, Ill.: Interstate, 1963.
What insights resulted from this "psychotherapy"?
10. Johnson, W. "Some Practical Suggestions for Adults Who Stutter." *Speech Pathology and Therapy,* I (1961), 68–73.
What are his five basic suggestions?
11. Johnson, W., Brown, S. F., Curtis, J. F., Edney, C. W., and Keaster, J. *Speech Handicapped School Children,* 3d ed. New York: Harper & Row, Publishers, 1967.
Read pp. 298–329 and tell how the classroom teachers can help the stutterer.
12. Kent, L. R. "A Retraining Program for the Adult Who Stutters." *Journal of Speech and Hearing Disorders,* XXVI (1961), 141–44.
Describe the basic kind of therapy advocated by this author.

13. Kinstler, D. B. "Covert and Overt Maternal Rejection in Stuttering." *Journal of Speech and Hearing Disorders,* XXVI (1961), 145–55.
What kinds of rejecting behaviors were shown by the mothers of these stuttering children?

14. Luper, H. L. and Mulder, R. L. *Stuttering Therapy for Children.* Englewood Cliffs, N.J.: Prentice-Hall, Inc., 1964.
Summarize the story of Mike, pp. 92–110.

15. Marland, P. M. "Shadowing—A Contribution to the Treatment of Stammering." *Folia Phoniatrica,* IX (1957), 242–45.
Describe shadowing and how it is used.

16. McDonald, E. and Frick, J. "Store Clerks' Reaction to Stuttering." *Journal of Speech and Hearing Disorders,* XIX (1954), 306–34.
How did these people respond to the simulated stuttering?

17. Martin, R. R. and Siegel, G. M. "The Effects of Simultaneously Punishing Stuttering and Rewarding Fluency." *Journal of Speech and Hearing Research,* IX (1966), 466–75.
Summarize the authors' findings.

18. Murphy, A. T. and Fitzsimons, R. M. *Stuttering and Personality Dynamics.* New York: The Ronald Press Company, 1960.
Read pp. 234–78 and analyze the basic principles of the treatment of these five cases.

19. Perkins, W. H. and Curlee, R. F. "Clinical Impressions of Portable Masking Unit Effects in Stuttering." *Journal of Speech and Hearing Disorders,* XXXIV (1969), 360–62.
How effective was this instrument?

20. Rickard, H. C. and Mundy, M. B. "Direct Manipulation of Stuttering Behavior." In L. P. Ullmann and L. Krasner, eds., *Case Studies in Behavior Modification.* New York: Holt, Rinehart & Winston, Inc., 1964.
What types of contingent reinforcement were used, and what was the final result of this operant conditioning therapy?

21. Robinson, F. B. *Introduction to Stuttering.* Englewood Cliffs, N.J.: Prentice-Hall, Inc., 1964.
Read pp. 77–102 and describe the different kinds of clinical problems presented by the stutterers mentioned.

22. Shames, G. and Sherrick, C. "A Discussion of Nonfluency and Stuttering as Operant Behavior." *Journal of Speech and Hearing Disorders,* XXVIII (1963), 1–3.
How does stuttering start, and how is it reinforced?

23. Shearer, W. M. and Williams, J. D. "Self-recovery from Stuttering." *Journal of Speech and Hearing Disorders,* XXV (1965), 288–90.
What are the characteristics of these stutterers who seemed to have outgrown their disorder?

24. Sheehan, J. G. and Martyn, M. M. "Spontaneous Recovery from Stuttering." *Journal of Speech and Hearing Research,* IX (1966), 121–35.
How many recover, and to what do they attribute their relief from stuttering?

25. Soderberg, G. A. "Delayed Auditory Feedback and the Speech of Stutterers: A Review of Studies." *Journal of Speech and Hearing Disorders,* XXXIV (1969), 20–29.
Summarize the author's conclusions.

26. Soufi, A. "One-month Stutterer." *Journal of Speech and Hearing Disorders,* XXV (1960), 411.

Was this boy's stuttering really due to imitation?

27. Speech Foundation of America. *Conditioning in Stuttering Therapy.* Memphis, Tenn.: Fraser, 1970.
   This small book presents the case for operant and classical conditioning together with pertinent criticisms of these methods.

28. ———. *Stuttering: Its Prevention.* Memphis, Tenn.: Fraser, 1966.
   Summarize the basic principles for preventing stuttering.

29. ———. *Stuttering: Successes and Failures in Therapy.* Memphis, Tenn.: Fraser, 1968.
   Several well-known clinicians each present one stutterer with whom they succeeded and another with whom they failed.

30. ———. *Treatment of the Young Stutterer in the Schools.* Memphis, Tenn.: Fraser, 1964.
   Outline the contents of this booklet.

31. St. Onge, K. "The Stuttering Syndrome." *Journal of Speech and Hearing Research,* VI (1963), 195–97.
   What is this author's basic challenge?

32. Travis, L. E. and Sutherland, L. D. "Suggestions for Psychotherapy in Public School Speech Correction." In Travis, L. E., ed., *Handbook of Speech Pathology.* New York: Appleton-Century-Crofts, 1957.
   What kinds of psychotherapy activities could be used in the public-school setting?

33. Van Riper, C. "A Clinical Success and a Clinical Failure." In Fraser, M., ed., *Stuttering: Successes and Failures in Therapy.* Memphis, Tenn.: Speech Foundation of America, 1968. Pp. 99–129.
   What seemed to be the factors which were responsible for the successes and failures in these two cases?

34. ———. "Historical Approaches." Chapter 2 in Sheehan, J. C., ed., *Stuttering: Research and Therapy.* New York: Harper & Row, Publishers, 1970.
   What are the past and present trends in the treatment of stuttering?

35. Vette, G. and Goven, P. *A Manual for Stuttering Therapy.* Pittsburgh: Stanwix House, 1965.
   Outline this workbook.

36. Wallen, V. "A Stutterer With a Low IQ." *Journal of Speech and Hearing Disorders,* XXVI (1961), 392–93.
   Summarize this case.

37. Williams, D. E. "A Point of View About Stuttering." *Journal of Speech and Hearing Disorders,* XXII (1957), 390–97.
   What does he say about the stutterer's feeling that he is blocked and has a speech impediment?

38. Wingate, M. E. "A Standard Definition of Stuttering." *Journal of Speech and Hearing Disorders,* XXIX (1964), 484–89.
   Summarize this attempt to identify the essential nature of stuttering.

39. ———. "Recovery from Stuttering." *Journal of Speech and Hearing Disorders,* XXIX (1964), 312–21.
   What are the author's conclusions?

40. Wohl, M. T. "The Electronic Metronome—An Evaluative Study." *British Journal of Communication,* III (1968), 89–98.
   How does the author answer the usual objections that such a device is a mechanical crutch and a distraction?

41. Wyatt, G. and Herzan, M. "Therapy with Stuttering Children and Their Mothers." *American Journal of Orthopsychiatry,* XXXII (1962), 645–59.
What were the authors' conclusions?

Texts

42. Barbara, D. A. *Stuttering: A Psychodynamic Approach to Its Understanding and Treatment.* New York: Julian Press, 1954.
A provocative and readable book which presents stuttering as a neurosis.
43. Beech, H. R. and Fransella, F. *Research and Experiment in Stuttering.* London: Pergamon Press, 1968.
Critically evaluates some of the research on stuttering.
44. Bloodstein, O. A *Handbook on Stuttering.* Chicago: National Easter Seal Society for Crippled Children and Adults, 1969.
An excellent summary of the nature and treatment of stuttering.
45. Brutten, E. J. and Shoemaker, D. J. *The Modification of Stuttering.* Englewood Cliffs, N.J.: Prentice-Hall, Inc., 1967.
Presents the two-factor conditioning explanation of stuttering.
46. Freund, H. *Psychopathology and the Problems of Stuttering.* Springfield, Ill.: Charles C Thomas, Publisher, 1966.
This book presents a review of the European writings on stuttering together with the author's view that it is essentially an expectancy neurosis.
47. Gray, B. and England, G. eds. *Stuttering and the Conditioning Therapies.* Monterey, Calif.: Monterey Institute for Speech and Hearing, 1969.
A series of papers from an international conference on conditioning therapy for stutterers.
48. Hunt, J. *Stammering and Stuttering: Their Nature and Treatment.* New York: Hafner Publishing Co., Inc., 1967.
First published in 1867, this reprint contains most of the early theories and therapies for stuttering.
49. Johnson, W. *Stuttering and What You Can Do About It.* Minneapolis: University of Minnesota Press, 1961.
Written to the adult stutterer or to the parents of a young stutterer, the author presents this semantic and interaction approach.
50. Luper, H. and Mulder, R. *Stuttering Therapy for Children.* Englewood Cliffs, N.J.: Prentice-Hall, Inc., 1964.
This book brings together much of the current information on the treatment of stuttering in childhood.
51. Murphy, A. and Fitzsimons, R. *Stuttering and Personality Dynamics.* New York: The Ronald Press Company, 1960.
A very readable book, this text is slanted toward the view of stuttering as maladjusted behavior due to interpersonal conflicts.
52. Robinson, F. B. *Introduction to Stuttering.* Englewood Cliffs, N.J.: Prentice-Hall, Inc., 1964.
A short book which surveys our knowledge of stuttering as a disorder. Noteworthy for its presentation of the common types of clinical problems that confront the therapist.
53. Sheehan, J. G. *Stuttering: Research and Therapy.* New York: Harper & Row, Publishers, 1970.

Summaries of the physiological, sociological, and psychological studies of stuttering are given, together with the author's view of its nature as a false-role conflict.

54. Van Riper, C. *The Nature of Stuttering*. Englewood Cliffs, N.J.: Prentice-Hall, Inc., 1971.
Summarizes most of the information concerning the nature, but not the treatment, of the disorder.

55. Weiss, D. *Cluttering*. Englewood Cliffs, N.J.: Prentice-Hall, Inc., 1964.
The classic book dealing with this disorder and its treatment. Weiss believes that all stuttering begins in cluttering and marshals much information in support of that thesis.

8

The Organic Disorders

of Speech

While we have previously considered certain speech disorders (such as those associated with laryngectomy and brain injury in children) that reflect organicity, in this chapter we deal with a set of disorders—aphasia, cleft palate, and cerebral palsy—in which the speech therapist works closely with the physician, the physical therapist, the occupational therapist, and others. In each of these disorders, teamwork is required since multiple problems are encountered. The aphasic person has speech and language problems, but he may also have seizures and other difficulties that require medical attention. The physical therapist will need to deal with the paralyzed limbs. The occupational therapist must enable the person to develop capacities and skills so that he can find some meaningful role in our society. The speech therapist, whose basic responsibility is to help the patient recover verbal and visual comprehension and the ability to speak and write again, must constantly be aware of these other problems and services. Formally or informally, the speech therapist is a member of a team.

The same situation exists with respect to persons with cleft palates. Here we work with the plastic surgeon, the orthodontist, the prosthedontist, and other specialists. These rely upon us not only for helping the person with cleft-palate speech to be more intelligible, less nasal, and free from nasal grimaces, but also in evaluating the effects upon speech of surgery or the fitting of speech appliances. In cerebral palsy, we find a set of problems due to brain injury that require physical therapy, medical care, and special education along with other services; and again, the speech therapist constitutes only one member of a team. With all of these individuals whose basic problems are organic in origin, we find ourselves dealing with the families of the patients. Speech pathology can never be an isolated profession, and the set of disorders discussed in this chapter makes that point very clear.

APHASIA

Approximately two million Americans are handicapped as a result of strokes. While about 200,000 die each year from this cause, those who survive are disastrously crippled, and not the least important part of the disability is the impairment in the ability to use language. They have what is called *aphasia,* or more accurately, *dysphasia.*[1]

The Disorder. Aphasia is the general term used for disorders of symbolization. The aphasic has difficulty in (1) formulating, (2) comprehending, or (3) expressing *meanings.* Often there is some impairment in all of these three functions. Along with these difficulties there may be associated problems of defective articulation, inability to produce voice, and broken fluency; but the basic problem in aphasia lies in handling *symbolic* behavior. Aphasics not only have difficulty in speaking, they also find it hard to read silently, to write, to comprehend the speech of others, to calculate mathematically, or even to gesture. Let us illustrate some of this behavior in a severe case of aphasia.

> Mr. A. was fifty-five when he had his "stroke." Some blood vessels in his brain had ruptured. As a result of this injury, his right arm and leg became paralyzed, his face pulled to one side a little, and he had many symptoms of aphasia. For example, he was unable to tell time even when he looked at his watch. He was still able to speak a little, but often he spoke a gibberish or his meanings were very difficult to understand. Here is how he asked for a cigarette: "Me me my . . . ah . . . go come . . . no . . . me go . . . no no no . . . um . . . suck now . . . suck, smuck, smoker . . . scum . . . oh my . . . smoker me smoker . . . oh dear . . . goddamm . . ."
>
> And this is how he wrote to his wife. We found that this was the best of his methods for communicating, although the script was very poor because he had to use his left hand. "I want you you come now see mmy. Butter I am. (He meant "better.") I love tell John. I come well sssssn."
>
> But Mr. A. could not write his name, not even in his checkbook, not

---

[1] C. R. Willis, ed., *Vocational Rehabilitation Problems of the Patient with Aphasia* (Washington, D.C.: U. S. Dept. of Health, Education, and Welfare, Rehabilitation Services Administration, 1967).

even from copy. He could print from copy, but the letters were often reversed. He seemed unable to read and had no interest in doing so, but he spent much time looking at the pictures of an illustrated magazine and enjoyed the television. Most of the gestures, and he gestured a lot, were fairly easy to understand, but at times he would shake his head vertically when he really meant "No!"

We had known Mr. A. before his stroke and knew him as an extrovert, a pleasant, highly verbal person. He was a crack salesman for a life insurance agency. When we saw him some six months after the stroke, he seemed markedly different. He cried frequently and did not seem to be able to stop crying once he had begun. Often he was profoundly depressed, confused, and withdrawn. Occasional bursts of profanity and vile language appeared in many inappropriate situations, and this behavior was very unlike his former manner.

There are some terms which are commonly used to describe some of this behavior. Mr. A.'s inability to write is termed "agraphia"; his inability to read, "alexia"; his inability to handle mathematics, "acalculia"; his jumbled sentences, "paraphasia." The inability to stop crying, the repetition of words in speaking or letters in writing is called "perseveration." His inability to remember or find a necessary word is called "anomia." Recovered aphasics tell us that often they can see the letters but that they appear to have no meaning, or they see the picture of an object but cannot tell what it is. This is termed a "visual agnosia." Or they can hear someone talking to them but cannot comprehend. The speech sounds "jumbled." This is called an "auditory agnosia." There is one other major term we must, reluctantly, provide you: "apraxia." This refers to an inability to command a part of the body to make a willed movement. An aphasic who may understand perfectly what you mean when you ask him to protrude his tongue or to pick up a pencil may not be able to command his tongue or hand to do so. Perhaps he lacks the inner speech that determines voluntary movement. At any rate, this inability to make a voluntary movement is termed "apraxia." There are many other technical words, but these are the most common.

Different aphasics show different patterns of impairment. The case we cited, Mr. A., was severely affected not only in the *expressive* and *receptive* aspects of handling meaningful symbols but also in their *formulation*. Most aphasics show some general loss in language ability, and it becomes more marked under fatigue or stress. However, certain aphasics may show their difficulty *primarily* in only one area. One of our cases after an automobile accident could speak fairly well but she could not read even a child's primer. Another could read magazines and newspapers readily but had much paraphasia in speaking.

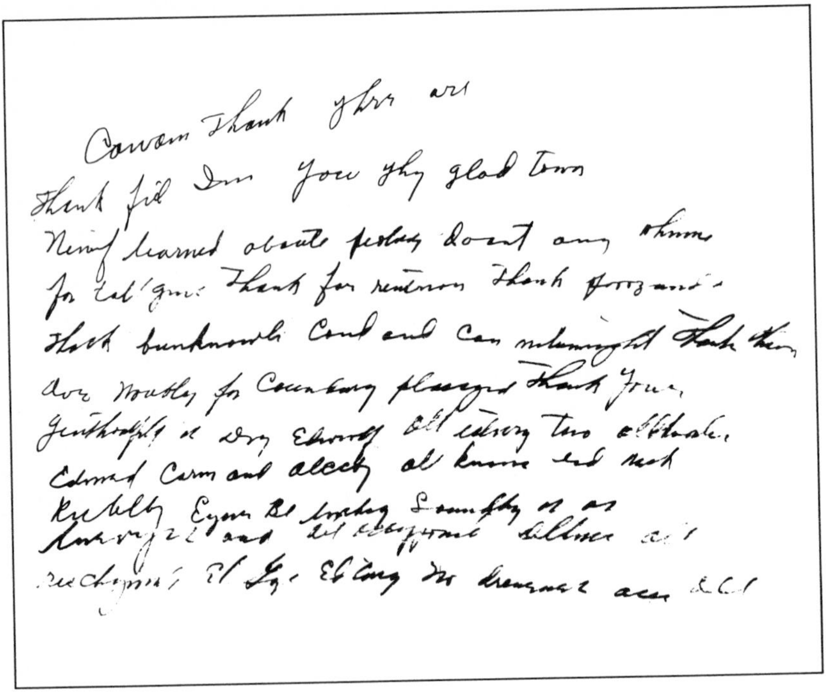

FIGURE 29: A *Thank You* Note *Written by an Aphasic to His Therapist,* Miss Josephine Simonson

This difficulty in comprehension is one of the major features of aphasia; and some impairment is usually present in one or another of the sense modalities, though in some patients it appears only under stress. A clear picture of this receptive disability is provided by Boone:

One man who recovered fully from aphasia described his inability to understand spoken language in this way: he knew that his wife was talking to him as he could hear her voice, but all the words she said were meaningless. When she asked him if he wanted a cup of coffee, he said it sounded like "ba boo la cakka somma ba boo?" It was without sense. When she finally poured him a cup of coffee and pointed to it, he knew immediately what she meant. The same thing was true when he tried to read the morning paper. He remembered the name "Johnson," which was the only word he could recognize. He could see the various letters and even the grouping of the letters into words, but the words didn't mean anything to him. It was like trying to read a foreign language. As he improved, he was able to understand a spoken command if it were simply stated. Then, if his wife said, "Have a cup of coffee?" he could understand it. But had she said something more complex like "The coffee pot's on the stove; why don't you let me pour you a cup?" he would not have been able to understand all that she had said.[2]

Causes. In adults, most of the causes of aphasia are due to some impairment in the blood supply that nourishes the brain, to tumors, or to traumatic injuries which destroy brain tissue. The blood supply impairment (termed "stroke" or "cerebral vascular accident") can occur as the result of (1) an embolus in which a bloodclot forms in one of the blood vessels and blocks off the nourishment of some area in the brain; or (2) a thrombosis in which a clot arising in some other area of the body such as an injured limb travels upward and lodges in one of the blood vessels supplying the brain; or (3) a hemorrhage in which an essential blood vessel breaks. Most of the aphasias caused by direct head injury are the result of automobile accidents, gunshot wounds, or brain surgery. Certain diseases of the brain may also produce aphasia.

It is necessary to explore each case individually to determine the areas of language and symbol functioning that are impaired. Generally speaking, the aphasic can handle concrete concepts better than abstract ones. Aphasics may be able, for example, to tell what a cup is named, yet be unable to *tell* you what it is used for, though they may show they know by going through the gesture for drinking. One other characteristic should be mentioned. Aphasics often seem to be able to handle what is termed "automatic speech" and social gesture better than speech which is highly communicative. For example, they can sing the words of a simple song when they cannot say them meaningfully. They might be able to say "Hello" and "Fine" or "Nice day," when they can't tell you the names of their children. They may be able to count only if they begin with "one, two, three"; never if they begin with "five" or have to count backward. They can often curse when they cannot talk at all. Aphasia is a complicated disorder because it deals with symbolic meanings, the most complex of all human achievements.

Tests for Aphasia. The first task of the speech therapist who seeks to help the person with aphasia is to determine the extent of his disability. While there are many tests which can be used to assess the language deficits of aphasics, three of those most frequently used are Schuell's *Minnesota Test for Differential Diagnosis of Aphasia*, Eisenson's *Examining for Aphasia*, and *The Language Modalities Test for Aphasia* by Wep-

[2] D. R. Boone, *An Adult Has Aphasia* (Danville, Ill.: Interstate, 1965), pp. 4–5.

man and Jones.[3] The Schuell test evaluates the aphasic's performance in five major areas: auditory disturbances; visual and reading difficulties; speech and language difficulties; visuomotor and writing disturbances, and deficits in handling mathematical concepts. A brief and incomplete outline of the subtests in each area may be illustrative.

Auditory Disturbances: The examiner evaluates the patient's abilities in recognizing common words; understanding sentences; following directions; repeating digits and sentences.

Visual and Reading Difficulties: This part examines the patient's ability to match forms, letters, pictures, and words with visual symbols, and checks for comprehension of silent and oral reading passages.

Speech and Language Difficulties: This section of the test explores the aphasic's difficulties in expressing himself in oral language. Speech movements and articulation patterns are checked, and the presence or absence of dysarthria and dyspraxia are confirmed.

Visual and Writing Difficulties: This section requires writing numbers, spelling, copying, and other such activities.

Mathematical Deficits: The testing here examines the patient's ability to handle the simple mathematical skills, knowledge of coin values, ability to tell time, and other similar skills.

The Eisenson test is less structured and is designed primarily to assess the aphasic's difficulties in reception and expression. It is primarily a screening test consisting of two parts. The first part tests auditory and visual comprehension and seeks to determine what auditory, visual, and tactile agnosias exist. In the second part of the test we find tasks that reveal nonverbal and verbal apraxias. The patient is asked to write numbers, letters, and words from dictation, to spell, to do arithmetic problems, oral reading, and clock-setting.

The *Language Modalities Test for Aphasia* (LMTA) by Wepman and Jones uses film strips to present the stimulus materials, though they are also supplemented by words spoken by the examiner. It was based upon extensive research and explores the patient's deficiencies in being able to translate from visual to oral symbols, aural to oral, aural to graphic, and visual to graphic. The test also explores the ability to do arithmetic and to comprehend language symbols. By analyzing the responses, the examiner is able to place the patient in one or another of the

---

[3] H. Schuell, *Differential Diagnosis of Aphasia with the Minnesota Test* (Minneapolis: University of Minnesota Press, 1965); J. Eisenson, *Examining for Aphasia: A Manual for the Examination of Aphasia and Related Disturbances* (New York: Psychological Corporation, 1954); J. M. Wepman, and L. V. Jones, *Studies in Aphasia: An Approach to Testing; Manual of Administration and Scoring for the Language Modalities Test of Aphasia* (Chicago: Education Industry Service, 1961).

following types of aphasic categories: syntactic, semantic, jargon, para-digmatic, and global aphasia. A brief description of the essential charac-teristics of these "types" of aphasia would run as follows:

Syntactic aphasia: The person speaks telegraphically, omitting many of the function words. Often has a moderate receptive loss.

Semantic aphasia: The patient has difficulty finding or recalling the words he needs. He seems to be searching, often frantically, for these words. Some difficulty in understanding spoken messages, especially when they are long or complex.

Paradigmatic aphasia: The patient has moderate to severe problems in comprehension and thus cannot respond appropriately.

Jargon aphasia: The patient has great difficulties in auditory reception, not only for the speech of others but also for his own speech. His utter-ances are garbled often to such a degree that communication is impossible, and yet he does not seem to be aware of what he is saying. He thinks he's making sense.

Global aphasia: Both receptive and expressive language are so greatly impaired that the handicap is almost total. Despite this, the person often seems alert and tries to understand and to speak.

There are other tests besides these three for diagnosing and appraising the extent of the aphasic involvement, but these are representative. Our brief description of their content should be sufficient to indicate the kinds of impairment shown by aphasics. What the tests do not show are the frustrations, anxiety, and helplessness experienced by people who have suffered a loss in the ability to handle symbols. They are lost souls. Speech therapists must also explore these areas if they hope to help the aphasic person. The text by McKenzie Buck entitled *Dysphasia* can provide much of the needed understanding.[4]

Most aphasics also show a one-sided paralysis (hemiplegia) or weak-ness of one arm and leg on the side opposite the brain injury, usually the right side. This may persist in some patients, but usually the patient re-gains the use of the leg enough to permit walking. Aphasics sometimes show *hemianopia*, a visual disturbance that makes it impossible for them to see more than half of the field of vision. Some of them have convulsions. For these reasons, no speech therapist will work with aphasics without consultation with the physician. Some patients show personality changes, an outgoing happy person becoming despondent and moody, while others become aggressive and controlling; but usually the basic personality traits persist despite the tremendous frustration and change in self-concepts which take place. Some laugh or cry without reason. They all fatigue very easily, find it difficult to concentrate, and tend to perseverate.

[4] M. Buck, *Dysphasia* (Englewood Cliffs, N.J.: Prentice–Hall, Inc., 1968).

Not long ago a wife of an aphasic patient said that it was not the situation or the familiarity of the words which would determine if her husband could understand, but rather that he might fail because sudden fatigue occurred. Surely we see many of the aphasic adults performing well, and then with a sudden clogging of the circuits they are deprived of the ability to understand or to express an idea. The aphasic seem to experience sudden momentary disorganization.[5]

Prognosis.   Immediately after the injury, the patient often shows a picture of extreme helplessness; but much of the impairment may subside within three or four months when what is known as "spontaneous recovery" occurs, though it is seldom complete and residual. Signs of aphasic disturbance can usually be found even in those who apparently have become well. Most authorities feel that spontaneous recovery seldom can be expected after six months and any improvement thereafter must be viewed as due to the relearning efforts of the patient himself or the teaching efforts of his therapists. The younger and the more intelligent and the more motivated the person is, the better are his chances for regaining his place in a communicative world. Wise handling of these patients immediately after the injury is absolutely essential if the terrific frustration that produces depression and defeatism is to avoided. Often the attitudes of the members of the family, doctors, and nurses can create unfavorable prognoses. With professional speech therapy and the cooperation of all those who tend the patient, many individuals suffering from the milder forms of aphasia can regain much of their ability to communicate.

Treatment.   In the section of this chapter devoted to diagnostic testing, the various deficits and impairments in reception, formulation, and expression were explored. In therapy we begin with those functions that have remained comparatively unaffected—we begin with what the patient can do. If he can gesture but not talk, we would start by strengthening that gesture language, then seek to attach simple verbalizations to the gestures. If he cannot write but has less difficulty in reading simple material, we would begin with reading and then later have him start copying. If there is a pronounced difficulty in word-finding, we may instead have him identify pictures or words by pointing. Or we may start with the automatic speech that remains—"How are you?" "Good morning," "bread and butter," or counting or naming the days of the week. If he has difficulties in comprehension, as most aphasics do, we make sure that we speak simply and slowly, though naturally. Aphasics are very susceptible to time

[5] J. Simonson, "Associated Social Problems of the Aphasic Patient . . . ," in C. R. Willis, ed., *The Vocational Rehabilitation Problems of the Patient with Aphasia* (Washington, D.C.: U. S. Dept. of Health, Education and Welfare, 1967), p. 43.

pressure. We make sure that we make silence comfortable so that he has time to search. Often he may get only one or two words of a sentence we say to him, and he must have time to guess how they are related. When we repeat what we say, we wait, and then repeat it exactly so that he will not have to decode a new message when he's just beginning to comprehend the old one. We avoid abstractions as much as we can. We talk about the things related to his major interests. Discovering one day that one of our patients had been a racing buff—a fact that had not appeared in our case history or family interviews, we procured some racing forms and had him help us select the horses to win, place, and show. At first he could only point, but from this nucleus we were eventually able to help him recapture some of the speech and mathematical skills he had lost.

Aphasic therapy consists of building bridges from the things the patient can do to those he cannot do. One of the surprising features of aphasic therapy is that when the patient begins to progress in one area of his language-handling, that progress often spreads to other areas. We do not have to teach these people new skills of symbolic processing; we have to help them *find* the ones that they have lost. We have to teach them to search without becoming frantic and frustrated. Our role is that of an immensely patient guide and companion to one lost in a wilderness not of his own making.

Although it is often difficult to get the person with aphasia, so overwhelmed is he by the catastrophe of the sudden change, to accept some responsibility for his own recovery of language, it is of paramount importance that this be done. As soon as we can, therefore, we try to encourage him to do his homework, setting up the tasks which he can perform by himself or with the help of his family: copying, writing, memorizing, naming pictures in a catalog, describing, echoing—whatever is within his capacity and can be reinforced. The Language Master is a useful tool for this purpose, but the daily newspaper and television have been used by some of our aphasics in their determined effort to regain some of their speech and comprehension. In achieving this self-therapy, the speech therapist must work closely with the family of the patient. As McKenzie Buck says, "aphasia is a family illness as well as a family catastrophe." By helping the members of the family understand the nature of the problem, by helping them make the necessary adjustments, they can aid the aphasic greatly in his self-therapy.

It is very difficult to describe the treatment for aphasia in general terms because the patterns of disability vary so much from case to case. As we have said, most of our early work with these patients consists of strengthening and improving the symbolic skills which are least impaired so that they can feel that they are not helpless and hopeless but beginning to improve. But we also work hard on the whole general language disability, building foundations for improvements in all areas; and it is this that we wish to consider next.

Stimulation. The world of an aphasic must be a most confusing place. Depending upon the particular functions affected, he may hear sounds or people talking to him but be unable to comprehend them; he may pick up the morning paper and see only meaningless squiggles running across the page. He may try to write his name in his checkbook and be unable to do so. He tries to ask for a cigarette and either he cannot remember its name or he speaks gibberish. He looks at the clock and cannot tell the time. He puts his hand in his pocket and feels something but does not know that what he feels is a coin. It is a blooming, buzzing confusion without rhyme, reason, or meaning. Here and there are moments of clarity, but they flit by too swiftly or are lost in frustration and depression.

One of the major tasks of the therapist is to provide islands of consistency in this sea of uncertainty. Patiently she explores her case to determine the things he can do. Perhaps he can copy letters from the alphabet; or if he cannot, perhaps he can trace over those she provides. Very well, she begins with this activity and continues with it until he knows that this function at least is within his powers. Then she stimulates him with other things. She may have him echo her words, animal noises, or gestures. They (therapist and patient) may put their spoons in their coffee cups in unison and stir the sugar and cream. She may ask him to point predictively to which one of the objects—knife, fork, or spoon—she will use in a moment to spread his bread. She may ask him to read her lips as she stimulates him with the number "three" for the three peanuts in her hand, then help him count them aloud. She may guide his hand in writing a few sentences to his wife. She will take his hand and touch it to his nose, his ears, his mouth, his feet, saying these names as she does so. Always she uses self-talk and parallel talk in very simple words, phrases, or sentences, providing the spoken symbols for every experience, for every activity. Day after day, she reviews this patient stimulation, tolerant of failure and happy when success comes. For success will come as the confusion subsides and the aphasic begins to find the functions he has lost.

Inhibition. Brain injury makes it hard to inhibit oneself. The lower centers of the brain miss their old brakes, as we see in the frequent overflow of emotion in the form of crying and laughing spells or catastrophic responses. Perseveration continues too long. One of our aphasics, once he had begun a sentence with "I think" could not stop saying these two words, over and over, over and over, over and over. Another was unable to speak what he desired to utter because all speech attempts began with "Yes, yes, yes," and the broken record went round and round on that single word. Accordingly we train our cases to inhibit themselves, to stop doing what they are doing, first upon our command, and then upon their own. We train them to inhibit any attempt to speak until we give the signal, or until they tap their foot five times. We teach them to wait, to pause, to say "No more that." We give them time to reorganize. We have them wait until we smile before they try again. We ask them to rehearse silently or in a mirror or in pantomime what they are about to do or say. We have them duplicate on purpose their crying or laughing jags and to stop them when the second hand of the watch points down. For the aphasic who can read, we provide "inhibition cards" which might, for example, read as follows: "Stop laughing!" "Wait!" "Whisper first!" We have them confess and cancel the perseveration which does occur.

Translation. The aphasic often gets blocked in formulating receiving, or sending messages because he keeps going up the same blind alley over and over again. We must teach him to shift when he meets these dead ends, to try another tack. Basic to this is translation training. By this we mean that we train the aphasic to shift from one type of symbolization to another. We may ask him to spell aloud, then print the name of the animal he hears meowing on the tape recorder. We have him count to three by the taps, again by drawing vertical lines, again by clapping hands, again by tracing the numeral, and finally by saying it. We say "Sit down!" and he must try to point to the appropriate picture, then to pantomime it with his lips silently, then to act it out, then to find the phrase on a card. We don't overwhelm him with too many translations at first; we let him lead us; but we always work to give him experiences in shifting from one set of symbolic meanings to another.

Memorization. One of the best ways of creating islands of consistency in the hurly-burly world of the aphasic is to teach him to memorize. Often we begin by having them memorize sequences of movements as in a calisthenic exercise or a sequence of lines to be drawn or the selection of a set of objects in a definite order. We demonstrate such sequences as opening the window, then closing the door, then saying "Too hot!" and then ask them to duplicate our performance. We have them find us three desired objects in a catalogue in the order in which we write them on the board. We arrange wood block letters in a row on the table so that they spell his name. We have him memorize the cards of different sizes and shapes which have written upon them such phrases as: "Good morning," "Nice day," "How are you?" "Goodbye," so that he can show them to us appropriately long before he can say these things. We have him write from memory, draw from memory, using flash cards to stimulate him and varying the exposure and delay time so he succeeds more than he fails. Finally, we ask him to learn by rote such passages as this:

I have been sick. I had a stroke. I must learn to read and write and speak again. Getting better. Takes time. Must work hard. No use feeling sorry. Get to work now.

Later on, we have the aphasic memorize poems and prose passages of increasing complexity. These not only help to provide associations between words, but also help in relearning the basic syntax of language.

Parallel Talking. We emphasize stimulation with simple materials, not complex ones. We speak simply and clearly, suplementing with gesture or written or pictured materials when needed. We do a great amount of parallel talking in this stimulation, telling him, simply and in short phrases or sentences, what he is doing, feeling, or perceiving. We use not only this sort of commentary but also prediction and recall. Often, as we do this parallel talk, we find the patient will almost unconsciously join in and say a word for us on which we fumble or postpone the utterance. This technique we have come to make the basic part of our therapy. It is a bit difficult to learn to do this well, for the therapist must make sure that he does the appropriate verbalization and hesitates at exactly the moment when the patient is experiencing the thought expressed. It is also necessary to keep from making too much of the case's spontaneous utterance when it does occur under these conditions. We merely say yes, and then restimulate him with what he has spoken in the context of the entire utterance. This is especially effective with the *expressive* aphasic, but we have also used a whispered or pantomimed form of parallel talking to help those who have trouble understanding spoken speech to read our lips. Often these individuals, if they learn to pantomime the speech they *see*, can then comprehend it, and some of the auditory agnosia subsides. The wife and other associates of the patient can be taught to do much of this parallel talking. We have found it most useful.

Scanning and Concentrating. The aphasic is like a man who suddenly finds himself in a strange country. He is overwhelmed by strange sights and sounds. He may hear people talking and be unable to understand what they are saying. He cannot write their language. He does not know what purposes some of the objects about him serve. Even a spoon is something strange. What he must do, in such a situation, is learn to observe and scan for meanings and consistencies. He must come to concentrate on things that look alike or on meaningless words which always seem to appear in the same context. Only in this way can such a person, suddenly transported to a strange land, come to find a place in it. But it is difficult for him to concentrate and difficult for him to observe closely. He needs help in scanning and concentration.

Accordingly, the therapist assists him to create order out of his chaos by training him in sorting out things that look alike, feel alike, sound alike.

She may give him a magazine and ask him to find all the pictures in which shoes are portrayed, to tear them out, and to put them under one of his own shoes. She may say some words for him and ask him to signal every time he hears one that begins with an *s* sound. She may have him feel a series of objects with his eyes closed and select those which are smooth to the touch. She may work with opposites: big things and little things; hot foods and cold foods. She asks him to choose, to match, to classify. He needs categories. She helps him acquire them again.

Organization. The aphasic needs order in his disordered cosmos. He needs definite routines of daily living, consistent schedules of events. When we come to our daily sessions with an aphasic, we use the same greeting each time and begin our therapy with the same sort of activity before we try something new. The other people about him must help in this same ordering of his life so that a portion of it will become familiar and organized rather than confused.

But he must also learn to organize his own life, his own thoughts, and outward behaviors. He needs help in patterning his consciousness. Accordingly we train him to make patterns of all types. We may begin by merely asking him or showing him how to set the table, or to turn the pages of a magazine left to right, or to arrange a few scrambled numbers in the proper order. We may have him raise his arm in a series of gradual steps. We may ask him to count the number of windows in the room, to draw a house, to roll a clay model of the cigarette he cannot ask for. We give him form boards to assemble. We give him some cards, each with a word on it, and ask him to place them serially so they make a sentence which commands us to do something. We get him to sing some old tunes. We ask him to read aloud a sentence through the window of a shield which exposes only one word at a time. We ask him to correct our mispronunciations, our use of wrong words, his own mistakes. All these activities require scanning and concentration. The therapist helps, always using her self-talk and parallel talk to provide a running commentary for his thinking.

Formulation. The aphasic often has trouble not only in sending his messages or in receiving them; he also cannot formulate them with precision. Sometimes he cannot find the exact word he needs; and instead of searching for another almost as good, or revising the whole utterance, he stops right there, helplessly, fixed on the thorn of his frustration. Basically, what he needs is the freedom to make new wholes, to try it again in a different way so that this different way also makes sense.

Although, as we have indicated, we use self-talk and parallel talking constantly throughout all of these various approaches to therapy with the aphasic, we use these techniques with greatest effectiveness in helping him to formulate. Here is a brief excerpt from such a therapy session:

Therapist: All right, John. Let's begin. Talk to yourself. Say what you do. Like this. (*Therapist opens her purse, takes out pencil, writes his name. As she does so, she speaks in unison with her activity.*) Open purse . . . here pencil . . . write name. (*She hands him the purse and signals him to repeat her behavior.*)

Aphasic (*opens purse*): Open puss . . . no . . . poos . . . no . . . oh dear oh my . . . (*gives up*).

Therapist: OK. You got mixed up on "purse". . . . Purrrrrse . . . Never mind. Say the whole thing. (*She repeats action.*)

Aphasic: Open puss . . .

Therapist: And here pencil . . .

Aphasic: Pencil . . . and now I write mame . . . no . . . mama . . . no . . .

Therapist: Write name . . . name . . . like this. (*Demonstrates.*)

Aphasic: Write name like . . . (*writes John*) . . . John . . . John . . . Write no good . . .

Therapist: Fine! You did it. Now let's do it again. Talk to yourself. Say what you're doing.

A thousand experiences of this sort, based on the experiences of daily living, cannot help but aid the patient to improve in formulation. His wife and his children can easily learn to do these things. They should use simple self-talk whenever he can hear them so he knows what they are doing, perceiving, or feeling. Through parallel talking, they can put the words in his ears at the moment he needs them, thus reauditorizing his thinking and giving them the verbal symbols that have become lost or scrambled. Sooner or later, the aphasic will begin to talk to himself as he does things, sees things, or feels things. This should be highly rewarded by all about him. He may even begin to use parallel talk as he views the behavior of others. We have found no difficulty in having this vocalized thinking persist in inappropriate situations because later, as he becomes facile in their use, we have him learn to do his self-talk and parallel talking in a whisper or in pantomime.

We may also help him to formulate in other ways. We ask him to complete unfinished figures, to assemble toys, to repair a broken electric cord, to weave a rug, to complete the writing of unfinished sentences, to prewrite what he is about to say, or to rehearse it in pantomime. We have him do simple description and exposition on paper or aloud. We teach him to fill in the hands of a series of blank clock faces to indicate the hours. We teach him to make change; to do mental arithmetic, or if he cannot do so, to do the operations on paper. We give him simple problems to solve. We teach him to paraphrase, to tell us what he has read in the paper or heard on the radio. The fascinating thing about all of this is to discover how each new achievement seems to unlock the doors to new achievements. If this therapist could begin over again, he would specialize in aphasia.

Body Image Integration.   It is not only the outside world which is strange to the aphasic. He also is a stranger to himself. He has changed. He is not the person he used to be. The various members of his family often show this by their reactions. They treat him like a child or as a nuisance or as though he were an imbecile. Good counseling can prevent much of this, but it is difficult for a family to become adjusted to a handi-capped stranger in the house.

We have said that the aphasic is also a stranger to himself. Often there is paralysis of the arm or leg. A part of him will not obey his bid-ding; he has suddenly sprouted a dead limb. Any one of us who has lain too long on an arm in bed and awakens to find it "gone to sleep," a strange inert thing there in bed with him, will vaguely understand how important this experience must be. But there are a thousand other changes in the person too. He has trouble reading, writing, talking, telling time, comprehending, counting. Who is this person who suddenly has come to inhabit his skin? It is the therapist's job to help him become acquainted, to introduce him to his new self and to get him to like this new person. It isn't easy but it can be done.

We begin by introducing him to his body. We massage his feet and name them as we do so. We lift his arm and tell him what we are doing. We have him stroke his face and find his eyes and ears and mouth. We get him to move his lips and his tongue as we do. We do much of our work with the body image in front of the mirror. We command the help-less hand to squeeze on the exercise ball, and we squeeze it. We take his picture in all sorts of therapeutic activities and show them to him. We look together in old albums at the snapshots of his childhood and youth. Perhaps all the king's horses couldn't do it, but a good therapist can put Humpty Dumpty together again.

Psychotherapy.   It should be obvious by now that these patients need psychotherapy. They meet many penalties, experience frustrations so intense they would break up almost any physical normal person. They find their cups overflowing with anxiety, guilt, and hostility. They worry about the hospital bills, about the paycheck that is no more, about their possible future in a nursing home. They become furious with anger, often over trifles. And yet, fortunately, the same brain injury that creates these storms of emotion also makes them transient. They do not last, do not reverberate. Furious one moment, the next moment he is laughing.

Such an outline of therapeutic activities is far from being compre-hensive, but it may provide a starting platform. It does not indicate how the therapist works especially on the functions of one area in which progress seems most likely to occur. And it does not show, except by implication, the need for ingenuity and, above all, the patient perseverance needed to rehabilitate these persons. Personally, we have found our work with aphasics to be more fascinating and rewarding than that with many other communicative disabilities. This is true not only with children with aphasia but also with the many adults who have been brought to us for help. To see a person who has been stricken down at the entrance to the valley of death rejoin the human race, and to feel that perhaps you have had a humble part in that rejoining, is reward enough for all the failures and frustrations aphasia therapy brings.

Speech Problems Associated with Cleft Palate

Another set of speech disorders primarily organic in origin are due, not to brain damage, but to deficiencies and abnormalities of the peripheral structures needed for normal speech. We have already considered one of these, the problem presented by laryngectomy. The speech therapist also encounters occasional individuals whose articulation is impaired by the loss of a tongue (*aglossia*) or by grossly deformed jaws and teeth. In this section, however, we are primarily concerned with the speech problems associated with clefts of the lips and palate. Most of these clefts are embryonic in origin, but some few persons are seen in whom the clefts were produced by accidents or other injuries. They present a problem that requires the speech therapist to work closely with other specialists.

Speech Problems. Clefts of the lip and palate affect speech in two major ways: the voice quality becomes deviant, and the articulation is impaired. With regard to the voice quality, the most prominent impression is that of excessive nasality. The person seems to be speaking through his nose, but this perception should not be confused with the nasal twang heard in certain dialects. Moreover, when closely analyzed, the voice quality differences shown by cleft-palate speakers are not confined entirely to excessive nasality.[6] Denasality also occurs, and the listener will often hear it first on the nasalized continuant sounds such as *m*, *n*, and *ŋ* when these are spoken by persons with cleft palates. There are also other rather unique types of articulation errors present in cleft-palate speakers. They have more trouble with the plosives and fricative sounds since these require the storing up of air pressure behind the closure or the narrowed opening. Voiced sounds seem to be easier than the unvoiced ones, but the consonant blends present considerable difficulty. In contrast to the errors made by young normal children, young cleft-palate children (and often

---

[6] A good discussion of these voice quality differences is given in H. Westlake, and D. Rutherford, *Cleft Palate* (Englewood Cliffs, N.J.: Prentice-Hall, Inc., 1966), pp. 34–44.

adults) tend to substitute glottal stops and pharyngeal fricatives for the standard sounds. Their speech seems to be punctuated by the little "catches of the breath" they use instead of such sounds as *p, b, t, d, k* and *g,* or clearing-of-the-throat noises which replace the fricatives.[7] The distortion errors are almost unique to the cleft-palate speaker. They are primarily due to nasal emission, the person snorting the sounds out of his nose. One of our adults with a cleft palate who, despite surgery and prostheses, still showed very deviant speech summed it up this way when he heard himself on tape: "Jeez, that's terrible. I knew it was bad, but not that bad. I can hardly understand what I was saying with all that honking and snorting." In severe cases the intelligibility is very poor, and often one of the major tasks of the speech therapist is to help the cleft-palate speaker to be understood. Fortunately, even without therapy, many cleft-palate speakers manage to discard some of their gross errors and improve their intelligibility somewhat as they grow older. The problem however is a complicated one, and the speech therapist must know the basic information about clefts and their rehabilitation if he is to help these persons.

Types of Clefts. Although classifications differ, there are three major problems involved: clefts of the prepalate, clefts of the palate, and clefts which include both palate and prepalate. All of these stem from embryological failure, or more rarely, from accidents. The two halves of the lip, or of the bony upper-gum ridge (alveolar process), or the two halves of the hard and soft palate fail to grow together and unite as they do before the third month in normal children. As a result, when the baby is born, it shows clefts of the upper lip, the upper-gum ridge, the hard palate, or the soft palate. These clefts may be complete or incomplete, but the right and left sides of these structures have not come together as they should have done.

Clefts of the Prepalate. These include clefts of the upper lip and also those of the alveolar process (upper jawbone beneath the upper gum). They may be unilateral and show a cleft on one side which if *complete* extends up into the nostril on that side. Or they may be bilateral or double clefts, each of which (if complete rather than incomplete) runs up into the nostril above it. These clefts of the lip in some children are also accompanied by similar clefts in the alveolar process; in other children the rift is in the lip alone. Although the majority of clefts are right-sided, left-sided, or both, a few rare median clefts (in the middle) are found.

Clefts of the Palate. Clefts in both the soft and hard palates are included in this category. The opening in the muscular soft palate may

---

[7] For a more detailed description of these articulation errors, see D. C. Spriestersbach, F. Darley, and V. Rouse, "Articulation of a Group of Children with Cleft Lips and Palates," *Journal of Speech and Hearing Disorders,* XXI (1956); M. Morley, *Cleft Palate and Speech* (Edinburg: Livingstone, 1958).

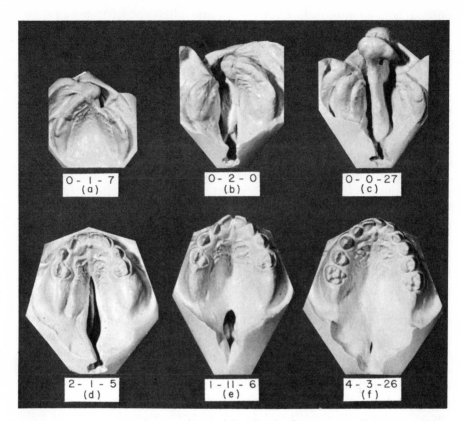

FIGURE 30: *Representations of the Most Common Clefts of the Lip and Palate.* All of these casts (of the upper surface of the mouth) were obtained from infants prior to any surgery. The numbers refer to the child's age in years, months, and days. They may be interpreted as follows: (a) Complete unilateral cleft of the lip and alveolar process; (b) Complete unilateral cleft of both the lip and palate; (c) Complete bilateral cleft of the lip and palate; (d) Cleft of the hard and soft palate; (e) Cleft of the soft palate; (f) Bifid uvula. From Samuel Pruzansky, "Description, Classification and Analysis of Unoperated Clefts of the Lip and Palate," *American Journal of Orthodontics,* XXXIX (1953), 590–611. By permission of the author.

show itself merely in a split (bifid) uvula or may extend upward and forward all the way to the edge of the bony hard palate. In this case we speak of a complete velar (or soft-palatal) cleft. There are also soft-palate clefts which extend only partially toward the hard palate.

Clefts of the Hard Palate. The bony roof of the mouth cavity formed by palatal shelves which grow together and join long before birth, also may be cleft, creating an opening into the nasal cavity. These clefts are along the midline, but one of the edges of the cleft may be attached to the base of the *vomer* (the bony partition that separates the right and left chambers of the nasal passages above). Usually, if the hard palate is cleft, the soft palate is also, since in the embryo the two halves of the roof of the mouth unite in stages proceeding from the front toward the rear.

Submucous Clefts.　Some children show no apparent signs of clefts when their mouths are visually inspected, and yet clefts may be present under the mucous linings of the mouth cavity. Those of the soft palate cannot be discovered except by radiography. The child's speech can be affected by such submucous clefts.

Clefts of Both Palate and Prepalate.　Unfortunately frequent are these clefts that run through both the palate and prepalate. There are some children who show total clefts: bilateral complete clefts of the lip and upper-gum ridge and an opening which runs from these all the way back to the division of the uvula. Some cases show no uvula. These babies with total clefts are not pretty to look at when they are born.

Causes.　When the cleft is in the prepalate or in both prepalate and palate, the cause seems to lie mainly in heredity. When the palate alone is cleft, we find other causal factors such as malnutrition, certain drugs such as cortisone, fetal anoxia (lack of oxygen in the blood, probably due to incompatible blood groupings), and mechanical injuries. The genetic factor is probably recessive. Other types of congenital abnormalities often seem to be found in the same familial lines, but it should be stressed that all clefts do not show hereditary influence. The inability of the embryonic structures to unite has also been explained in terms of the failure of the tongue to descend from the nasal cavity in which it resides before the embryonic palatal shelves begin their growth toward the midline. Not only humans, but mice, lambs, dogs, and goats have been born with clefts. Scientists have been able to produce clefts along with other abnormalities by depriving the animal mothers of riboflavin, a vitamin found in large amounts in the liver, by inducing calcium deficiency, and by irradiation. The exact origin of clefts is as yet not completely understood.

Effects of Clefts.　As we have indicated earlier, when a baby is born with a cleft, special services are required to combat the many problems which arise. Among other problems are those involving feeding. The baby must be fed more carefully, held in a special position, burped more often, and fed more frequently. The family must finance trips to all the special services and spend the time necessary. Many psychological problems arise, silent accusations leading to friction between the father and mother, sacrifices of the needs of other siblings to the cleft-palate child's needs, problems in social adjustment. Since often the speech therapist must serve as a general, long-time counselor for these families, she should know the nature of these difficulties.

Surgery. Surgery for the prepalate is accomplished early, within the first three months in a healthy baby. Scars remain which will diminish as the child grows, and these can often be removed or concealed by later plastic surgery. The double and complete prepalate clefts present more difficulty than the incomplete or unilateral ones and may require more than one operation.

The age for palatal surgery is still the subject of conflict. Critics have shown that early surgery has sometimes been responsible for distortions of head growth and for some of the facial, dental, and palatal malformations which contribute to the cosmetic handicap and that of speech. The defenders of early surgery have attributed such failures to poor surgical technique or to insufficient tissue or other reasons; and they point out that with proper surgery, no head malformations occur, and the child is enabled to learn his initial speech without the handicap of the open cleft which otherwise would produce abnormal speech habits. Fortunately, the speech therapist is able to stay out of these arguments. His job is to help with surgical failures at any age. While some surgery is now being carried out as late as four and five years, often after a temporary prosthesis has enabled the child to have a chance to develop a good speech from the beginning, the majority of initial operations take place early.

In cases of extensive clefts, the surgery is performed in several stages, necessitating two or even three operations. The first is to effect closure or partial closure of the cleft palate, the others to create a muscular mechanism capable of shutting off the pharyngeal (throat) passageway to the nose. Several different types of operations are employed that need not be described here since this information is available in other texts and articles, but the student should at least know that the "push-back" operation requires an incision along the inside of the gum ridge so that the tissue can be moved rearward to effect a better closure, and that the "pharyngeal flap" operation creates a living bridge of tissue taken from the rear wall of the throat and joined to the soft palate in front. In other operations, the side walls of this part of the throat are narrowed. It should be kept in mind that what is intended in all these operations is the provision of a mechanism which can direct the airflow and sound through the mouth rather than the nose.[8]

Each year major advances in surgery seem to occur, and great strides have been made in providing the structures needed to shut off the nasal

[8] See R. B. Yules, and R. D. Chase, "Pharyngeal Flap Surgery: A Review of the Literature," *Cleft Palate Journal,* VI (1969), 303–8.

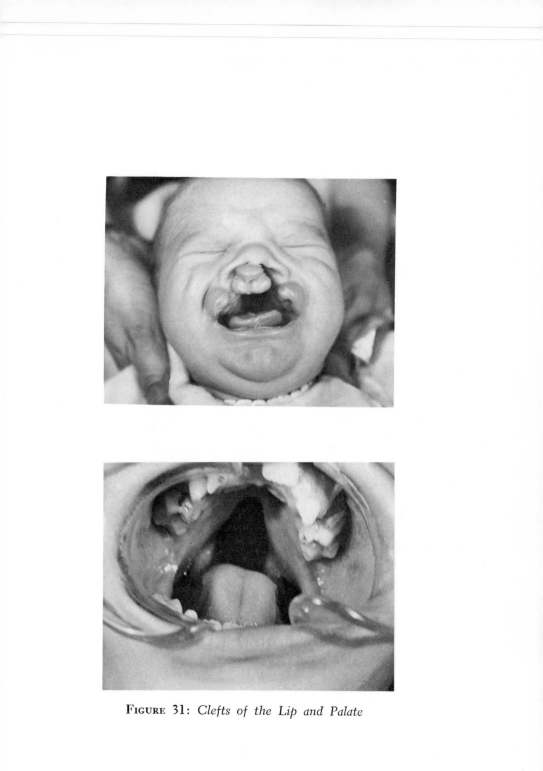

FIGURE 31: *Clefts of the Lip and Palate*

airway.[9] We are not seeing nearly as many persons with cleft-palate speech as we did twenty years ago, and those we do see do not show the facial deformations and grossly deviant speech that were common then. Nevertheless, not even the best surgeon using the most modern techniques can help all these persons.

Prostheses. There are certain cases of cleft palate for whom surgery is not the wisest course. Certain clefts are so large or the tissue remaining so scant or poorly developed that the prognosis for good speech, easy swallowing, and a good facial appearance is very poor. A real controversy has raged for many years between the dentists (prosthodontists) and the surgeons. Surgeons claim that living tissue is always preferable to any artificial means for closing the mouth from the nose. They point to the unsanitariness of prostheses, the inconvenience, the difficulty of fitting, the lack of a movable-at-will valve, the inability of small children to tolerate them until after poor speech habits have been formed. The prosthodontists, on the other hand, point to the numerous instances of surgical failure, the interference with facial growth and the poor cosmetic appearance, the pain and mortality, the short palates that do not work, the tearing of tissues and perforations, and the defective speech that often results from surgery. The argument still rages in many quarters, but recently the development of teams of specialists to fit the treatment to the needs of the particular child rather than to the disorder has resulted in a most hopeful compromise. Often the speech therapist is called upon to referee, and so he had better know enough about protheses to play his part.

Essentially, prostheses are artificial substitutes for a missing part. In the past the term was synonymous with "obturator"; but so far as cleft palates are concerned, obturators are now used to mean fixed appliances that are more or less permanently inserted into clefts of the hard palate, whereas prostheses are detachable appliances consisting of an artificial hard palate (perhaps bearing also some artificial teeth) and a bulb. The latter is designed to close the nasopharynx (partially rather than completely), and to serve as an object to be gripped by the constrictor muscles of the pharynx to create a valve.

Prostheses have been made of many materials. There are accounts in ancient Greek literature of cleft-palate individuals filling their clefts of the hard palate with fruit rinds, cloth, leather, tar, and wax so that they could eat and drink. Passavant made a stud-shaped obturator which he inserted into a slit in the palate after it was sewed up, but it did not work too well. Others injected wax or inserted silver plate projections into

[9] For a description of the newer forms of surgery and the team approach to cleft-palate habilitation, see R. B. Stark, ed., *Cleft Palate: A Multidisciplinary Approach* (New York: Harper & Row, Publishers, 1968).

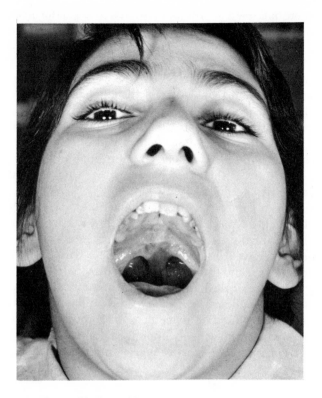

Figure 32: *Pharyngeal Flap*

the back wall of the pharynx. In the late 1800s artificial hard palates anchored to the teeth were provided with hinged gates, rubber bulbs, rubber tubes, silver balls, and other devices to plug or narrow the nasopharyngeal airway. All of these were very unsanitary, often prevented nasal breathing or interfered with it, and at times produced marked denasality on some sounds while failing to eliminate the nasality on others. Some of these devices were painful and caused gagging and choking. Ear infections were common.

Modern appliances use an acrylic resin that can be molded and worked by the designer so that it will fit any opening. They are highly sanitary, easily cleaned, and are very light in weight. Plastics opened the way for truly effective cleft-palate prostheses. They can even be modified without the need for new impressions to be taken or new casts made.

Design of Prostheses. There are two parts to the usual prosthesis, the palatal part and the bulb. The former is designed through the taking of impressions to conform to the contours of the hard palate. Frequently, if there is a cleft in the hard palate, the palatal part of the appliance is raised to fit into this cleft to provide some of the retention. Besides this, clasps to fit around the teeth are provided. Even in very small children, as soon as their first teeth have been cut, small orthodontic bands on the molar teeth can be used to keep the prosthesis in place. In most instances, the palatal part of the appliance is made first and fitted into place to close the cleft. Gradually an extension is added to the rear part of this palatal section as the individual learns to tolerate it and larger and larger bulbs are used until finally the desired size and shape has been reached. Some very young children are thus fitted with these prostheses when study of their case indicates that surgery should be postponed until they are five and six years old.

The location of the bulb in the nasopharynx often is critical. In general, the bulb should be placed in the area of greatest nasopharyngeal construction. This is usually determined by taking X-rays in the production of a sustained [u] vowel, or by observation in a dental mirror, which is less satisfactory. Often the fitting of these bulbs is tedious, and the speech therapist is sometimes called upon to use his critical ear to determine the extent of nasality and nasal emission in the various trial positions. If the bulb is placed too high, some denasality may appear, and reducing the size of the bulb will not affect the amount very much. Instead of shaving the bulb, it is sometimes wiser to change its position.

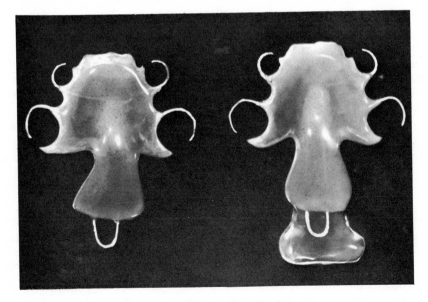

FIGURE 33: *A Prosthesis*

It is often difficult to predict the shape or size of bulb required, and only patient fitting with judgments of speech adequacy and tolerance in swallowing, yawning, and blowing will help. At times altering the shape of the bulb may be even more important than the cross-sectional area, since the constrictor muscles may require a larger vertical surface to grip for adequate closure. Usually the first bulbs used are larger than those required later, since the bulb itself stimulates muscle activity, and as these muscles develop, the bulb may need to be shaved if denasality or interference in breathing is to be prevented.

In the fitting of the prosthesis it is sometimes unavoidable that a secondary operation be performed to create a better shaped cleft so that the prosthesis can be made suitable to the needs of the case. Many surgeons tend to oppose this, but if the tissue is not functioning and the scar tissue or perforations are preventing the proper positioning of the appliance, it is wise to accept the necessity. There are also times when some of the taut musculatures may move along with the constrictor muscles which squeeze upon the bulb and displace the palatal part of the appliance with their residual movement. In these instances, operations on the tensor muscles may eliminate this movement, though care must be taken to insure that they not be cut completely since their upper ends seem to play a part in the opening of the Eustachian tube to the middle ear.

With regard to the cost of prostheses, it seems that they are seldom any less expensive than surgery. Repeated visits are necessary, and when the prosthesis is fitted to a small child, the costs mount up. However, if costs are calculated in terms of pain, the appliance certainly will win. We should not expect that the use of a prosthesis will immediately produce normal speech, though some reduction in nasality and nasal emission usually does occur. The patient must be taught to use the prosthesis in speech and in swallowing.

Summary

When should a prosthesis be recommended?

1. In cases of unilateral and bilateral clefts of the palate which have been surgically closed anteriorly but the constrictor muscles left unscarred and still functional.
2. In cases of postsurgical failure in which excessive scar tissue or loss of tissue or perforations have produced a nonfunctioning closure so far as speech or swallowing are concerned.
3. In cases of acquired clefts.
4. Where any operation would be likely to interfere with the centers of growth or tend to produce marked malformations of the maxillary bone.

5. Where operations cannot be performed because of health conditions or psychological hazards.
6. When three stages of operations have already been performed.

When should we refuse to recommend a prosthesis?

1. Where there is a floating premaxilla that will dislodge the appliance until it is removed. Also a protruding premaxilla.
2. Where the hard palate is depressed or so full of scar tissue that the palatal part of the appliance would be unlikely to be retained.
3. When there are not sufficient teeth in good condition to hold the appliance.
4. When surgery seems to be the better course.

What are the requirements of an adequate prosthesis?

1. It should be so designed as to create sufficient closure for good speech.
2. It should have good retention, bracing, and support.
3. It should be comfortable after adaptation.
4. It should improve, where necessary, the facial appearance.

Speech Therapy with Prostheses. When the prosthesis is finally finished, the speech therapist's work has just begun. If the case has been properly prepared, he will realize that the appliance itself will not solve his speech problem but that he must learn to use it. If the prosthodontist is wise he will have made the acrylic bulb so it can be temporarily detached, though it will be fixed later.

The speech therapist will begin with warming up exercises for pharyngeal constriction and oral airflow, then insert the bulb and duplicate these. We use silent air sucking through the mouth in the supine position first, then gradually raise the head. Then we run through all of the other activities which involve no phonation but airflow control. Next we use pantomimic speech while holding the breath; then whispered (soft) vowel sequences, omitting the *i* and *u*. Then we use the same with soft voice, often returning to the silent airflow activities between trials. Then we begin with the consonants, first of all the loose-contact *p* and *t*, then the *b* and *d* sounds. Then the *f* and *v*, and then the *ch* and *j*, the *l* and *r*, and only finally the *z* and *s*.

Only after the case has worked with each of these sounds successfully with the prosthesis and has used them not only in isolation but in nonsense syllables and in isolated words, should he be permitted to begin to speak short phrases or simple sentences, and these at first should have no *m*, *n*, or *ng* sounds in them. Much checking with a recording device and amplification of nasal airflow or voice should be used during the training sessions.

Gradually, the muscle control will improve, and better closures will be obtained. We have seen cases who made steady gains for more than two years. But the beginning of therapy is vital. Unfortunately, many prosthodontists do not understand how important it is to build new habits from the start. If the first speech attempts with prosthesis in place are done without guidance of a trained speech therapist, the case may learn how to continue his habitual nasality and nasal emission despite the appliance.

Evaluation of Velopharyngeal Competency. Surgery and prosthetic appliances unfortunately do not always guarantee that normal speech can be obtained even with the best of speech therapy. The person may come to us with a closure mechanism that will not close sufficiently to permit adequate speech no matter how long and hard we work. We may be able to improve the person's articulation and intelligibility, but he will still sound hypernasal and abnormal. We have known therapists and cases who struggled for years to do the impossible, years which might better have been spent in designing a better prosthesis or in new surgery. How can we be sure that this case of ours can really close the rear passageway to the nose? How can we know that he has a competent velopharyngeal valve?

In the past, speech therapists have used such simple tests as the ability to suck liquids up a straw or to blow a horn or a feather or to say a series of isolated vowels to determine this capacity for closure. Or they visually observed the uvular movement or the constriction of the pharyngeal wall. Unfortunately, tests of this nature are far from being adequate. At times it is possible to procure from the cleft-palate clinic some evidence from X-ray films that the closure is sufficient. Still pictures, however, are not as good as those procured by fluoroscopic movies, since the former require the prolongation of sounds and do not show what happens in a plosive sound such as *p* or *k*. It is also possible to determine the competency of velopharyngeal closure by comparing the amount of air pressure which can be produced with the nostrils open and with them closed. The oral manometer is one of the instruments used to measure the air pressure under these two conditions. In normal blowing, we get the necessary oral airflow by closing the velopharyngeal opening enough to prevent the airstream from leaking out of the nose. The air-pressure values with the nose occluded should be approximately the same as when the nasal airway is open. If the person does better with the nostrils shut, then we suspect that the velopharyngeal valve is not working right.

There are various other devices and techniques which help us deter-

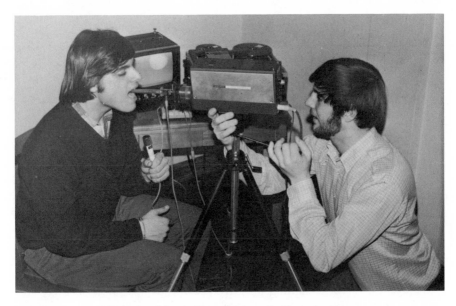

FIGURE 34: A *Panendoscopic Examination*

mine whether the person really has the capacity to close off the nasal airway—pressure transducers, airflow sensors, the nasendoscope, and the oral panendoscope. We will describe only the last of these. The panendoscope is essentially a tiny camera fitted into the end of a slender probe tube that is inserted into the mouth and then back into the opening of the pharyngeal cavity. By combining this instrument with a videotape recorder, the image of the velopharyngeal area can be displayed during certain speech activities, thus permitting the viewer to observe directly whether closure is occurring.

However, we can also get some impression concerning the adequacy of the closure mechanism by analyzing the speech itself. First of all, we should check the articulation errors. If we find key words in which all of the defective sounds or most of them are used correctly, we can be pretty sure that enough closure is present. Again, if at times these errors are not accompanied by nose twitching or nasal emission of air, we can feel that the valve is all right. If the person can speak very well with his nostrils closed but has much nasal distortion when they are open, we would suspect inadequate closure. Finally, if the consonants that require extra mouth pressure (*p-b; t-d; k-g; s-z; ch-j*) are those which are nasally distorted while the *r* and the *l* or *f* and v are quite adequate, we would feel that the closure was poor.

It is impossible to outline a program of speech therapy techniques which would be applicable to all cleft-palate cases, or even a majority, since the problems presented by the cases are so different. Individual diagnoses are absolutely essential. We deal with speech that reflects the personality of the case, with his concept of self. The basic attitude of a case who feels that, because he has an organic disability there is nothing which can be done to alter his speech, has a profound effect upon therapy. Often little speech therapy can be accomplished until psychotherapy has produced some reality testing, until some hope has been provoked, until the case can trust the therapist when he cannot trust his own parents or closest friends. Most of these cases know little about the nature of their problem or the possibilities for improving speech. They come as passively and as unenthusiastically as they go to the surgeon, the prosthodontist, or the orthodontist, because they have been told they should. Few of them feel any powerful urge to accept some of the responsibility for their speech improvement. Like the stutterer, the cleft-palate case has detached himself from his speech because it is too painful to confront. As in stuttering, we meet with strong resistance when we are forced to demand the active cooperation of the cleft-palate person in confronting his nasal emissions, his nasality, and his poor articulation. Without this control, without this monitoring, it is almost impossible to make any but perfunctory gains. Like the normal speaker, the cleft-palate person does not hear himself speaking; he hears his expressed thoughts. It is difficult for the normal speaker to concentrate on self-hearing. In the cleft-palate person, this self-hearing is not only burdensome but also painful. Unless the speech therapist understands this basic psychology, he can hardly hope to be effective.

It is also necessary, quite apart from the individual's attitudes toward his speech and its therapy, to take into account the actual organic disability which may be present. Some cleft-palate persons with very defective speech may have complete closures and the potential for completely normal speech. Some of these are already using their closures in activities other than speech or on other speech sounds save those which are defective. Others of the same group may have the potential to use their soft palate or pharyngeal musculatures but have not learned to do so. But we must also recognize that there are some cleft-palate cases whose structures or prostheses are not adequate for normal speech, and for whom we may be able to do very little except in the improvement of intelligibility. Again, let us state our melioristic philosophy of speech therapy: We make the person's speech better and we make him a happier person. We do not have to make his speech perfect or make him a completely happy human. Within the limits of our time and energy and knowledge, and with an awareness of the limitations which the case also possesses, let us do our utmost and be content with that. They must learn to speak as well as they can, with as little interference to communication as possible and as little abnormality as possible.

Aims of Speech Therapy for Cleft-palate Speech.   Our basic points of attack are these: We must decrease the nasal emission, the hypernasality, and the defective articulation. We must improve the oral air pressure and oral airflow. We must eliminate abnormal foci of tension and abnormal nostril contractions. We must activate the tongue tip, lip, and jaws. We must improve the respiratory rhythms of speech, and their rate and control. We must improve velar and pharyngeal contraction.

We once examined a complete, unilateral cleft of both the hard and soft palates who had completely normal speech. How he managed this we were unable to tell, but he did use wide jaw movements, slow speech, short phrases, and dentalized most of his frontal sounds. All plosives were made with very loose contacts. He spoke softly and did become nasal when he spoke loudly. So far as we could ascertain, this person operated his speech with very little air pressure, and it flowed out of the larger mouth opening rather than the smaller nasal opening merely because it was larger. He was not tense, but very relaxed, and perhaps this accounted for his lack of hypernasality, since certain authorities feel that the characteristic tone of nasality is due to a *constricted* open-ended tube rather than to the open tube itself. At any rate, he demonstrated how much we might be able to do in speech therapy. This case also illustrates an important principle. We should work for altering the direction of airflow so that it flows outward toward the mouth rather than upward through the nose. And we should teach the cleft-palate person to articulate with a minimum of oral air pressure.

Air-pressure Controls.   Air pressure within the mouth varies with the various speech sounds. The plosives and the sibilants require the most air pressure. Voiced sounds require less than do the unvoiced sounds due to the increased audibility of the former. The *t* and *d* require less than *k* and *g*. People vary widely one from another in the degree of closure used in producing the plosives and the fricatives. Certain individuals use very tight closures and sudden releases; others do not. Cleft-palate cases often use very tight closures and sudden releases. This is very unwise since much more air pressure is required for such plosives than for the loose-contact, slow-release type. We experimented once by inserting a small air hose into the corner of the lips and had the subjects, both normal and cleft-palate, articulate a series of plosives and fricatives. They then held their breath and pantomimed the various sounds both with tight contacts and with loose ones. Less air pressure was required to produce clear sounds when the loose contacts were used. In the cleft-palate cases, little air escaped from the nose when loose contacts were used; but it was very evident when tight contacts were used. The cleft-palate person whose velum is functioning also reacts very characteristically to a tight contact either of tongue tip or lips. These tight contacts almost seem to act as triggers to cause a lowering of the palate and a relaxation of the superior constrictor in much the same way as they tend to set off stuttering tremors in the stutterer.

This occurs not only with the plosives. The fricatives, which employ a narrow opening or channel for the airflow, are also produced differently by different people. Certain ones use a very narrow channel; others a broader one. Cleft-palate individuals tend to use the narrower ones that require a greater air pressure, and so nasal emission tends to occur. We therefore should teach them differently.

Much of the stimulus value of a sound can be increased by prolonging its duration. If cleft-palate persons are to soften their contacts in order to make use of the lessened air pressure in the mouth due to the palatal air leak, they must prolong these sounds somewhat, to gain the same intelligibility. Weaker s sounds should be held longer. A slightly prolonged *f* in the word *fish* even if weaker in airflow will be understood as readily as a quicker, stronger one.

Concentration in therapy upon these factors also emphasizes the direction of airflow through the mouth rather than the nose. Cleft-palate people are nose-conscious as the contraction of their nostrils demonstrates. By concentrating on the longer, slower, looser contacts and the shallower channels of articulation, the airflow tends to go mouthward. This emphasis upon the mouth, rather than the nose as the major channel for speech and airflow, is among the major objectives of any speech therapy. It is in large part a psychological problem as we have indicated. We have known cleft-palate children to speak much better as soon as they held a megaphone to their lips or thought that we were going to hold their noses. We have had several cases who were able to blow trumpets very well and yet could not manage a simple *p* sound without having it come through their nose. For this reason, most speech therapists do much lip and tongue training along with blowing exercises. We have given lip exercises with profit to cleft-palate cases who already had perfect lip control, primarily so that they would become mouth-conscious. We have had then talk through fringed holes in a sheet of paper, through various sizes of slits and blowing tubes, with their fingers in their mouths, with their mouths to ears, through fringed paper mustachios, into the vibrator mouthpiece of toy musical instruments, with their mouths held under water, into cones whose apex flickered a candle flame. One of our children spoke much better when he put on a clown's mask that had a monstrous big mouth which he watched in a mirror. He just became more mouth-conscious, and the air came out of that opening. We have improved the speech of cleft-palate cases by teaching them to read lips and to help in training deaf children in lipreading. One of our majors got better speech from a cleft-palate girl by putting lipstick on her mouth and having her watch it in the mirror. We have darkened a room and put a little flashlight focused on the outside of the mouth in a narrow beam, and also within the mouth, and improved the speech by having the case watch it in the mirror. Cleft-palate cases must think of speech as coming out of the mouth.

Many speech therapists teach their cleft-palate cases to open the mouth widely in speech, as far as they can without appearing abnormal. This is often difficult to teach, and resistance is almost sure to be found; but when it can be used it does seem to improve speech markedly. It does this first because any larger opening attracts airflow. Air must take a tortuous course when it must go upstairs through the filters of the nasal caverns and then down and out through the narrow slits of our nostrils. It would much rather come out of a side door, especially if that side door is open. Moreover, larger mouth openings for the vowels tend to produce looser contacts of lips and tongue, and they certainly increase the consciousness of the mouth rather than the nose.

The source of the air pressure and airflow is, of course, in the contractions of the muscles that lower the chest and contract the abdomen and these muscles, with a relaxing diaphragm, create a condition of pressure upon the lungs. Many cleft-palate cases require training in breath control for speech. Their breathing records show many instances of air wastage, speaking on residual air, opposition, and staircase breathing. They often start speaking with a very strong pulse of air which goes up through the pharynx or cleft because of its pressure, and then creates the path for whatever air is left to follow. They often inhale too deeply prior to utterance (which causes tension all along the airway) to produce this initial strong blast or pulse. With much of the air wasted in the first few syllables, the person then must speak on residual air or opposition breathing, both of which increase tension everywhere. It is possible to improve the speech, the nasal emission, and the hypernasality by teaching the case to inhale a normal amount of air and to start his utterance gradually rather than suddenly and to monitor the amount of air used. Cleft-palate speakers must learn to watch their phrasing, which means their breathing.

Muscle Training. It is also possible of course, in many cases, to improve the state of air pressure within the mouth by shutting off the air leak, by improving velopharyngeal closure. Many of the muscles are weak and can be strengthened through appropriate exercises if surgery or prosthesis has been successful in creating the conditions for a possible closure. If the cleft-palate case can blow up a balloon or whistle, or if inspection with a dental mirror shows good occlusion of the nasopharynx, we should be able to help him use some closure in speech. Even when this is not possible but when, in phonation, yawning, or other activities, we can see the velum lift or the side walls of the pharynx contract or the rear wall come forward slightly, we must presume that we can improve this functioning until we find otherwise. (This last statement may not be true if the velum is too short or taut or the pharynx so enlarged that no closure seems possible.)

Such muscle training requires two major items besides devoted practice: location of the musculatures by the patient and perception of their movement. In physical therapy where comparable tasks are present, the physical therapist, through massage, positioning, and passive movement, is often able to get movement of muscles as inert as those of the cleft-palate patient's repaired velum. Unfortunately a limb is easier to manipulate than is a palate. Nevertheless, speech therapists have employed some of the same principles of physical therapy in activating the velar and pharyngeal muscles. Light massage with a finger cot (covering of rubber) first along one side of the uvula, then on the other, and then with two fingers straddling the midline, has helped to localize the area. The stroking must be done very lightly and both away from the midline in a horizontal direction, and anteroposteriorly. Care must be taken that the child does not gag or bite your fingers off. These exercises must also be done with caution lest tissues be injured; but when they are done lightly and the patient attempts to feel and predict the location and direction of movement, they can be very effective. Only a little of this can be done at a time since the patient tires quickly. Another procedure involves the tapping of these structures in the same areas, the patient being requested to tell the number of taps and their intensity. We also may slightly depress the surface of the palate or tickle it or the pharyngeal wall if the gag reflex is not present or is weak. These techniques all involve the location of the structures by the tactual sense.

We may also use the visual sense. Many cleft-palate cases have no visual imagery of their palates with which to correlate movement. They should study and describe the action of the therapist's palate in action. They should watch both their own and their therapist's palate in mirrors. They can be shown large pictures of the palate on charts and be taught to point to the area which the therapist touches. When there is residual movement, it should be viewed visually, and then imagined. A very clear picture should be possessed by every cleft-palate patient of the nature of his problem. Even little children can be given this in imaginative terms: "the little red gate or door."

Since most repaired cleft-palate cases have some movement of the levator and tensor muscles as well as of the constrictor muscles in certain activities, they must be taught to isolate and to identify the experience. Certain key words should be conditioned to palatal activity: "up . . . down . . . squeeze . . . let go . . . open . . . shut." These must be used by the therapist only when the activity actually occurs. They should first be used by the case when observing the therapist's palatal movements, then when observing his own, then with intermittent eye-closing with attention to kinesthesia.

It is also possible to become aware of palatal movement by other sensations. With the mouth open, try to get the case to feel some air pressure in his middle ear, to feel it click or pop. This must be done while holding the breath. The palatal tensor, when it contracts, has some effect upon opening the Eustachian tube. Also in yawning, the palatal muscles tend to contract and can be felt in action. Closed-mouth yawning is especially effective in developing kinesthesia, and it can be combined with the middle-ear pressure cues. Also use different mouth openings.

Some of the tactual sensations can also be achieved with a syringe by blowing a stream of air or "warm water" against certain parts of the soft palate. The child may also explore his own mouth with his own finger, using the fingers cut from sterilized rubber gloves. Loud snoring (with the nose held so that all inhalations are made through the mouth) will vibrate the uvula, and research has shown that in this snoring the palate is raised. It is possible to snore on the various vowels and with different tongue positions or lip postures. Tight closures of the tongue and velum in silence as in the position for a *k* sound will, if the release is very sudden, provoke some upward movement of the palate at the same time that the tongue is jerked downward. The sound-play known as "gibbegadong" is also effective when the case can do it, since it is based upon the last-mentioned principle.

Weak palatal movements, when present, can be made more effective in closure by having the patient lie on a cot with his head held far backward so that the force of gravity aids rather than resists the palatal movement. When there is asymmetrical pull on the palate, turning the head or the jaw to one side seems to be of some assistance.

Dry swallowing, when repeated, often helps the patient to activate and localize the velopharyngeal contractions. Often a state of localized strain or fatigue may help the case to become aware that he has such muscles. Very slow chewing may also produce certain muscular contractions of the pharynx and velum. Sudden sucking of air through various sizes of tubes will also initiate velar activity. Tubes of different sizes and shapes will produce more palatal contraction than others, but the sucking must be sudden.*

Blowing Exercises. Perhaps blowing exercises have been used more frequently than any other single device for strengthening the palate. Blow-

* An interesting device for improving velopharyngeal closure is a palatal exerciser invented by E. C. Lubit and R. E. Larsen. See their article "The Lubit Palatal Exerciser: A Preliminary Report" in *Cleft Palate Journal*, VI (1969), 120–133.

ing takes air pressure, and if the air is to come out of the mouth, a velo-pharyngeal opening will reduce that pressure enough to reduce the airflow through the mouth to a considerable degree. We must be certain, how-ever, that we are having an increasingly greater ratio of mouth airflow to nasal airflow if we can hope that the palate is being strengthened. Various devices have been employed to demonstrate this ratio: double shelves to be placed under nose and mouth openings with feathers or fringes to indicate airflow, tubes from the nose to the ear, contact microphones, the phonodeik and phonoscope, polygraphic recording, candle flame affected by tubes from the nose and mouth, clouded mirrors, and many others. Usually it is necessary that the patient become familiar with the two air channels by sucking air in through the nose, then through the mouth, then exhaling alternately through each channel. By using different mouth openings and palpating the nostrils during the blowing or interrupting the oral airflow with vibrating palms across the orifice, the case can come to have a clear idea of these channels. We must not expect him to already have such a concept. Also by having the case alternate nasal and oral airflow while he holds his fingers in his ears, he can hear a difference in the pitch of the two blowings. The oral airflow can be made to vary markedly in pitch by changing the lip protrusion or mouth opening; the nasal airflow is pretty well fixed in pitch. By attending to the different palatal and pharyngeal sensations during the different airflows, a more adequate control of the velopharyngeal musculatures can be achieved.

We should emphasize that blowing exercises performed with great tension and the constriction of the nostrils are most unwise. They merely inform the case that palatal contraction is too laborious to be used in speech. Besides, they often can cause ear infections. We also doubt the efficacy of blowing air out of the mouth while holding the nose shut, since we may raise the air pressure too high in the middle ear and make the case too nose-conscious; and in any event, closure of the nostrils does not help the velopharyngeal valve to shut. Indeed, there seems to be a sort of inverse reciprocal reaction in the action of the nares (nostrils) and the velar musculatures. Even in normal speakers, voluntary contraction of the nares often produces an increase in nasality. As the front door shuts, the back door opens. Often there is very little transfer of training from blowing to speech. This is especially true if the blowing is too strained, if air pressures far exceeding those used in normal speech are used, and if set mouth openings and passive tongue postures are employed. We could hardly expect much transfer with so many variables in the training. Never-theless, others have shown that the palatal and pharyngeal activity in blowing (especially in soft blowing) is more like that used in speech than is shown in such activities as yawning, swallowing, and so on. We must not throw the baby out with the bath. Blowing exercises can help the case to become mouth-conscious; they can help him discriminate the two air-flow channels; they can help him to increase the amount of oral air pressure needed for good articulation; and they can improve the contraction of the velar and pharyngeal muscles. But they must be used wisely rather than indiscriminately.

Many ingenious devices and activities have been invented by speech therapists to make the blowing activities interesting to children. Paper boats have been blown across pans of water. Ping-pong balls have been blown across miniature football fields or golf courses. Balloons have been blown up and burst. Bubble pipes, huffer-puffers, bean shooters, uncoiling paper tubes, flame throwers, vibrating wind instruments, mouth organs, holding tissue paper against a mirror with the breath, air-writing on the therapist's hand, cooling wet fingers, drying nail polish, blowing dry cereal or feathers on a string—all these are but a few of the activities used.

While many of these may be used for motivation or as transitional techniques, we feel that the most effective types of blowing exercises are those that alternate oral and nasal blowing done at fairly low levels of pressure, have a greater fraction of oral rather than nasal emission, and are combined with phonation, tongue protrusion and movement, or lip protrusion and movement. These transfer much more adequately to speech, and improve velopharyngeal closure. All blowing exercises under pressure may tend to cause dizziness and must not be maintained for more than short periods of time.

We conclude this section on velopharyngeal closure training by mentioning two other techniques which we have used with some success with adults. In the first, a large balloon is blow up (preferably by the case while holding his nose) and then held shut by the therapist's fingers on the stem as the case holds a tube leading from the stem with his lips. The therapist gradually releases his grip and allows some of the air to escape into the case's mouth. The latter tries, while holding his breath, to keep from letting the balloon collapse; this requires velar closure or the air will leak out of the nostrils. Another variation of this technique has the outlet to the balloon enter a Y-tube, the arms of which are attached to nasal olives inserted into the case's nostrils. He tried to retard the collapse of the balloon as he produces various vowels or merely contracts his palate in silence.

Articulation Problems. The backward playing of samples of speech of various degrees of nasality has demonstrated that the listener judges a given sample as being more nasal if it has poorer articulation. The voice quality itself seems more nasal when it is played forward than when it is played backward. Thus, the improvement of articulation can produce a decrease in perceived nasality. We have also seen that the majority of cleft-palate speakers have speech sounds which are defective.

The basic problems in articulation are three: lalling, the substitution of glottal stops and fricative for the standard stops and fricatives, and the nasalization or nasal emission of most of the consonants.

Lalling. The treatment for lalling requires training in increasing the mobility of the tongue tip; in raising the points of anterior contact for the *t, d, n, l, ch,* and *j,* sounds; and the differentiation of tongue-lifting from simultaneous jaw movement.

Exercises for increasing the mobility of the tongue include sensitization of the tongue tip—curling, grooving, lifting, lowering, thrusting, arching, tapping, sustaining postures, pressing, scraping, fluttering, and many others. These should not be practiced while holding the breath but while blowing gently both voice and unvoiced air if the training is to generalize to speech. Undue tension is to be avoided. Speed gains should be made in terms of rhythmic patterns. Different sizes of mouth opening and lip postures should be also practiced with the tongue-training. Many of these cases have never explored the many possibilities of tongue movement or action. It is wise to use these exercises as warm-up periods for consonant practice. Often the production of certain consonants is sandwiched between two tongue-training exercises.

The localizing of the focal articulation points higher and more forward in the mouth than those normally used can be done only by identifying those ordinarily used and searching for higher points while continuously articulating the sounds. This "stretching" of the phonemes in terms of height of contact will at first seem unpleasant and will seldom be used at their extremes, but practice will cause the necessary compromise. Most cleft-palate persons also have certain scar tissue, indentations, or bulges on the alveolar ridge that can be used as landmarks; but they must be found and localized. Tactual feedbacks must be sharpened. The teeth, especially the lower teeth, must come to lose their functions as the basic contact point. Silent practice in touching these new focal articulation points should be done. With one of our cases, we inserted a bit of toothpick or dental floss between the upper incisors and used this as the guide. An immediate improvement in speech occurred.

The differentiation of tongue movement from the accompanying jaw movements can be done by immobilizing the jaw with various heights of tooth props until enough independence is achieved to permit the activity without this aid. Frequent checking is necessary. Visual feedback from a mirror is also useful. Lateral movements of the mandible during tongue-tapping and consonant production will also be useful. The use of the first two fingers forked to monitor the location of both lips will help. Also, if the case will place one finger on his nose and his thumb under his chin, any accompanying movement of the jaw will be noticed immediately. Ventriloquism often provides an interesting motivation for these cases, and aids in the freeing of the tongue.

Glottal Stops. The use of the glottal stop or fricative substitutions requires a state of localized tension in the larynx, and some relaxation in this area often provides the optimal conditions for retraining. The use of slight coughs to teach a *k* sound is therefore very unwise. The back of the tongue must be raised, and this can be accomplished more easily on the *k* and *g* sounds by pressing hard with the tongue tip against the lower teeth and closing the jaws partially. Ear training is essential. We have also been able to eliminate this difficult error by having the case produce the consonants on inhalation, a procedure which improves much of the articulation of cleft-palate cases. The subsequent use of donkey breathing (inhaled, then exhaled) in the production of the sounds often solves the glottal problem.

Decreasing Nasality and Nasal Emission. While much of the success of articulating the consonant sounds without nasality or nasal emission will depend upon the success of establishing oral airflow and better velopharyngeal closure, we find that by teaching the plosives with very loose contacts, great improvement can be made. Too hard contacts seem to trigger off a lowering of the velum and a relaxation of the superior constrictor.

For the fricatives, the use of wider mouth openings on the following or preceding vowels tends to decrease the nasality. We also suggest the prolongation of these sounds with decreasing air pressure, thus using the duration rather than the clear quality of the fricative as the message-carrying feature.

It is important, of course, to use the usual ear training to identify the defectiveness of a given sound and to contrast it with the correct sound. Then we must teach the proper production of the isolated sound, strengthening and stabilizing it. We have mentioned before that cleft-palate cases often speak very rapidly so as to conserve the breath pressure. Slowing down the speed of utterance with proper phrasing and breathing often produces immediate improvement in all of the articulation even when little attention is paid to the isolated sounds.

Perhaps the most pronounced of all the ticlike mannerisms which characterized cleft-palate speech is the nostril contraction or flaring. This often serves as an equivalent for velar contraction, and often prevents the latter from taking place. It is cosmetically unattractive, often interferes with the utterance of the labial plosives, and helps to produce the snorting snuffling which is so unpleasant in these cases. It has no effect upon nasality or nasal emission except to make them worse. We therefore always do as much as we can to eliminate this habit. We first attempt to bring this nostril tic up to consciousness, to help the case to become aware of its unpleasant stimulus value, and then through negative practice, canceling, pull-outs, and preparatory sets to eliminate it. Usually it is responsive to this treatment, especially when mirror work is used. In the more severe cases a nucleus of nonnostril-contraction speech can be achieved by contracting the lips in a wide tight smile, stretching them so far that the upper teeth are bared. The therapist must be sure that he does not penalize contraction and thus suppress it before it is weakened.

Many cleft-palate cases have as poor eye contact as do stutterers, a behavior which makes the speech and condition more noticeable. They also may have unusual head postures and lip bitings, or they may cover their mouths in speaking. All these should be reduced.

Speech therapy with cleft-palate cases is usually long-term therapy. Few of these children show any dramatic improvement in a short time. There are many problems to be solved and many avenues to be explored. The work is time-consuming and often difficult. Nevertheless we can do much to help the person with cleft-palate speech to speak better.

CEREBRAL PALSY

The speech therapist is bound, sooner or later, to be asked to help someone with cerebral palsy to learn to speak better. The kinds of problems encountered vary widely and involve voice, articulation, fluency, language, or any combination of these. Yet when we work with persons who have cerebral palsy, we always find ourselves not working alone, but cooperating with other specialists and teachers and parents. Basically a motor disorder, cerebral palsy may also be accompanied by perceptual and learning disabilities. The speech therapist therefore finds himself a member of a team that may include any or all of the following: a pediatrician, an orthopedic surgeon, a psychologist, a social worker, a special education teacher, a physical therapist, and an occupational therapist. It is therefore important that the speech therapist understand the nature of the group of disorders generally classified as cerebral palsy.

We have said that cerebral palsy is a general term for a group of motor disorders; Westlake and Rutherford make the point: "Cerebral palsy is not a single type of neuromuscular disorder, but a group of disturbances which occur as a result of involvement of cortical or subcortical motor control areas. The cerebral insult may involve areas of the brain in addition to those whose primary function is motor control however. While the speech difficulties of children with cerebral palsy often are due to impaired functioning of muscle groups used in breathing, phonation, and articulation, some of the most severe communication handicaps are the result of damage to neural centers other than those associated with motor control." [10]

Most cerebral palsy has its origin in injuries to the brain at birth. The trauma may be due to extreme pressures on the skull that cause abnormal molding and cerebral damage. Strangulation by the cord or other causes of cyanosis or oxygen lack may produce destruction of brain tissue. Certain diseases with high fevers such as pneumonia or jaundice can also cause cerebral palsy. Many soldiers with gunshot wounds in the head develop spastic or athetoid symptoms, as well as aphasia.

Although the term *spastic paralysis* has come to be used as the popular designation for all types of cerebral-palsy cases, there seem to be four major varieties: the athetoids, the ataxic, the myasthenic, and the spastic. Usually more than one of these four symptom complexes are found in the same case. According to Phelps the athetoid and spastic varieties make up more than 80 percent of all cases.

Spasticity itself has been defined as the paralysis due to simultaneous contraction of antagonistic or reciprocal muscle groups accompanied by a definite degree of hypertension or hypertonicity. It is due to a lesion or injury to the pyramidal nerve tracts. The muscles overcontract; they pull too hard and too suddenly. Slight stimuli will set off major contractions. The spastic who tries to move his little finger may jerk not only the hand, but the arm or trunk as well. The spastic may have a characteristic manner of walking—the typical "scissors gait." The hands may be clenched and curled up along the wrists in their extreme contraction, or the whole arm may be drawn upward and backward behind the neck. The spastic tends to contract his chest muscles and thus enlarge the thoracic cavity during the act of speaking, which compels him in turn to compress the abdomen excessively in order to force out some air. He thus may be said to inhale with the thorax at the same time that he exhales with the abdomen. Great tension is thereby produced and this reflects itself in muscular abnormality all over the body. It also shows up in speech in the form of unnatural pauses and gasping and weak or aphonic voice. Many of the "breaks" in the spastic's speech are due to this form of faulty breathing.

Since it is difficult for the spastic to make gradual and smooth movements, the speech is often explosive and blurting. Often the extreme tension that characterizes spasticity will produce articulatory contacts so hard as to resemble or engender stuttering symptoms. The sounds involving complex coordinations are, of course, usually defective; and the tongue

[10] H. Westlake, and D. Rutherford, *Speech Therapy for the Cerebral Palsied* (Chicago: National Society for Crippled Children and Adults, 1961). This reference also provides a clear outline for the examination and assessment of the speech problems of the cerebral palsied.

tip sounds which make contact with the upper-gum ridge are very difficult. Where there is some facial paralysis, the labial sounds are much more difficult than might be expected. In cases where there are both symptoms of spasticity and athetosis, the articulation is prone to be more distorted than if spasticity alone is present. Finally, the diadochokinetic rate of tongue-lifting is a pretty good indication of the number of articulation errors to be found in any one case.

Cerebral-palsy cases are also classified in terms of how much of the body is affected. If one limb is spastic or athetoid, the term *monoplegia* is used; if half the body (right or left) is affected, the word *hemiplegia* designates the condition. *Diplegia* refers to involvement of both upper *or* both lower limbs; *quadriplegia* to spasticity or athetosis in all four limbs. The greatest number of articulatory errors are shown in quadriplegia involving combined athetosis and spasticity, and the fewest errors are evidenced in spastic diplegia.

By *athetosis* we refer to the cerebral-palsy cases with marked tremors. In these the injury is to the extrapyramidal nerve tracts. Athetosis may be described as a series of involuntary contractions that affect one muscle after another. These contractions may be fast or slow, large or small. The head may swing around from side to side. The arm may shake rhythmically. The jaw and facial muscles may show a rhythmic contortion or repetitive grimaces but in some athetoids, these movements disappear in sleep or under the influence of alcohol. There seem to be two major types of athetoids, the nontension type and the tension athetoid, who is often mistaken for a true spastic. The tension athetoids are those who have tried to hold their trembling arms and legs still by using so much tension that it has become habitual. The latter may be distinguished from true spastics by moving their arms against their resistance. The tension athetoid's arm tends to yield gradually; the spastic's releases with a jerk.

Athetoid speech often becomes weak in volume. The final sounds of words and final words of phrases are often whispered. A marked tremulo is heard. Monotones are very common, and in the tension athetoids the habitual pitch is near the upper limit of the range. Falsetto voice qualities are not unusual. Another common voice quality is that of hoarseness, especially in the males. Like the true spastics, athetoids make many articulation errors; and the finer the coordination involved in producing the sound, the more it is likely to be distorted. Tongue-tip sounds are especially difficult. Breathing disturbances are common.

Other Varieties of Cerebral Palsy. The other subvarieties of cerebral palsy are encountered only rarely. *Ataxia* manifests itself mainly in a lack of ability to balance oneself or to coordinate the muscles and these appear to have a low tonicity. This condition seems to be due to a lesion in the cerebellum. In myasthenia or flaccid paralysis we find the same weakness of the muscles but no primary loss of balance. Also, a variety of cerebral palsy which is marked most conspicuously by sustained tremor is occasionally seen. The student should understand that many of these features may appear in any one individual and that few pure types exist, although the spastic variety tends to show more consistency.

Intelligent cerebral-palsied individuals meet so many frustrations during their daily lives that they tend to build emotional handicaps as great as their physical disabilities. Fears develop about walking, talking, eating, going downstairs, carrying a tray, holding a pencil, and a hundred other daily activities. These often become so intense that they create more tensions and hence more spasticity or athetosis. Thus one girl so feared to lift a coffee cup to her lips that she could not do so without spilling and breaking it, yet she was able to etch delicate tracings on a copper dish.

Many of these children are so pampered and protected by their parents that they never have an opportunity to learn the skills required of them for social living. Their parents are constantly afraid that they will hurt themselves, but as one adult tension athetoid said to us, "My parents never let me try to ride a bicycle and now at last I've done it. Better to break your neck than your spirit." Many spastics come to a fatalistic attitude of passive acceptance of whatever blows, kindnesses, or pity society may give them. Others put up a gallant battle and succeed in creating useful and satisfying lives for themselves.

Speech Therapy.   Very often the cerebral-palsied child is first presented as a case of delayed speech. These children often do not begin to talk until five or six, but many of them could learn earlier with proper parental teaching. In general, the same procedures used on other delayed-speech cases and in teaching the baby to talk are employed.[11] Imitation must be taught. Sounds must come to have meaning and identity. Words must be taught in terms of their sound sequences and associations. Babbling games using puppets are especially effective in getting a young spastic child to talk. It is especially necessary that the child be praised for all vocalization, since he is likely to fall into a whispered or mere lip-moving type of speech. When possible, the first speech teaching should be done when the child is lying on his back in bed. Phonograph records with singing and speech games are very useful in stimulating these children.

In most cases of cerebral palsy the physiotherapist and occupational therapist will have done a great deal of work with the child before the speech therapist is called in. Many of the activities used in physiotherapy can be made more interesting to the child if vocalization is used in conjunction with them. Thus one child whose very spastic left leg was being

---

[11] The urgent need to give the cerebral palsied child some useful language as early as possible is well described by T. Trombly, "Linguistic Concepts and the Cerebral Palsied Child," *Cerebral Palsy Journal*, XXIX (1968), 7–8.

passively rotated in a whirlpool bath was taught to say "round and round; round and round" as the leg moved. He was unable to say these words at first under any other condition; but soon he had attained the ability to say them anywhere, and the distraction seemed to ease some of the spasticity. In some programs, general relaxation of the whole body forms a large part of the treatment of the spastic and tension athetoid, and even these exercises may be combined with sighing or yawning on the various vowels. Relaxation of the articulatory or the throat muscles seems to be very difficult for these cases, and we often indirectly attain decreases in the tension of these structures by teaching the child to speak while chewing.

Among several interesting new approaches to the treatment of the cerebral palsy is that advocated by the Bobaths.[12] Instead of using the traditional methods to induce general relaxation, the Bobath method, essentially a physical therapy approach, seeks first to inhibit the pathological reflex activity by holding the child firmly in a posture that prevents the usual abnormal motor activity. Then the primitive but normal reflexes are stimulated and facilitated and finally voluntary motor control is evoked. Some very surprising changes occur when this sequence is successfully carried out. We have seen young cerebral-palsied children who were thrashing around and unable to produce anything but strangled bursts of tortured vocalization become quiet and relaxed and able to babble normally when treated by a skillful Bobath practitioner.[13]

Rhythms of all kinds seem to provide especially favorable media for speech practice, if the rhythms are given at a speed which suits the particular case. In the following these rhythms it is not wise to combine speech with muscular movements because of the nature of the disability. Visual stimuli such as the rhythmic swinging of a flashlight beam on a wall are very effective in producing more fluent speech. Tonal stimuli of all kinds are also used. Many cerebral-palsied children can utter polysyllabic words in unison with a recurrent melody whether they sing them or not.

In general, the spastic's articulation disorder is of the lalling type. Most of the sounds that require lifting of the tongue tip are defective. When the *t*, *d*, and *n* sounds are adequate, it will be observed that they are dentalized. The tongue does not make contact with the upper-gum ridge but with the back surface of the teeth or it may be protruded. Several of these cases were able to acquire good *l* and *r* sounds without any direct

[12] For further information on these, see G. McDonald, and B. Chance, *Cerebral Palsy* (Englewood Cliffs, N.J.: Prentice-Hall, Inc., 1964).

[13] The book by Marie Crickmay, *Speech Therapy and the Bobath Approach to Cerebral Palsy* (Springfield, Ill.: Charles C. Thomas, Publisher, 1966) presents a clear picture of this kind of treatment.

SUPINE POSITIONS DESIGNED TO BREAK UP REFLEX PATTERNS OF EXTENSION:

PRONE POSITIONS DESIGNED TO BREAK UP REFLEX PATTERNS OF FLEXION.

→ = force applied to counteract reflex.

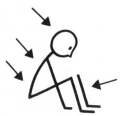

1. A position of total flexion—diametrically opposed to reflex patterns of extension.

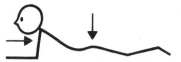

1. A position of total extension—diametrically opposed to reflex patterns of flexion.

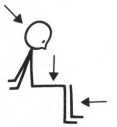

2. A position introducing some extension (of spine and arms) but flexion of neck, hips and knees.

2. A position introducing some flexion (of elbows) but with spine and hips still extended.

3. A position introducing greater extension, but controlled so as not to provoke former reflex pattern of total extension.

3. A position introducing greater flexion of hips and knees, but with spine and arms extended.

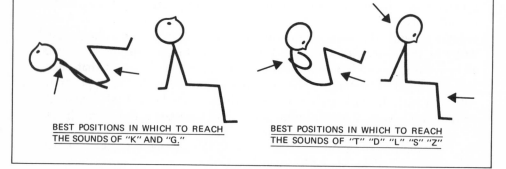

BEST POSITIONS IN WHICH TO REACH THE SOUNDS OF "K" AND "G."

BEST POSITIONS IN WHICH TO REACH THE SOUNDS OF "T" "D" "L" "S" "Z"

FIGURE 35: *Reflex-Inhibiting Patterns for Cerebral Palsy*

teaching. Instead, we taught them to make the *t, d,* and *n* sounds against the upper-gum ridge, and the tongue-tip lifting carried over into the *l* and *r* sounds immediately.

In most of these cases, the essential task is to free the tongue from its tendency to move only in conjunction with the lower jaw. The old traditional tongue exercises have little value, but those that involve the emergence of a finer movement from a gross one are very useful. Just as we have been able to teach spastics to pick up a pin by beginning with trunk, arm, and wrist movements, so we can finally teach him to move his tongue tip without closing his mouth.

Phonetic placement methods in the teaching of new sounds are seldom successful. The auditory stimulation and modification of known sounds are much better. Babbling practice has great value in making the new sounds habitual. We have found that it is wise to make a set of tape recordings for each case that provides him with material appropriate to his level and with which he can speak in unison when alone.

It should be obvious that no speech therapist can hope to solve the many problems of giving the cerebral-palsied child usable speech unless the parents and other professional members help in the process. Much of the work of the speech therapist will involve demonstration and consultation. We cannot simply tell others how to facilitate speech. We must show them. In turn, in our work we also must reinforce the treatment being provided by other members of the team.[14]

At times one of the major obstacles in achieving useful speech in the cerebral-palsied person is the inability to produce voice without great struggle. When he tries to talk, he may exert great physical effort; and this may induce closures of both the true and false vocal folds. The little mountain labors, but only a tiny mouse of sound is produced. We rarely work directly on voice production for this reason. Instead we try to combine sounds and movements, or we vibrate the child's chest with our hands as he is vocally exhaling and as we stimulate him with pleasant sounds. We do a lot of singing and humming in our early speech therapy with these children, making speech pleasant, making sound production desirable. Often the breathing of the cerebral-palsied child shows great abnormality, especially when he tries to produce speech. He may inhale far too deeply, then exhale most of this air prior to speech attempt or in the utterance of just one syllable, and then strain from that time onward. He may even try to speak while inhaling, an activity which will evoke strain even in a normal speaker. These persons must be trained to eliminate these faulty procedures.[15]

[14] The following reference will help the speech therapist to understand the need to deal with parents: P. R. Wildman, "A Parent Education Program for Parents of Cerebral Palsied Children," *Cerebral Palsy Journal*, XXVIII (1967), 5–8.

[15] Chapter VII in M. Crickmay, *Speech Therapy and the Bobath Approach to Cerebral Palsy, op. cit.,* offers some very valuable suggestions.

The breaks in fluency which are so characteristic of the spastic are often eliminated by this training but it is usually wise to teach these children a type of phrasing that will not place too much demand upon them for sustained utterance. The pauses must be much more frequent than those of the normal individual, and they should be slightly longer. Thus the sentence: "Practice about thirty words involving the *s* blends according to the following models" might be spoken as a single unit by an adult normal speaker, but the adult cerebral-palsy case should pause for a new breath at least three or four times during its course. If he trains himself to speak short phrases on one breath, his fluency will improve. Moreover, since no untimely gasps for breath will occur, his voice will be less likely to rise in pitch, or to be strained, and the final sounds of the words will be better articulated. Spastics frequently omit the puff of their final plosives and use lax vowels and continuant consonants because they run out of breath so easily.

Fluency may be improved also by giving the child training in making smooth transitions between vowels or consecutive consonants. Thus, he is asked to practice shifting gradually rather than suddenly from a prolonged *u* to a prolonged *e* sound to produce the word *we*. At first, breaks are likely to occur, but they can be greatly improved through practice; and the child's general speech reflects the improvement. Again the plosives often cause breaks in rhythm because the contacts are made too hard and consequently set up tremors. We have had marked success in treating these errors with the same methods we use for the stutterer's hard contacts. In one case, who always "stuck" on his *p*, *t*, and *k* sounds and showed breaks in his speech, we were able to solve the problem by simply asking him "to keep his mouth in motion" whenever he said a word beginning with these sounds.

It is, of course, necessary to supplement this speech therapy with a great deal of informal psychotherapy, especially in adult cerebral-palsied individuals. They must be taught an objective attitude toward their disorder. They must whittle down the emotional fraction of their total handicap; they must increase their assets in every way. As fear and shame diminish, the tensions will decrease. In many cases, greater improvement in speech and muscular coordination will come from psychotherapy than from the speech therapy itself.

REFERENCES: Aphasia

Articles

1. Berman, M. and Peelle, L. M. "Self-generated Cues: A Method for Aiding Aphasic and Apractic Patients." *Journal of Speech and Hearing Disorders*, XXXII (1967), 372–76.
    How do these self-generated cues really help the aphasic?
2. Biorn–Hansen, V. "Social and Emotional Aspects of Aphasia." *Journal of Speech and Hearing Disorders*, XXII (1957), 53–59.
    What are the impacts of brain injury on the person who has lost his speech because of a stroke?
3. Buck, M. "The Language Disorders: A Personal and Professional Account of Aphasia." *Journal of Rehabilitation*, XXIX (1963), 37–38.
    Summarize Buck's experiences and feelings.
4. Brain, L. *Speech Disorders: Aphasia, Apraxia, and Agnosia.* 2d ed. Washington, D.C.: Butterworth, 1965.
    What are the basic distinctions between these three disorders?
5. Culton, G. L. "Spontaneous Recovery from Aphasia." *Journal of Speech and Hearing Research*, XII (1969), 825–32.
    What is meant by spontaneous recovery in aphasics, and when is it most likely to occur?
6. Eisenson, J. "Developmental Aphasia: A Speculative View with Therapeutic Implications." *Journal of Speech and Hearing Disorders*, XXXIII (1968), 3–13.
    What are the basic difficulties shown by children with developmental aphasia?
7. Gargan, W. *Why Me?* New York: Doubleday & Company, Inc., 1969.
    Describe Gargan's reactions to the loss of his larynx and how he learned to speak again.
8. Greene, M. C. L. "Differential Diagnosis of Developmental Aphasia." *Speech Pathology and Therapy*, VII (1964), 84–94.
    Describe the two cases.
9. Hall, W. A. "Return from Silence—A Personal Experience." *Journal of Speech and Hearing Disorders*, XXVI (1961), 174–77.
    Describe the experiences of this aphasic.
10. Holland, A. L. "Some Current Trends in Aphasia Rehabilitation." *ASHA*, XI (1969), 3–7.
    How does the author apply operant conditioning principles to aphasia therapy?
11. Johnson, B. "Cookbook Therapy for the Aphasic." *Rehabilitation Record*, VIII (1967), 20–22.
    What were the experiences of the family of this aphasic?
12. Keenan, J. S. "A Method of Eliciting Naming Behavior from Aphasic Clients." *Journal of Speech and Hearing Disorders*, XXXI (1966), 261–66.
    How did the author do it?
13. ———. "The Nature of Receptive and Expressive Impairments in

Aphasia." *Journal of Speech and Hearing Disorders,* XXXIII (1968), 20–25.
   What's wrong with the usual classification of receptive-expressive disabilities in aphasia?

14.   La Pointe, L. L. and Culton, G. L. "Visual-Spatial Neglect Subsequent to Brain Injury." *Journal of Speech and Hearing Disorders,* XXXIV (1969), 82–86.
   Describe the perceptual problems of this aphasic and his therapy.

15.   Leche, P. "Speech Therapy with Adult Brain-damaged Patients." *Occupational Therapy,* XXXI (1968), 20–21.
   List ten suggestions regarding the treatment of these persons.

16.   Malone, R. L. "Expressed Attitudes of Families of Aphasics." *Journal of Speech and Hearing Disorders,* XXXIV (1969), 146–51.
   How is the family life of an aphasic changed by the injury?

17.   Rolnick, M. and Loops, H. R. "Aphasia as Seen by the Aphasic." *Journal of Speech and Hearing Disorders,* XXXIV (1969), 48–53.
   What were the major difficulties reported by these six aphasics?

18.   Sefer, J. and Schuell, H. "A Year of Aphasia Therapy: A Case Study." *British Journal of Disorders of Communication,* IV (1969), 73–82.
   Describe the course of treatment.

19.   Sies, L. F. and Butler, R. "Personal Account of Dysphasia." *Journal of Speech and Hearing Disorders,* XXVIII (1963), 261–66.
   Summarize this aphasic's account of his experiences.

20.   Simonson, J. "Associated Social Problems of the Aphasic Patient Which Interfere with Vocational Rehabilitation." In Willis, C. R., ed., *The Vocational Rehabilitation Problems of the Patient with Aphasia* (Washington, D.C.: U.S. Dept. of Health, Education, and Welfare, Social Rehabilitation Service, Rehabilitation Services Administration, 1967), 42–46.
   What are the eight bits of information every employer of an aphasic should know?

21.   Stein, L. and Curry, F. "Childhood Auditory Agnosia." *Journal of Speech and Hearing Disorders,* XXXIII (1968), 361–70.
   Describe the history of this person's symptoms and the therapy she received.

22.   Van Riper, C. "Case Study of an Aphasic." In Berg, I. A., and Pennington, L. A., *An Introduction to Clinical Psychology,* 3d ed. (New York: The Ronald Press Company, 1966). Pp. 344–54.
   Outline the sequential steps used in examining this patient.

Texts

23.   Buck, M. *Dysphasia: Professional Guidance for Family and Patient.* Englewood Cliffs, N.J.: Prentice-Hall, Inc., 1968.
   An excellent short book which reveals much about the inner world of an aphasic.

24.   McBride, C. *Silent Victory.* Chicago: Nelson-Hall, 1969.
   How did the wife of this aphasic help him to recover the ability to use language?

25.   Sarno, J. E. and Sarno M. *Stroke: The Condition and the Patient.* New York: McGraw-Hill Book Company, 1969.

Explains in fairly simple terms what aphasia is and its effect upon the patient.

26. Schuell, H., Jenkins, J., and Jiménez–Pabón, E. *Aphasia in Adults: Diagnosis, Prognosis, and Treatment*. New York: Harper & Row, Publishers, 1964.

The most comprehensive book in the field. The research is summarized, and the theories and methods of testing and treatment are given.

REFERENCES : Cleft Palate

Articles

27. Blakeley, R. W. "The Complementary Use of Speech Prostheses and Pharyngeal Flaps in Palatal Insufficiency." *Cleft Palate Journal*, I (1964), 194–98.
How do prostheses supplement surgery?

28. ———. "The Rationale for a Temporary Speech Prosthesis in Palatal Insufficiency." *British Journal of Disorders of Communication*, IV (1969), 134–39.
Explain the uses of the temporary speech appliance.

29. Bluestone, C. D., Musgrave, R. H., and McWilliams, B. J. "Teflon Injection Pharyngoplasty–Status." *Laryngoscope*, LXXVIII (1968), 558–64.
For what kinds of cleft-palate patients is Teflon injection unwise?

30. Bzoch, K. R. "The Effects of a Specific Pharyngeal Flap Operation upon the Speech of Forty Cleft-Palate Persons." *Journal of Speech and Hearing Disorders*, XXIX (1964), 111–20.
What were the good and bad effects of this operation?

31. Chase, R. A. and Jobe, R. P. "Rehabilitation Literature of the Forgotten Cleft Child." *Rehabilitation Record*, X (1969), 10–14.
Summarize this article.

32. Coccaro, P. J. "Orthodontics in Cleft-palate Children: A Continuing Process." *Cleft Palate Journal*, VI (1969), 495–505.
What were the problems encountered in the three children with cleft lips and palates during the five years?

33. Morris, H. L., Spriestersbach, D. C., and Darley, F. L. "An Articulation Test for Assessing Competency of Velopharyngeal Closure." *Journal of Speech and Hearing Research*, IV (1961), 48–55.
What sorts of articulatory errors indicate a lack of velopharyngeal closure?

34. Shelton, R. L. and Lloyd, R. S. "Prosthetic Facilitation of Palatopharyngeal Closure." *Journal of Speech and Hearing Disorders*, XXVIII (1963), 58–66.
How are prostheses for cleft-palate persons made and fitted?

35. Smith, J. K. "Contraindications for Speech Therapy for Cleft-palate Speakers." *Cleft Palate Journal*, VI (1969), 202–4.
When is it unnecessary to offer speech therapy to cleft-palate speakers?

36. Van Demark, D. "Misarticulations and Listener Judgments of the Speech of Individuals with Cleft Palates." *Cleft Palate Journal*, I (1964), 232–45.

How does misarticulation affect the judgment of deviancy in cleft-palate speech?

37. Yules, R. B. "Pharyngeal Flap Surgery: A Review of the Literature." *Cleft Palate Journal,* VI (1969), 303–8.
    How effective is this type of surgery?

Texts

38. McDonald, E. T. *Bright Promise.* Chicago: National Society for Crippled Children and Adults, 1959.
    The basic information needed by parents of a cleft-palate child is given in this book.
39. Morley, M. *Cleft Palate and Speech.* Edinburgh: Livingstone, 1958.
    This book contains much of what the speech therapist needs to know about clefts and their management.
40. Spriestersbach, D. C. and Sherman, D., eds. *Cleft Palate and Communication.* New York: Academic Press, 1968.
    While rather technical, this collection of articles covers most of the aspects of cleft-palate disorders. The chapter on hearing problems associated with cleft palate is especially valuable.
41. Stark, R. B., ed. *Cleft Palate: A Multidisciplinary Approach.* New York: Harper & Row, Publishers, 1968.
    The relationships between different professional members of the cleft-palate team and the contributions of each are clearly presented.
42. Westlake, H. and Rutherford, D. *Cleft Palate.* Englewood Cliffs, N.J.: Prentice-Hall, Inc., 1966.
    A survey of the nature, causes, and symptoms of cleft-palate disorders and how to deal with them. Especially valuable are the sections on examining the patient and the relationships with others on the cleft-palate team.

REFERENCES: Cerebral Palsy

Articles

43. Hoberman, S. E. and Hoberman, M. "Speech Habilitation in Cerebral Palsy." *Journal of Speech and Hearing Disorders,* XXV (1960), 111–23.
    Summarize the authors' suggestions.
44. Huber, M. "Letters to the Parents of the Cerebral-Palsied Child." *Journal of Speech and Hearing Disorders,* XV (1950), 154–58.
    What suggestions regarding speech are given?
45. Irwin, O. C. "A Talk with Parents." *Cerebral Palsy Review,* XXIV (1963), 3–5.
    What advice does the author have concerning their attitudes toward the child with cerebral palsy or brain damage?
46. Jones, M. V. "Breathing Therapy for the Cerebral Palsied." *Journal of Speech and Hearing Disorders,* XXVI (1961), 294–95.
    What techniques are described and how useful are they?
47. Lencione, R. M. "Speech and Language Problems in Cerebral Palsy."

In Cruikshank, W. M., ed., *Cerebral Palsy*, 2d ed. (Syracuse: Syracuse University Press, 1966).
Summarize her three-stage program for developing speech in these children.

48. Plotkin, W. H. "Situational Speech Therapy for Retarded Cerebral-Palsied Children." *Journal of Speech and Hearing Disorders*, XXIV (1959), 16–20.
Describe the sorts of activities used.

49. Snidecor, J. "The Speech Correctionist on the Cerebral-Palsy Team." *Journal of Speech and Hearing Disorders*, XIII (1948), 67–70.
What functions do the other professionals perform, and what are the specific responsibilities of the speech therapist?

50. Trombly, T. "Linguistic Concepts and the Cerebral-Palsied Child." *Cerebral Palsy Journal*, XXIX (1968), 7–8.
Why does the author suggest we do little therapy on the misarticulation of these children?

51. Wehrle, P. F., ed. *Services for Children with Cerebral Palsy*. New York: American Public Health Association, 1967.
Outline the contents of this booklet.

52. Wildman, P. R. "A Parent Education Program for Parents of Cerebral-Palsied Children." *Cerebral Palsy Journal*, XXVIII (1967), 5–8.
Outline this program.

Texts

53. Crickmay, M. C. *Speech Therapy and the Bobath Approach to Cerebral Palsy*. Springfield, Ill.: Charles C Thomas, Publishers, 1966.
A fascinating account of one of the newer approaches to the motor and speech problems of the cerebral palsied.

54. McDonald, E. T. and Chance, B. *Cerebral Palsy*. Englewood Cliffs, N.J.: Prentice-Hall, Inc., 1964.
Perhaps the best book available for therapists who must work with the cerebral palsied. Gives most of the basic information concerning the causes, nature, and treatment methods used for cerebral-palsied persons.

55. Westlake, H. and Rutherford, D. *Speech Therapy for the Cerebral Palsied*. Chicago: National Society for Crippled Children and Adults, 1961.
Most useful for diagnosing the multiple problems shown by the cerebral palsied.

9

Hearing Problems *

Since this text is primarily designed to survey the field of communicative disorders for the beginning student, it seems wise to include a chapter dealing with the problems that are caused by defective hearing. Speech pathology and audiology are twin disciplines; they share many commonalities. All speech therapists are expected to have some basic understanding of the way we hear and the difficulties experienced by those who do not hear well.

THE HEARING MECHANISM

Although we shall not describe the hearing mechanism in detail, we must at least present its three major parts: the outer ear, the middle ear, and the inner ear. When we ordinarily think of the ear we refer to the visible portion of it, the *auricle* or *pinna*. Some few of us can wiggle our auricles. As contrasted with certain lower animals, in humans the auricle makes only a minor contribution to hearing. If one's ears were cut off, their removal would result in a loss of hearing sensitivity of about five or six decibels, not enough to make any real difference. Cupping our hands to hear better increases our hearing sensitivity only by the same amount. Besides the auricle, the outer ear contains the external auditory canal, a short passageway leading to the ear drum. Sound waves are conveyed down this short funnel to impinge upon the tympanic membrane,

* The author was assisted in the preparation of this chapter by Dr. Albert Jetty, audiologist at Western Michigan University.

which separates the outer from the middle ear. The canal contains small hairs (cilia) and cerumenous glands, which secrete the "wax" found in the canal. The cilia and wax prevent dirt and insects from entering the canal, thus serving as a protective device for the tympanic membrane. The fact that the canal is not straight is also considered to be a protection for the tympanic membrane. The inner portion of the canal is bony and becomes narrowed in front of the tympanic membrane. At this constriction point foreign objects tend to lodge, and thus the canal provides added protection for the eardrum. In addition to this protective function, the external ear canal serves to keep the tympanic membrane at a constant temperature and humidity so that its vibratory function is maximal at all times.

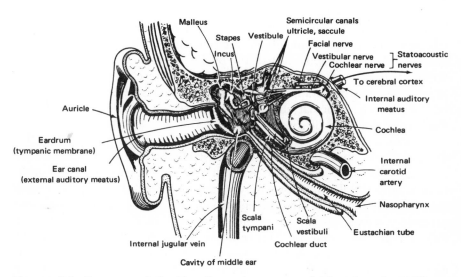

FIGURE 36: *Structure of the Ear.* From *Anatomy and Physiology* by William F. Evans. Englewood Cliffs, New Jersey: Prentice-Hall, Inc., 1971.

The second major part of our auditory mechanism is called the *middle ear,* or tympanic cavity. The middle ear is an irregularly shaped, air-filled space, which can be viewed as a six-sided figure. Imagine it as a tiny irregular room or chamber about the size of a garden pea having a ceiling, a floor, and walls. The tympanic membrane is situated on the lateral wall of this chamber and is composed of three layers of tissue. It is conical in shape with the tip facing inward. It is at the tympanic membrane that sound waves are transduced—that is, changed to a different form of energy. The acoustic energy in the air is changed to a vibratory or mechanical type of energy. This energy is then routed across the tympanic cavity by the ossicular chain.

The ossicular chain consists of three tiny bones arranged as a system of levers. These bones are the smallest in the body. The first bone in the chain is the *malleus*, or hammer, which is attached to the tympanic membrane by means of its manubrium or handle. Thus, when the tympanic membrane vibrates, the vibrations are immediately transferred to the malleus. The malleus is the largest of the three bones of the middle ear. The second bone is the *incus*, or anvil, which serves to link the malleus with the third bone, the *stapes*. The stapes, or stirrup, is attached at its footplate to the oval window. Thus, the sound energy is carried across the tympanic cavity to the oval window, which forms part of the boundary between the middle ear and the inner ear. Since sound waves striking the relatively large tympanic membrane are concentrated by the ossicular chain into the relatively smaller area of the oval window, and because the lever action of the ossicular chain probably adds some mechanical advantage of its own, our hearing is approximately thirty decibels better than it would be if we had no ossicular chain. In this sense the middle ear serves as a mechanical amplifier of sound.

Another important structure that we find within the middle ear is the opening to the *eustachian tube*. The eustachian tube forms a back-door connection between the middle ear and the nasopharynx. Its function is to aerate the middle ear so that the air pressure behind the ear drum equals that in front of it, an arrangement which lets it vibrate freely. We experience a feeling of fullness in our ears when we climb a mountain or make a rapid plane descent. This condition is due to differences in outside and inside air pressure and is relieved by yawning or swallowing, since during these activities the eustachian tube is then opened allowing air to pass into the middle ear.

The third major part of the auditory mechanism is called the inner ear, also known as the labyrinth because of its complexity. It contains three *semicircular canals* which help us balance ourselves, a snailshell-shaped structure called the *cochlea* which contains the nerve endings of the eighth cranial nerve essential for the transmission of auditory information to the brain, and the *vestibule* which connects the cochlea with the semicircular canals. Since one of the tiny bones of the ossicular chain within the middle ear fits into an opening of the vestibule known as the *oval window*, its vibration excites the nerve endings in the cochlea; and the nervous impulses thus set off travel to the auditory cortex of the brain to produce the sensations we call hearing.

CLASSIFICATION OF HEARING LOSS

Since the auditory mechanism is composed of three distinct sections, lesions manifest themselves differently depending on their location. The outer and middle ear are the sound-conducting part of the mechanism. That is, these parts convey or relay the sound to the inner ear, which is the sound-perceiving part of the mechanism. Normally we hear other people talking by means of air conduction, whereby the sound travels through the outer and middle ear and into the inner ear. When we speak, we hear ourselves by air conduction and also by bone conduction. In bone-conduction hearing, the stimulus is conveyed directly to the inner ear by the vibrations of the bones of the skull. It is because we normally hear ourselves by both air and bone conduction when we speak that many people are quite amazed to hear how their voices sound the first time they hear a tape recording of themselves. The reason they sound so different is because they are hearing themselves strictly by air conduction for the first time.

In examining hearing, the audiologist tests both by air conduction and by bone conduction. The air-conduction testing is accomplished through earphones, whereas bone conduction is tested by by-passing the outer and middle ears and testing the inner ear directly with a bone vibrator placed at some point on the skull. Formerly the mastoid was the usual choice, but other placements such as the forehead and teeth are becoming more popular as the site for the vibrator.

When testing reveals a loss of hearing sensitivity by air conduction and the bone-conduction thresholds are normal, then the hearing loss is classified as *conductive*. A typical audiogram for a conductive hearing loss is shown in Figure 37. In a conductive type loss, the inner ear is normal and the breakdown lies in either the outer or middle ear. The problem is with the "conduction" of the sound to the inner ear.

When a loss of hearing is found by both air conduction and bone conduction and the bone-conduction thresholds are essentially at the same level as the air-conduction thresholds, the loss is classified as *sensori-neural*. A typical audiogram for a sensori-neural hearing loss is shown in Figure 38. In this instance, the outer and middle ears are normal and the breakdown is in the cochlear sense organ itself, or in the auditory nerve. The problem is with the "perception" of sound in the inner ear or beyond.

A third major classification of hearing loss is termed a *mixed type* of loss. As the term implies, this type of loss is a combination of a conductive and a sensori-neural type loss. There is a loss of hearing by both air conduction and bone conduction, but the loss by bone conduction is not as

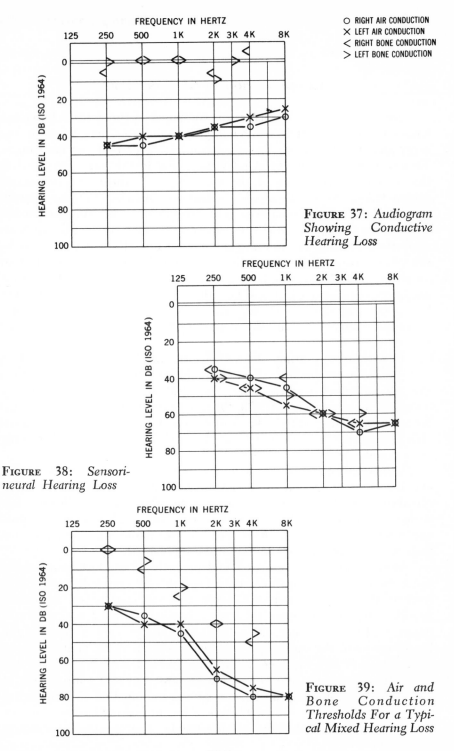

FREQUENCY IN HERTZ

○ RIGHT AIR CONDUCTION
× LEFT AIR CONDUCTION
< RIGHT BONE CONDUCTION
> LEFT BONE CONDUCTION

FIGURE 37: *Audiogram Showing Conductive Hearing Loss*

FIGURE 38: *Sensorineural Hearing Loss*

FIGURE 39: *Air and Bone Conduction Thresholds For a Typical Mixed Hearing Loss*

great as the loss by air conduction, thus producing in what is termed an "air-bone gap" at certain test frequencies. A typical audiogram for a mixed type hearing loss is shown in Figure 39. With this type of loss the bone-conduction thresholds show the presence of a sensori-neural loss, but, since air-conduction thresholds are much worse, there is also a conductive component to the hearing loss. This type of loss could result from any number of factors.

Conductive Impairments. Hearing loss can, of course, occur at any time. Losses occurring before birth are said to be congenital. One kind of congenital hearing loss involving the outer ear is atresia of the external ear canal. Atresia means that a natural canal has been blocked. When this blocking occurs in the ear canal, it results in a conductive type hearing loss. Atresia of the ear canal is usually not found as an isolated defect, but usually in conjunction with a small or deformed auricle or with middle-ear abnormalities. The following case illustrates the classic symptoms of this kind of conductive hearing impairment:

> Judy, age six, had a hearing loss due to congenital bilateral microtia of the auricle and bilateral atresia of the external auditory canal. She had a moderate, bilateral, conductive hearing loss. At the time of the audiological evaluation, the extent of middle-ear involvement had not been determined, and she had undergone several operations for restoration of the auricles. Her speech was quite good, and she had only a few minor articulation errors.
>
> Since surgery to correct her hearing loss would entail several years, steps had to be taken to insure that she would not be handicapped educationally, as well as having a hearing handicap. Further testing revealed speech reception thresholds of 52 dB in the right ear and 50 dB in the left ear. Her ability to understand speech was normal when speech was presented at an intensity level sufficient to overcome the conducive barrier.
>
> Persons with conductive losses are generally excellent candidates for hearing aids. Judy was no exception, and a hearing-aid evaluation with a body-type hearing aid employing a bone-conduction receiver yielded a speech reception threshold of 8 dB—she had normal understanding of speech.
>
> Because of her excellent performance with a hearing aid, provisions were made for her to remain in the regular classroom and to obtain instructions from a homebound teacher during the times she had to miss school following an operation on her ears. Judy was placed in a regular second grade in her home community, and the follow-up report indicated that she was a "good student, attentive and in the best reading group."

Another congenital defect resulting in a conductive hearing loss is the *Treacher–Collins Syndrome*. This syndrome is marked by deformities of the facial bones resulting in a small receding lower jaw and eyes that are slanted downward in an antimongoloid fashion at the lateral corners. The auricles are deformed, and usually both external auditory canals and eardrums are missing bilaterally, along with ossicular chain deformities.

> Vivian, age five, was born with Treacher–Collins Syndrome. There was malformation of both auricles, along with complete atresia of the left ear canal and marked stenosis (narrowing or stricture) of the right ear canal. Audiological evaluation revealed normal, bilateral inner-ear function with a moderate to severe loss by air conduction in the right ear. The left ear was not tested by air conduction due to the complete absence of an ear canal. A sound field (loudspeaker) speech reception threshold of 55 dB was obtained, and understanding of speech was normal when it was presented at a sufficient loudness level to overcome the conductive barrier. Further testing revealed that Vivian was considerably retarded in her language development and had markedly defective articulation.
>
> Remedial procedures included an air-conduction hearing aid fitted to her right ear by a special earmold. In addition, Vivian was placed in a special school where she could receive an intensive program of academic instruction and remedial assistance in speech, language, and auditory training. Later, corrective surgery would be performed in an attempt to alleviate her conductive hearing loss.

Acquired Hearing Losses. Hearing losses occurring at any time after birth are referred to as acquired losses. One of the most common acquired losses involving the outer ear is that of simple blockage of the ear canal by foreign objects or impacted wax. Children have been known to put into their ears such things as beans, color crayons, small ball bearings, wads of paper, and just about anything else small enough to fit into their ear canals. Foreign objects cause a mild conductive loss if the blockage is complete. They are readily visible on otoscopic examination and should be extracted by the otologist.

The most common blockage is a result of impacted wax. Well-meaning mothers can cause this type of loss by cleaning their children's ears with cotton swabs. Since the cotton tip just fits the ear canal, it cannot get behind the wax and instead forces it back and may impact it against the tympanic membrane. One otologist, an acquaintance of the author, is very vehement in his objection to mothers using cotton swabs to clean their children's ears. If he had his way, cotton swabs would be taken off the market. He maintains that it is unnecessary to clean wax from the ears, since old accumulations will dry up and fall out naturally if left alone.

Impacted wax should be removed by the otologist since there is always danger of perforating the tympanic membrane unless it is done by a skilled person and with proper instruments such as a cerumen spoon. Often it is necessary to soften the wax with some type of softening agent before the wax can be removed. After the wax is softened the ear is syringed and the wax flushed out. Syringing of the ear must also be done carefully, since a forceful stream of water directed at the tympanic membrane could rupture it. For this reason, the water is usually directed at the canal walls, so that only reflected water hits the membrane. Although impacted wax results in only a mild hearing loss, it often enough causes a youngster to have difficulty in school. This is the child who often becomes what the teachers refer to as a "behavior problem." Any child who does not seem to pay attention in school or suddenly changes in alertness should be suspected of having a hearing loss.

There are a number of other problems involving the outer ear which come under the broad title of *external otitis*. These would include erysipelas, seborrheic dermatitis, eczema, and other inflammatory conditions. The hearing loss resulting from these conditions resembles the loss from simple blockage of the ear canal. These conditions result in a swelling of the external ear canal so that it is closed or nearly closed, or the collection of scaly debris in the canal. These types of conditions are treated medically and may involve other areas of the body as well as the ear canal and auricle.

A common type of otitis externa is called otomycosis or "swimmers ears," since it is often found in people who are habitual swimmers. It consists of a fungus growth in the external canal which results in irritation and itching. Secondary infection can be set up by scratching in attempts to relieve the itching. The following case is an example of this type of ear problem:

Mr. J. V., age forty-three, was seen for an audiological evaluation. Although he complained of some loss of hearing, his chief complaint was the itching in his left ear canal. He attributed the itching to an accumulation of wax. (The average person tends to lay the blame for all hearing problems or ear conditions on excessive amounts of wax.) In attempts to rid his left ear canal of what he thought was an acculation of wax, Mr. J. V. poured hydrogen peroxide into it since this can be used to soften wax. This procedure resulted in a pain deep in the left ear and left him dizzy and nauseous.

Audiological evaluation showed evidence of air-borne gaps in the low frequencies, indicating the presence of a conductive hearing loss. In addition, a mild high-frequency sensori-neural hearing loss was present bilaterally. Physical examination of the left ear revealed a fungoid external otitis and a perforated tympanic membrane. Thus, the pain experienced upon application of the hydrogen peroxide was due to the fact that the peroxide was getting into the middle ear through the perforated tympanic membrane. By carrying the bacteria from the ear canal with it, a middle-ear infection could have resulted. Mr. J. V. was referred for otologic treatment, and medication was prescribed to eliminate the fungus and to relieve the itching in his ear canal.

The foregoing case points up the danger of self-treatment combined with ignorance. Since Mr. J.V.'s hearing loss in the high frequencies was mild, further rehabilitation was deemed unnecessary.

Middle Ear Abnormalities and Problems.   Congenital malformations can also be found in the middle ear. These take the form of deformed ossicular chains, missing ossicles, replacement of the tympanic membrane by a primitive bony plate, fixation of the stapes in the oval window, and breaks in the ossicular chain. As indicated earlier, these abnormalities are usually found with congenital atresia of the outer ear, but they can also be restricted to the middle ear itself. The following is a case of congenital middle-ear deformities resulting in a conductive type hearing loss:

Miss T. W., a university student eighteen years old, was seen for an audiological evaluation, which showed the presence of a severe, bilateral, conductive hearing loss. Case history information revealed that Miss T. W. had a bilateral, congenital middle-ear problem for which surgery was being contemplated. Both outer ears were normal, and she wore a binaural hearing aid built into glasses. With this type of amplification, speech reception thresholds and understanding of speech were well within the normal range. The left corner of her mouth was pulled to the side slightly, indicating a possible paralysis of the facial nerve. She also had a distorted *s* sound.

Subsequent surgery on the left ear revealed a normal tympanic membrane but a defective ossicular chain consisting of a deformed incus and a rudimentary stapes. In addition, the oval window could not be identified. The operation was not successful from the audiologic standpoint because air-conduction thresholds in the left ear were not improved.

Since she was already wearing a binaural hearing aid, from which she appeared to obtain substantial benefit, Miss T. W. was enrolled in therapy for correction of her defective *s* sound and strengthening of muscular control around the mouth area. Within two semesters she was dismissed from therapy, but she continued to receive periodic hearing evaluations. She is scheduled for further ear surgery, which hopefully will prove to be more successful.

Acquired middle-ear problems resulting in conductive hearing loss can result from many causes. One very common problem associated with this type of hearing loss is caused by a ruptured eardrum. The tympanic membrane can be penetrated by any number of sharp objects. In attempts to relieve itching or to dig out the wax from the ear canal people use hair-pins or paper clips, and any slip can result in the penetration of the tympanic membrane. The tympanic membrane can also be ruptured by a sharp blow across the ears and is one of many very good reasons why children should not be struck on or about the head. Nature has provided a much lower and safer target for such disciplinary measures. Sharp objects should never be introduced into the external ear canal and an old cliché still carries the best advice, "Never put anything into your ears smaller than your elbow."

The eardrum can also be perforated from within by the build-up of fluid in the middle ear. The size and location of the perforation will indicate how serious the problem is. Fortunately, small perforations will tend to heal spontaneously once the middle-ear infection has been removed. Other persistent perforations may indicate the presence of a more serious problem.

Otitis Media. Otitis media is an inflammation or infection of the middle ear. There are a number of types, the most common cause of conductive hearing loss in children being due to eustachian tube malfunction. Most often the tube is swollen so that it can no longer open properly. This swelling may be due to allergies or upper respiratory infection or to the growth of a large amount of adenoidal tissue around the opening. This excessive growth of adenoidal tissue is probably the most common cause of otitis media. Since the middle ear is aerated through the eustachian tube, blockage of the latter results in the eardrum bulging inwards and secretion of a clear, watery fluid from the mucous lining of the middle ear. As a result of this retraction of the eardrum, the ossicular chain is impeded and a conductive hearing loss results. This condition is then known as *serous otitis media.* The term serous refers to the fluid or serum that may partially or completely fill the middle-ear cavity.

Treatment of serous otitis media consists of ridding the ear of fluid by *myringotomy* in which the eardrum is cut to allow the fluid to drain or to be pumped out, and by tonsillectomy and adenoidectomy (T & A). If the condition persists after adenoidectomy, small polyethylene tubes may have to be inserted in the eardrums in order to aerate the middle ear until further growth restores the proper functioning of the eustachian tube. The following is a case of serous otitis media in need of medical attention:

David, age seven, had been enrolled in speech therapy for correction of an articulation problem. After about two months of therapy, it was decided to have his hearing evaluated. It was readily apparent that David was a mouth breather, and when asked to close his mouth and breath through his nose, he was unable to do so because of the congestion. Oral examination revealed such extremely large tonsils we wondered how the child was able to swallow his food.

Audiological evaluation showed a mild, bilateral, conductive type of hearing loss. The child, however, did not complain of pain in his ears, which would be the case with serous otitis media. Treatment called for a T & A and myringotomy as well as investigation of a possible allergic condition that might account for the chronic nasal congestion. Following the T & A the child's congestion diminished, and he actually became much more understandable, since the denasality in his speech disappeared. Hearing returned to the normal range. Further speech therapy could then be expected to correct his misarticulations.

Acute otitis media is the problem which is usually experienced by a child or adult as a result of an upper respiratory infection such as a cold or an allergy attack. Coughing, sneezing, or blowing the nose forces secretions containing bacteria through the eustachian tube into the middle ear. Infants and children are particularly susceptible to this type of infection because their eustachian tubes tend to lie on a horizontal plane. In the adult this relationship changes, the tube becoming more vertical, and thus it is more difficult for infected material to be forced into the middle ear. Acute otitis media is accompanied by the earache familiar to all of us. The fluid in the ear may initially be clear but it soon changes to pus and the pressure of this fluid causes the eardrum to bulge outwardly to produce pain.

If the condition is caught in time, medical treatment with antibiotics may be all that is needed. Once the infection has cleared up, the debris will be absorbed. However, it is interesting to note that some otologists feel that their work has increased because of antibiotics. The drug clears up the infection, but the fluid is left in the middle ear. If left there over a period of time, the fluid will turn into a thick, mucous, sludgelike material resulting in even greater loss of hearing. This condition is often referred to as "glue ear."

Chronic otitis media is a condition where there is a continuous infection of the middle ear over a long period of time. It is not a recurring infection, but one that is never completely cleared up. In it we usually find a perforated eardrum and an accumulation of fluid in the middle ear which gradually erodes the ossicular chain. The combination of these factors may result in a severe conductive hearing loss. If the mastoid process becomes infected and the infection is allowed to persist, it could result in an infection of the brain.

G. O., age forty-nine, suffered from chronic otitis media for years. The infection was not properly controlled and resulted in infection of the mastoid bones. Eventually the infection travelled to the brain and resulted in some tissue damage. G. O. is now subject to epileptic-like seizures and is under constant medication for control of them. In addition, he has a severe conductive hearing loss due to the erosion of his middle-ear structures.

Discharge from the ear or complaints of earaches from children should never be ignored. The speech therapist in the public schools can do much to help the teachers understand conductive type hearing losses, refer children for proper medical treatment, help the otologist with follow-up, and provide the child with the extra help he may need until an infection can be cleared up.

Otosclerosis. Another disease of the middle ear that accounts for a great number of conductive type hearing losses is *otosclerosis*. In it, the hearing loss is the result of a formation of spongy bone which fixates the footplate of the stapes in the oval window. The cause of this type of growth is unknown. There are, however, some interesting aspects of this disease. It is more common in females than males and is usually first noticed during the late teens or early twenties. The hearing loss is usually accompanied by tinnitus (ringing in the ears) and increases during pregnancy. Evidently the hormonal changes which take place in the body during pregnancy enhance the spongy bone growth.

There are no effective drugs for otosclerosis, and the medical treatment consists of a number of surgical procedures. One of the most popular and successful of these is called a *stapedectomy*. In this procedure the fixated stapes is removed and replaced by a prosthetic device. Speech therapists should know that there is a high percentage of success with this procedure and that hearing thresholds can be returned to within the normal range or at least be markedly improved.

Mr. D. G., age twenty-seven, has had otosclerosis since the age of sixteen. He underwent surgery on his right ear on two different occasions without any apparent success. He has worn several binaural hearing aids for a number of years, but complained that his present aid was not giving him satisfactory service.

Audiological evaluation revealed the audiogram shown in Figure 40. As shown by the audiogram, Mr. G. has a moderate conductive type hearing loss in his left ear and a severe, mixed type loss in his right ear. The surgical procedures performed on the right ear were not successful and had apparently resulted in some inner-ear damage.

Hearing-aid evaluation procedures indicated that Mr. G. was unable to use amplification in his right ear to any advantage because of the depressed speech reception threshold and poor understanding of speech in that ear. Since a hearing aid on the right ear was not feasible and a hearing aid on the left ear brought his hearing to within the normal range, he was fitted with a glasses type hearing aid in a Bi–CROS arrangement. With this type of aid a pickup microphone is located in each bow of the glasses, but the output of the one on the poorer ear is fed into the better ear. The abbreviation CROS stands for the contra-lateral routing of signals and is a fairly recent concept in amplification for the hearing impaired.

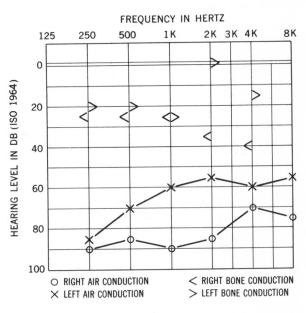

FIGURE 40: *Bilateral Otosclerosis Resulting in a Conductive Loss in the Left Ear and a Mixed Loss in the Right Ear*

Sensori-neural Impairments. Congenital sensori-neural hearing losses can result from hereditary factors or be caused by conditions affecting the mother during pregnancy. Relatively little is known about hearing loss suspected to be the result of a genetic defect. We do know that hearing loss tends to run in certain families and that deaf parents are more likely to have deaf children although the exact genetic mechanism for many of these losses is as yet undiscovered. The following family history of hearing loss illustrates a kind of loss that has no apparent etiology other than a possible genetic problem:

Patty, age twelve, Lois, age eleven, and Vanessa, age seven, are sisters who, as far as could be determined, were probably born with mild, bilateral, sensori-neural hearing losses. The hearing losses of the two older girls were discovered just before they entered school, whereas Vanessa's loss was known quite early, since hearing testing was carried out at a much younger age due to the family history of hearing loss. This type of progressive hearing loss can be very challenging in terms of therapy and educational placement. The two oldest girls progressed from mild-gain hearing aids worn on the head to high-gain body aids. Their gradually deteriorating hearing caused them to go through a series of educational placements from the regular classroom with the use of amplification, to regular classroom with extra help, to placement in a special class for the severely hard of hearing. In addition, because of educational considerations, these children needed remedial procedures to develop their speech and language skills.

A most interesting twist to this family's history is the fact that a fourth child, a boy, has completely normal hearing. This poses the possibility that the hearing losses experienced by the girls are due to some sex-linked genetic factor. The problem is further complicated by the fact that both parents have normal hearing, and there is no history of significant hearing loss on either side.

Congenital hearing loss can also occur as a result of illnesses, drugs, and accidents sustained by the mother during pregnancy. At one time it was thought that the placental barrier shielded the fetus to a great extent from infections of the mother, but it is now realized that a great many diseases are transmitted directly from the mother. This is also true of drugs taken by the mother. Such drugs as streptomycin and kanomycin are especially dangerous during pregnancy. Quinine and aspirin may also affect hearing, and alcohol and smoking are also suspect, especially if used excessively. It is probably a good rule for a woman not to take any type of drug during pregnancy that is not specifically prescribed by her physician and even then reluctantly.

One of the greatest causes of congenital hearing losses is maternal *rubella*. This is the name given to German measles occurring during pregnancy. Rubella is usually a rather mild disease in the child or adult, but it is extremely dangerous to the fetus. The greatest danger comes during the first three months of pregnancy, though there is evidence that defects can also be caused during the second three months.[1] In addition to hearing loss and deafness, rubella can also cause other defects such as blindness and heart problems. The disease is rather insidious since the symptoms are so very mild in the adult and a rash may not appear. Fortunately, a rubella vaccine has been developed, and a program to immunize all children in the lower grades in school was started in early 1970. Since children are the carriers of this disease, by immunizing them it can be stamped out. The following case is typical of the so-called "rubella babies."

[1] "Investigators Reveal Greater Rubella Risks During Pregnancy," *Washington Sounds*, III (1969), 3.

Doug, age four, is the youngest of four children. His two older brothers and a sister are normal in all respects. Doug's mother's pregnancy was uneventful, except that she contracted rubella during the early months. Doug appeared normal at birth; but as he developed, a slight heart murmur and an eye problem were discovered. He was also subject to occasional dizzy spells. His hearing loss was first noticed when he was two and a half years old. Later audiological evaluation showed a moderate to severe sensori-neural hearing loss in the left ear and a severe loss in the right ear.

Rehabilitation procedures consisted of fitting him with a body-type hearing aid and enrollment in a preschool nursery program for children with hearing impairments. Doug was fortunate that such a program was available in the area since usually there is a considerable lack of help for many preschool youngsters like him. He adjusted well to the program, and he has been able to make good use of his residual hearing and is now able to do some lipreading. His articulation skills are fairly good, and the speech he does use is intelligible. However, his vocabulary and language skills are below normal for children of his age. The preschool program appears to have been of significant value to Doug, and he will be entering special classes for the hard-of-hearing in a short time.

Unfortunately some children who have had rubella sustain much greater losses, and the prognosis is not as favorable as for the case just cited.

Having survived intrauterine life and birth trauma, the human being is still subject to a great many events that can cause hearing loss. Accidents, drugs, and diseases all take their toll and a complete discussion of all the possible causes of acquired hearing loss is beyond the scope of this chapter. However, there are some common causes which we can mention.

Effects of Drugs on Hearing. Just as drugs taken by the mother can be harmful to the fetus, so too can drugs taken by the individual be ototoxic to him. Some people, of course, are allergic to them. For instance, some people cannot take pencillin, since they are prone to allergic reactions that might prove fatal. Drugs such as dihydrostreptomycin, streptomycin, neomycin, and kanomycin are extremely ototoxic and must be given with great care. Usually the hearing should be monitored while a person is on these drugs, and any changes in thresholds should signal that the drug must be stopped. Even such drugs as quinine and aspirin may prove to be ototoxic in susceptible individuals. The hearing loss caused by drugs is usually bilateral and usually permanent, but not progressive. Ototoxic drugs are especially dangerous when used in conjunction with any kidney disease. The following is a case of sensori-neural hearing loss caused by a particular drug:

Tim, age seven, was being treated for tuberculosis and had been on streptomycin for the year previous to his hearing evaluation. Streptomycin is often used for treatment of tuberculosis because of its great effectiveness against this disease. Audiological evaluation revealed a bilateral, sensori-neural hearing loss as shown in Figure 41. There was mild to moderate loss in the lower test frequencies, with a severe loss in the higher frequencies. Understanding of speech was markedly reduced even when it was presented at intensity levels well above that at which conversation normally occurs.

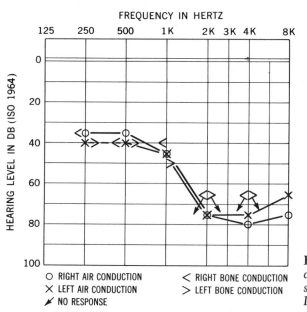

FIGURE 41: *Drug-Induced, Bilateral Sensori-neural Hearing Loss*

In addition to his problem with tuberculosis, Tim was now in need of rehabilitation for his hearing loss because of the injudicious use of an ototoxic drug. His hearing loss might have been avoided or held to a much milder degree had monitoring audiometry been performed while he was on the drug.

Tim was fitted with a hearing aid and enrolled in special classes for the hard-of-hearing where he could receive training in the use of a hearing aid, auditory training, and lipreading as well. In such cases it becomes a challenge to prevent a child from adding an educational handicap to the already existing hearing handicap.

The so-called "childhood diseases," that many people think have no serious consequences often cause hearing loss. Mumps, measles, chicken pox, scarlet fever, diptheria, and whooping cough can attack the end organ of hearing and cause sensori-neural hearing loss. Fortunately it is now no longer inevitable that a child undergo these diseases. Only recently vaccines have been developed to immunize children against measles, rubella, and mumps.

Hearing loss resulting from these diseases is usually bilateral, except for mumps. Mumps is the most common cause of unilateral hearing loss, and the loss is usually total. The following case illustrates hearing loss from mumps:

> John, age seven, is presently enrolled in therapy for an articulation problem that consists mainly of substitutions of one sound for another. At the age of five, he came down with a case of mumps that resulted in a profound loss of hearing in his right ear. His left ear was normal. His audiogram is typical of unilateral deafness due to this disease.
>
> In this youngster's case it would have been a mistake to think that his articulation problem was in any way related to his hearing loss. People with unilateral hearing are able to function fairly normally, although the sense of direction of sound may be somewhat impaired. With a child, however, even this tends to be something they are able to compensate for. In John's case, the important thing was to prevent any damage to his good ear either by illness or accident. All his teachers in school were told his loss, and he was given preferential seating. Speech therapy was continued, the therapist making sure she was working from his unimpaired side.

Effects of Noise.   A kind of hearing loss which is receiving a great deal of attention at this time is noise-induced hearing loss. Noise-induced hearing loss produces a gradual loss of hearing, and is due to exposure to loud noise over a long period of time. It should not be confused with "acoustic trauma," which is a sudden loss of hearing due to one exposure to a loud noise such as an explosion.

Since man is becoming concerned over pollution of his environment, the topic of "noise pollution" is a timely one. There is a growing concern over environmental noise as is indicated by the Conference on Noise as a Public Health Hazard held in Washington, D. C., on June 13–14, 1968.[2] We should also be concerned about the noise generated by the new "jumbo" jets, increased traffic, and new industry.

A more subtle danger to the ears of youth also exists. A number of studies have indicated that "hard rock" music can cause noise-induced

[2] W. D. Ward, and J. E. Fricke, eds., "Noise as a Public Health Hazard: Proceedings of the Conference," *American Speech and Hearing Association Reports,* IV (1969).

hearing loss.[3] Another study has indicated that the potential for damage is there, but that there is not the great danger that our youth is going deaf as many popular articles in the mass media would lead one to think.[4] This last study indicated that "rock" muscians who are exposed the most do not incur hearing losses of any great magnitude. Since this type of music does exceed the 85 to 90 decibels of sound that is considered safe, the exposure time is probably a critical factor. Young people just do not listen to loud music eight hours a day, five days a week, for years. However, the man working in the noisy environment of a foundry may be exposed to noise that exceeds safe intensity levels for a full working day for many years. The following case study illustrates this point:

> J. V., age forty-seven, stated that he was no longer able to hear birds sing or the tick of his watch. He complained of a "high-pitched ring-ing" in both ears. He also complained of difficulty hearing in group situations or in the presence of background noise. J. V. had worked in a drop forge for twenty-three years and was exposed to extremely loud noise for most of the working day. He had spent the last twelve years as a "hammerman" operating a huge hammer used to flatten steel bars. A subsequent hearing evaluation revealed the high-fre-quency, sensori-neural hearing loss shown in Figure 42.
>
> J. V. was fitted with a hearing aid that gave a high-frequency empha-sis and a special vented earmold that further emphasized the higher frequencies. Since he had worked in an environment which made normal communication almost impossible, he had become rather adept at speechreading. He was advised to wear ear-protective devices while working in order to prevent any further damage to his ears.

Noise-induced hearing loss causes damage to the higher frequencies first. The point of greatest loss is usually at 4000 Hertz, and this is referred to as an "acoustic trauma dip." Men such as J. V. usually get along quite well while they are working, since communication with fellow employees is difficult at best. However, upon retirement, they often find it impossible to enjoy a movie or the theater, and social groups also present difficulty. Thus, this person tends to withdraw from social contacts of any kind, and the well-known loneliness of the hearing impaired begins to take hold.

Presbycusis. The hearing loss that people incur with advancing age is called *presbycusis*. It is the most common single cause of sensori-neural

[3] C. P. Lebo, K. S. Oliphant, and J. Garrett, "Acoustic Trauma from Rock-and-roll Music," *California Medicine*, CVII (1967), 378–80; D. M. Lipscomb, "High Intensity Sounds in the Recreational Environment," *Clinical Pediatrics*, VIII (1969), 63–68; R. R. Rupp and L. J. Koch, "But, Mother, Rock 'n' Roll Has to be Loud: The Effect of Noise on Human Ears," *Michigan Hearing* (Spring, 1968), 4–7.

[4] W. F. Rintelmann, and J. F. Borus, "Noise-induced Hearing Loss and Rock-and-roll Music," *Archives of Otolaryngology*, LXXXVIII (1968), 377–85.

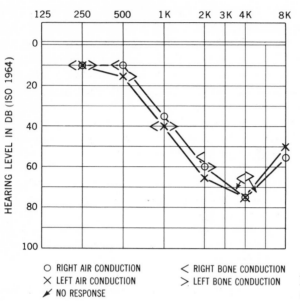

FREQUENCY IN HERTZ

○ RIGHT AIR CONDUCTION   < RIGHT BONE CONDUCTION
✕ LEFT AIR CONDUCTION   > LEFT BONE CONDUCTION   **FIGURE** 42: *Noise-In-*
↗ NO RESPONSE   *duced Hearing Loss*

hearing loss. The incidence of presbycusis seems to be increasing, but this is understandable when one considers that people live much longer than they used to and that we now have a substantial percentage of senior citizens in this country. The loss of hearing by presbycusis is a rather slow, insidious process and probably starts early in life, although the symptoms of hearing loss are usually not manifested until the person is over sixty years of age. The higher sound frequencies are affected first, and as the disorder gradually progresses, the person has trouble in hearing lower frequency sounds as well. Comprehension of speech may be affected to a much greater degree than would be expected from thresholds on a pure-tone audiogram. Even in the presence of a mild loss in pure-tone thresholds, the person may have extreme difficulty understanding speech. It is for this reason that an older person may be labeled as being inattentive or senile, when actually he just has presbycusis.

The cause of presbycusis are complex and little is known about them. There is apparently a degeneration of structures not only in the inner ear, but along the central pathways and in the cerebral cortex of the brain. It has also been stated that the hearing loss is due to the wear and tear on the ear from everyday living in our noisy society; studies on primitive tribes in Africa do not reveal nearly the amount of loss with age. Aging, of course, does not affect every person in the same way, and some people have relatively good hearing even into very old age. The following case is typical of the problems involved in presbycusis:

Mr. J. D., age sixty-seven was referred for an audiological evaluation and hearing-aid evaluation and selection following otologic consultation for his hearing problem. He was originally examined by the otologist upon the insistence of his daughter with whom he had been living since the death of his wife two years previously. The otologist diagnosed his disorder as presbycusis.

Mr. J. D. stated that he had noticed a decrease in hearing sensitivity for a number of years, but that it had become much worse during the past two years. He complained of difficulty hearing the radio and television, and he had to have the volume turned up beyond the comfort level of other family members. Consequently he had gradually lost interest in watching television. Conversation was also difficult for him to follow, and he found himself more and more frequently having to ask what was said. He felt that if other family members would not mumble or speak so fast he would be able to hear them without difficulty.

An interview with Mr. J. D.'s daughter revealed that she had become concerned for her father since he was showing an increasing tendency to isolate himself from other people. She also felt guilty. She worked outside the home and was usually tired in the evening. Talking with her father was a strain. She had to speak louder and often repeat what she said. This was annoying to her, so she found herself avoiding conversation with her father. It was at this point that she decided to seek professional advice and thought that perhaps a hearing aid might help them.

Audiological evaluation revealed the moderate, bilateral, sensori-neural hearing loss shown in Figure 43. Fortunately, Mr. J. D.'s understanding of speech, when it was presented at a fairly loud level, was good. A subsequent hearing-aid evaluation indicated that he received substantial benefit from wearing amplification.

The foregoing case, although it has its unique aspects, is typical not only of the hearing loss, but also of the family dynamics that are often involved. A hearing aid was not the total answer to this man's problem. He needed to have a greater understanding of his problem and so did the other family members. Rehabilitation in this type of case should involve family counseling so that its members can do their share in improving communications. For example, we often find improvement in communication by pointing out to the family that shouting at the hard-of-hearing person does no good, and that instead they should talk more slowly and

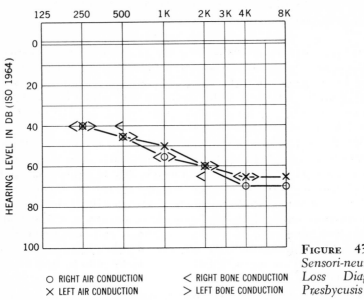

FREQUENCY IN HERTZ

FIGURE 43: *Bilateral Sensori-neural Hearing Loss Diagnosed As Presbycusis*

○ RIGHT AIR CONDUCTION   < RIGHT BONE CONDUCTION
✕ LEFT AIR CONDUCTION   > LEFT BONE CONDUCTION

distinctly. It is also important that the family realize the advantages and disadvantages of hearing aids and how they operate.

CENTRAL AUDITORY IMPAIRMENTS

The terms *central hearing loss* or *central deafness* are used to describe a hearing loss due to some problem in the auditory pathways in the brain stem or the auditory cortex itself. Audiologically this type of disorder shows itself as a sensori-neural problem on the pure-tone audiogram. However, even though the pure-tone audiogram may be normal, the person may be unable to use the incoming stimuli meaningfully. He may hear speech, but be unable to understand it.

One example of this type of auditory disorder is called *auditory agnosia.* As we have seen in our chapter on aphasia, in auditory agnosia the person hears but is unable to recognize meaningful sounds. Auditory agnosia often accompanies receptive aphasia and is a complicating factor in the rehabilitation of an aphasic patient. This type of auditory disorder is thus quite different from the hearing losses previously described that affect the peripheral hearing mechanism. When a central problem occurs in a child before the development of speech, it is extremely difficult to distinguish it from a peripheral hearing loss. Not enough is understood about these central problems, and their treatment is extremely difficult.

HEARING REHABILITATION

As in the organic speech disorders, the effective rehabilitation of a person with a hearing disorder is dependent on the skill, knowledge, and cooperation of a number of different specialists. Let us describe some of these professionals.

The Otologist. The otologist is concerned with the medical aspects of hearing impairment. He is first of all a physician who is concerned with the total well-being of a patient and secondly a specialist in the area of pathological hearing. The otologist is interested in determining if a hearing loss is present and in differentiating between conductive and sensorineural impairments. He may use various tuning fork tests or perform an audiometric evaluation. He may also check vestibular functioning by means of caloric tests since ear problems often manifest themselves through spells of dizziness or vertigo. He also has at his disposal the information that can be gained by laboratory procedures such as X-rays, blood tests, bacteriological tests, neurological examinations, and so on. In addition to the specialized techniques used to determine the medical status of a patient's ears, the otologist treats any aural pathologies he may find. This treatment may take the form of prescribing medication such as antibiotics for a middle-ear infection, or it may entail some type of ear surgery.

The Audiologist. Once the otologist has completed his medical treatment, or has determined that medical treatment is not feasible for a particular hearing loss, his basic responsibility is finished except for making the proper referral. It is precisely at this point that the audiologist becomes the primary person responsible for the patient's well-being. The audiologist's chief role is one of rehabilitation. This does not rule out the important job he may play in detecting hearing losses or referring patients for otologic consultation. He also supplies information based on certain special audiological tests which may help to determine the site of the lesion and thus aid the otologist in his differential diagnosis. The audiologist is also often able to obtain information about the hearing function of very young children or other difficult-to-test patients. He can detect malingering and pseudohypocusis. He may also work closely with the otologist in determining the amount of sensori-neural reserve in an ear when middle-ear surgery is being contemplated. In some settings the foregoing may, in fact, be his primary responsibilities.

The habilitation and rehabilitation aspects of hearing impairment are the essential domain of the audiologist. Through extensive clinical testing he is able to describe how a person's peripheral hearing functions and to plan the therapy needed to help the patient cope with his everyday communicative demands. This plan may incorporate hearing-aid evaluation and selection procedures as well as activities involving auditory training and speechreading. These will be discussed more thoroughly in the next section.

AURAL REHABILITATION

A complete program of aural rehabilitation would include auditory training, speechreading, hearing-aid orientation, speech correction, speech conservation, vocational guidance, and counseling. Any one hard-of-hearing person may not need all of these services, and we usually find that auditory training and speechreading form the core of the therapy with the hard-of-hearing.

Auditory Training. Auditory training teaches the hearing-impaired person to make the best possible use of his residual hearing. Even among those individuals classified as profoundly deaf there is usually some residual hearing for low-frequency sounds. Most hard-of-hearing persons often have a great deal of residual hearing that encompasses a relatively broad frequency range, and they may not be making full use of the hearing they possess. Auditory training is training in listening. Recently, we have begun to recognize that listening skills can be improved by training not only in the hard-of-hearing but even among normally hearing children and adults. To cite a simple example—a person learning to play the guitar usually has a difficult time tuning it since this requires the ability to tell when two strings sound exactly alike when they are held in a certain manner by one hand and plucked with the other. With a bit of persistent practice, the person is usually able to tune the guitar quite readily, since he becomes able to hear even a slight discrepancy between the tones and to make the proper adjustment. We don't usually refer to this discriminatory process as auditory training, but that is exactly what it is; and it illustrates the point that the discriminating ability of the ear can be improved.

Auditory training with the hard-of-hearing must vary according to age of the person, the age of the onset of hearing loss, and with severity of the loss. It need not be as intensive with adults who have previously had normal communication skills as it would be with a child who must learn to send and receive verbal messages despite a hearing loss. With children, auditory training may start at the level of gross sound discrimination. At this level the child is first taught to differentiate bells from whistles or whistles from horns by the noises they make. Identification training is begun by using only two objects at one time, and then gradually other noisemakers are added. This type of training is continued until the child is quite aware of the importance of sound in making the identification, and until he can make correct differentiations consistently without the aid of visual clues.

From this stage we progress to what is often referred to as "gross speech discriminations." Depending on the skill of the child, the discrimination of speech sounds can begin by first distinguishing between such words as *ball* and *car* and then proceeding to the harder contrasts of *bell* and *ball*. In the latter instance, although the discrimination is finer, we would still consider this gross speech discrimination since the distinctive differences are produced by dissimilar vowels. Finer speech discriminations are called for when two words such as *same* and *came* are contrasted because consonants do not have as much acoustic power or duration as do the vowels. The acoustic differences between them are even less detectable when such words as *same* and *shame* are contrasted. This pair of words would be particularly difficult for persons having a high-frequency hearing loss because much of the energy necessary for the intelligibility of [s] and [sh] is found in the frequency range of greatest loss. Nevertheless, through skillful auditory training most persons can make real gains.

After he is proficient in making discriminations of single words, the hard-of-hearing person should go on to sentences and paragraphs. Many clinicians feel that therapy should begin with the larger wholes and then work toward the finer discriminations in single words, the argument being that there are more helpful clues in a sentence. Single unrelated words are harder to identify than sentence strings. Therefore, key words are often used, and the patient is asked to repeat the sentence or write down what he hears. To be correct, he must hear the key words in the sentences.[5] Paragraphs can also be prepared that concern subjects or activities suitable for children or adults. After reading the paragraph, the therapist can ask prepared questions in order to determine how well the person was able to follow running speech. Since many hard-of-hearing persons have difficulty understanding speech in group situations or in the presence of a background noise, all of the above levels can be repeated by introducing varying levels of background noise. The therapist can make tape recordings of various types of noise or the babble of conversation and present this noise at gradually increasing intensity levels until the patient has increased his discrimination proficiency.

Speechreading. The term *speechreading* has now generally displaced the older term *lipreading*, doubtless because there is much more involved in comprehension through visual cues than in just watching lips. Facial

---

[5] Examples of these types of sentences are given in H. Davis and S. R. Silverman, eds., *Hearing and Deafness*, 3d ed. (New York: Holt, Rinehart & Winston, Inc., 1970), p. 491.

expressions, head movements, gestures—all of these can furnish important clues as to what is being said. Even normally hearing people use visual clues to a greater extent than they realize.

Numerous approaches in teaching speechreading have been advocated, but basically they can be divided into two broad categories: those advocating the analytic and the synthetic approaches. The analytic approaches stress careful analysis of phonetic elements, whereas the synthetic approaches advocate grasping the "whole" rather than one part at a time. Anyone who specializes in work with the hard-of-hearing will need to familiarize himself with the methods advocated by Nitchie, Bruhn, the Kinzies, and Bunger.[6] Few audiologists adopt only one of these approaches since our research does not seem to show that any one method is any better than the others. The better contributions of each method can be adapted to specific individuals in therapy by the hearing therapist.

Whatever approach is used, there are certain principles that must be followed. The stimulus material must be presented in a *natural* manner much as it would be encountered in a normal communication situation. Whenever material is presented pantomimically without voice, there is a tendency to exaggerate mouth movements. This is why we use a voice when stimulating the hard-of-hearing person in speechreading. However it is important, especially at the beginning of speechreading training, that the visual channel be emphasized as much as possible; for if the client can hear the clinician, he may be depending on his hearing too much and not obtaining enough practice in observing visual clues. For this reason we often speak very softly or whisper in the periods of speechreading. Through sufficient practice in front of a mirror, the clinician can learn to speak without exaggerated movements of his articulators even when pantomiming. Remember also, that in group work the patients must be seated so that all are able to see the clinician's face equally well.

Beginning lessons in speechreading for children should present the more visible speech sounds so that the child can experience some success right from the start. The child can be told how each sound is made, but care should be taken not to become too analytical. Each lesson should consist of (1) a list of vocabulary words with which children of certain age levels are familiar, (2) a series of practice sentences incorporating the words, and (3) a practice story or exercise that incorporates the words.

It must be remembered that speechreading alone is not a perfect substitute for hearing since many sounds of English are just not visible.

---

[6] E. B. Nitchie, *Lip-reading, Principles and Practice* (New York: Frederick A. Stokes Company, 1921); M. E. Bruhn, *The Mueller-Walle Method of Lipreading for the Hard of Hearing* (Washington, D.C., 1949); C. E. Kinzie, and R. Kinzie, *Lip-reading for the Deafened Adult* (Chicago: Winston, 1931); A. M. Bunger, *Speech Reading—Jena Method* (Danville, Ill.: Interstate, 1952).

For this reason a combination approach of auditory training and speech-reading is usually recommended. Also, a truly effective program of speech-reading must be geared to the interest of the patients involved. With children, lessons can be made enjoyable and interesting if they revolve around things which children tend to love, such as animals or fairy tales. School subjects such as arithmetic, history, and language can be incorporated into speechreading lessons. These kinds of lessons also have the advantage of preparing the child for the vocabulary encountered in the regular classroom.

Initially, speechreading lessons may revolve around matching the movements of the articulators to the names of common objects. However, progress must be made toward the goal of having the child grasp thoughts and concepts which are conveyed in more abstract language. Thus, speech-reading progress is from the concrete to the more abstract. Where we begin depends a lot upon the age and severity of the hearing loss. With the hard-of-hearing child who has a good deal of residual hearing and can learn some language through the auditory channel, it may not be necessary to begin at the simple matching level. Determining the needs of the individual child is all-important in good therapy.

HEARING AIDS

The modern hearing aid is an electronic device that changes acoustical energy into electrical current. The electric current is then amplified and changed back to acoustical energy with greater intensity.

A hearing aid consists of three major components: a microphone, a transistor amplifier, and a receiver. The microphone changes the sound waves into variations in electric current that are then fed into the amplifier where they are made more intense. The amplified current is then fed into the receiver, a miniature loudspeaker, where it is converted back to sound waves. The resulting acoustic energy is now, however, at a greater intensity level than originally. In the hearing aid, all three components mentioned above have been miniaturized; and with miniaturization, power and fidelity have usually been sacrificed for wearing comfort.

In addition to the main components, a hearing aid must have a source of power, which is usually a small carbon-zinc, silver oxide, or mercury battery. The hearing aid must also feed into the ear, and this is accomplished by a custom earmold which is individually fitted. Hearing aids can be classified into two distinct types according to where they are worn. Those aids worn on the head can be built into glasses, or suspended from the ears (auricle aids), or actually inserted into the ear. All of those which are worn on the head are collectively called ear-level aids.

Body hearing aids are usually larger and more powerful, and they are used with more severe hearing losses. The fairly large grill in the center of the case serves as the microphone, and the large button receiver is connected to the earmold. The cord connecting the receiver to the case is also readily visible. Since the cord plugs into each component, it can be disconnected, and different receivers can be used with the same instrument to achieve various frequency responses. Body-type aids also tend to have certain additional components not always found in ear-level aids. They usually have an on-off switch, whereas the ear-level aid may not, and a hinged battery compartment is swung out to break the battery contacts. The body-type aid also has a tone control whereby two or three settings enable one to change the frequency response characteristics of the instrument; the changes are usually made to obtain a low- or high-frequency emphasis or a flat response across the frequency range amplified by the instrument. A telephone pickup coil is also found on the body-type instruments. This enables the user to hear over a telephone without using the microphone of the aid.

Hearing aids are effectively used by people having various kinds of hearing losses. Some years ago it was a common belief that a sensori-neural hearing loss could not be helped by a hearing aid. This was probably quite true with the old carbon-type amplifiers because they introduced so much distortion into the instrument. Today, however, with the much more efficient transistor amplifier, some people with sensori-neural hearing losses derive substantial benefit from wearing hearing aids. In fact, the number of hearing aids used by people with conductive losses has declined because modern surgical techniques are often able to restore conductive hearing losses to a level where amplification is not needed.

After obtaining a hearing aid a person with a hearing loss is in need of some hearing-aid orientation sessions. In these he learns how to care for and use his hearing aid. This would include such things as changing batteries, cleaning the earmold, adjusting the volume control, and so on. He must also come to realize right from the beginning that he is not getting his ears back. For one thing, the quality of sound reproduction is not very good because a hearing aid is essentially a low-fidelity instrument, and hearing aid users often expect too much from their instruments. We must help such a person understand that a hearing aid is not usually the total answer to his hearing problem. Difficult listening situations such as those involving groups or background noise will also be difficult when wearing a hearing aid. In fact, he will learn that in some situations the hearing aid may even add to the confusion. Then too, the hearing aid may seem so unnatural to the person that he may tend to reject it too hastily. One reason for this is that with the instrument, he is now hearing sounds he hasn't heard for a long time, and so he feels bombarded by noise. This is especially true of the adult who has gradually lost part of his hearing over a period of time. Just as a person with normal hearing has to adapt to noise and to direct his attention to what he desires to hear, the hard-of-hearing person must also learn to ignore extraneous noises and to devote his attention to what is being said. At times a child or adult may complain that his hearing aid squeals whenever he turns the volume control up to where he is getting effective amplification. This particular squeal is due to amplified sound reaching the pickup microphone. It is the result of sound leaking out around a poorly fitting earmold. Either the earmold was not properly fitted in the first place, or the ear has changed so that the mold no longer fits. In the case of young children, the earmold may have to be changed every few months or even sooner, depending on growth patterns. A properly fitted earmold should allow the person to turn his aid up to full volume without obtaining the squeal that results from feedback.

The first few weeks of using a hearing aid will probably be the most difficult for the hard-of-hearing person. However, if he is helped to understand more about his particular problem, can manipulate the controls of the aid, and understands that the hearing aid is only as good as the effort he puts forth in learning to use it, he is well on his way to becoming an effective hearing-aid user.

REFERENCES

Articles

1. Bangs, T. E. "Training the Aurally Handicapped." Chapter 6 in Levin, N. M., ed., *Voice and Speech Disorders: Medical Aspects.* Springfield, Ill.: Charles C Thomas, Publisher, 1962.
   Summarize the new information given in this chapter.
2. Black, J. W., O'Reilly, P. P., and Peck, J. "Self-administered Training in Lipreading." *Journal of Speech and Hearing Disorders,* XXVIII (1963), 183–86.
   How is this self-training carried out?
3. Charklin, J. B. and Ventry, I. M. "Functional Hearing Loss." In Jerger, J., ed., *Modern Developments in Audiology* (New York: Academic Press, 1963).
   What are the causes and characteristics of functional hearing loss?
4. Egland, G. O. *Speech and Language Problems.* Englewood Cliffs, N.J.: Prentice-Hall, Inc., 1970.
   Read Chapter 9 and summarize what the classroom teacher can do for the hard-of-hearing child.
5. Giolas, T. G., Webster, E. J., and Ward, L. M. "A Diagnostic Therapy Setting for Hearing Handicapped Children." *Journal of Speech and Hearing Disorders,* XXXIII (1968), 345–50.
   How are diagnoses and therapy activities carried out in this setting?
6. ———. and Wark, D. J. "Communication Problems Associated with Unilateral Hearing Loss." *Journal of Speech and Hearing Disorders,* XXXII (1967), 336–42.
   If you can hear all right with one ear, why worry if the other shows a real loss?
7. Goeth, J. H. and Lounsbury, E. "Hearing Aids and Children in Elementary School." *Journal of Speech and Hearing Disorders,* XXXI (1966), 283–89.
   What are the problems concerning the use of hearing aids by school children?
8. Green, D. S. "The Peep Show." *Journal of Speech and Hearing Disorders,* XXIII (1958), 118.
   How do they test the hearing of children by this technique?
9. Harrison, A. "Practical Audiology." *Journal of Speech and Hearing Disorders,* XXXII (1967), 162–69.
   Describe the four cases presented in this article.
10. Johnson, W., Brown, S. F., Curtis, J. F., Edney, C. E., and Keaster, J. *Speech Handicapped School Children.* 3d ed. New York: Harper & Row, Publishers, 1967.
    Read Chapter 8 and list the bits of new information you discover.
11. Kowalsky, M. H. "Integration of a Severely Hard-of-Hearing in a Normal

First-Grade Program: A Case Study." *Journal of Speech and Hearing Disorders,* XXVII (1962), 349–58.
Describe Terry's problems and what was done to help her.

12. Leshin, G. "Childhood Non-organic Hearing Loss." *Journal of Speech and Hearing Disorders,* XXV (1960), 290–92.
Summarize this article.

13. Price, L. L. "Age and Normal Hearing." *Journal of Speech and Hearing Disorders,* XXIX (1964), 91–93.
How does hearing acuity vary with age?

14. Quizley, S. R. "The Deaf and Hard-of-Hearing." *Review of Educational Research,* XXXIX (1969), 103–24.
What is shown by the research on incidence, causes, and perception of these persons?

15. Sortini, A. J. "Importance of Individual Hearing Aids and Early Hearing Therapy for Preschool Children." *Journal of Speech and Hearing Disorders,* XXIV (1959), 346–53.
Summarize his argument.

16. Zink, G. D. and Alpiner, J. G. "Hearing Aids: One Aspect of a State Public School Hearing Conservation Program." *Journal of Speech and Hearing Disorders,* XXXIII (1965), 329–50.
Describe what the audiologist does in such a setting.

Texts

17. Davis, H. and Silverman, S. R. *Hearing and Deafness.* 3d ed. New York: Holt, Rinehart & Winston, Inc., 1970.
Covers the material on normal and abnormal hearing. An old classic, now revised.

18. DiCarlo, L. M. *The Deaf.* Englewood Cliffs, N.J.: Prentice-Hall, Inc., 1964.
Most interesting for its history of the treatment of the deaf.

19. Mykelbust, H. R. *Auditory Disorders in Children.* New York: Grune and Stratton, 1954.
Probably the basic text dealing with problems of diagnosis and treatment of children with hearing problems.

20. Newby, H. A. *Audiology.* 2d ed. New York: Appleton-Century-Crofts, 1964.
One of the major texts in the field.

21. O'Neill, J. J. *The Hard of Hearing.* Englewood Cliffs, N.J.: Prentice-Hall, Inc., 1964.
An overview of our essential knowledge concerning hearing impairments.

22. ———. and Oyer, H. J. *Visual Communication for the Hard-of-Hearing: History, Research, and Methods.* Englewood Cliffs, N.J.: Prentice-Hall, Inc., 1961.
Provides a clear summary of the information about lipreading.

10

Speech Pathology

as a Profession

Communication is the most complex aspect of human behavior. Impairments in the processes of communication—speech, language, and hearing—leave myriad problems in their wake. The child with a communication disorder may encounter overwhelming obstacles to learning and may find it difficult to establish the relationships with other children which are essential to growing up to healthy, stable adulthood. The adult who acquires a speech or hearing disorder may experience a variety of social problems. His livelihood may be endangered; he may withdraw from his friends and cease to be a participating member of his community. Speech Pathology and Audiology is the area of professional specialization which has developed out of concern for people in the processes of communication. The profession offers many opportunities for service to mankind.*

For many students this text will have been their first introduction to speech therapy as a professional field. We hope it has not been an unpleasant experience. We hope also that some of them may be interested in entering this new profession. But even those who have no personal interest in speech therapy as a career should know something of the qualifications required of those who do. They may desire to refer some child or their own child to a speech therapist some day.

Speech Therapist as a Profession. First, we must make it very clear that speech therapy is a very young newcomer to the family of the healing professions. Its professional organization, the American Speech and Hear-

* For a free copy of the information booklet describing this profession, write to the American Speech and Hearing Association, 9030 Old Georgetown Road, Washington, D.C., 20014 for *Careers in Speech Pathology and Audiology.* The above quotation comes from this source.

ing Association, is not even forty years old, whereas medicine, dentistry, and nursing have long histories. Nevertheless, this young profession has shown astounding growth both in membership and in its standards. Speech and hearing specialists are now to be found in almost every country of the world. The journals of this profession publish articles containing basic research and clinical methods in many languages. Certification standards require stringent preparation both in academic courses and in supervised casework, and they are constantly being raised. Parents who now refer their speech-defective children to a certified speech or hearing therapist can feel confident that they are in well-trained and competent hands.

The demand for trained workers in this field has constantly exceeded the supply and seems destined to continue in this accelerating fashion for some years. Training centers are finding it increasingly difficult to meet requests for newly trained clinicians to staff the many positions available. In part this is due to the fact that many college students still in search of a satisfying career never hear about this professional field, or, if they do, they hear about it too late. Speech and hearing therapists have probably been too busy with their cases and their research to blow their horns loudly enough to be heard over the masking noise of the other older professions. If the student who reads this finds some interest in such a career, or knows of other students who are still searching, he will find a cordial response from those who are actively engaged in the work. We have personally known speech therapists from all over the world. They form a devoted clan, still too young professionally to have become cynical or hardened to the troubles of those they serve. They are a bit idealistic. They are concerned about their cases. They care! They are still pioneering and exploring, still hungry to learn from each other and from their cases. A comradeship exists among them which is very warming.

Perhaps this spirit is due to the appreciation which speech therapists get from those who through them have finally become able to join the human race in that uniquely human function of speech. Teachers get affection and respect but not much appreciation. Businessmen get money —and ulcers. Speech therapists are paid more than teachers and less than businessmen, but they get more appreciation and have more fun than either. This is an intriguing profession in many ways. It uses information from many professional areas. The speech therapist, for example, who works with cleft-palate cases will need to know something about surgery, dentistry, orthodontia, prostheses, psychological counseling, family problems, and a host of other things. It is difficult to become bored in this field; there are too many new challenges. Indeed, each new case presents a different one. There are always new things for the therapist to discover, new skills to acquire, old skills to perfect, new roles to play. And, throughout the days of his professional career, the speech therapist enters many lives, shares many burdens, and heals many old wounds. In this life of ours there are belly pleasures and other pleasures. There are values of status and material possessions. But we know of none so thoroughly good as that of seeing some twisted life become untangled as the result of our efforts.

Perhaps another major feature of the attraction that speech therapy holds for its practitioners is that the work itself is usually pleasant work. These children we serve have been hurt in the mouth—and even deeper. They come to us feeling that speaking is unpleasant, that communication holds threat and rejection. Accordingly, one of the first tasks in therapy is to change this attitude; we must make speaking pleasant. No child can confront a speech defect long enough to modify it until he finds not only a permissive therapist but a pleasant one. With little children, much of our work is done through play. Even with adults, the interaction is usually flavored with humor and good-natured comradeship in experimentation. Relationships are close and warm. We deal with growth and change. We help the buds of potential to bloom.

To some people speech therapy work is very distasteful, and there seem to be certain personal qualifications which make all the difference between success and failure. In general, the nervous, impatient, high-strung individual does not make a good speech correctionist. Neither does the person who falls into routine, stereotyped methods and remains there contentedly. Successful teachers of speech correction possess the majority of the following traits to a high degree: a sense of humor, patience, curiosity, social poise, ingenuity in inventing and adapting techniques, professional enthusiasm, a sensitive and discriminating hearing, interest in the personalities of others, industriousness, objective attitude toward their own insecurities, calmness, ability to recognize subterfuge and mental mechanisms, and self-respect. Few people, of course, are born as virtuous as the above list of traits might imply, but speech therapy puts such a premium upon these characteristics that those who do not possess them try to acquire them as soon as possible. Speech therapists constantly seek to improve themselves in all of these traits. There is also one other highly essential qualification which must be developed if it is not already possessed: *empathy*. By empathy, we mean the ability to identify with the case, to understand how he feels, to predict his reactions—in short, to be able to get temporarily inside his psychological skin. The therapist must be secure enough herself so that she can make this identification and share the outward and inward behaviors of the case. She should understand herself, accept herself, and seek to improve herself.

All of these personal pronouns need some qualifying. Throughout this book, the author has referred to the therapist in the feminine gender, using the pronouns *she* and *her*. This was done not because speech therapy is a female profession, but merely as a literary convenience because the majority of the cases we had to mention were male. Speech therapy is rapidly attracting more men than women, perhaps because the latter get married and leave the profession until their children are grown, or they do private practice in their own homes while the men stay on the job. And the males marry the female speech therapists and put them to work teaching their own children to talk.

A *Career in Speech Pathology and Audiology.* Those students who have become intrigued by the kinds of problems we have presented in these pages and who are seriously considering entering the profession of speech pathology and audiology should know something about the American Speech and Hearing Association. This organization, to which more than 13,000 professional workers belong, publishes three journals, holds annual national conventions, and sets standards of ethics and competence. Through its boards of examiners, it is the accrediting agency both for the college centers which train speech and hearing clinicians and also for the service centers and clinics in which they work. It administers the examinations that are part of the requirements for its valued certificate of clinical competence. A House of Delegates made up of representatives from the various state speech and hearing organizations serves as the legislative body for the profession, while the executive business is carried out by the officers and committees of the association.[1]

Varieties of Professional Experience. One of the author's former students is employed by the State Department to teach English to officers in the Turkish army. Another ran the Crippled Children's Speech and Hearing Clinic in Alaska. Another operates a private preschool nursery for very young children with speech defects. Another is the speech therapist tutor of the stuttering son of a multimillionaire. Another works as a hospital therapist specializing in the diagnosis of aphasia. Another does nothing but laboratory research in voice science. Another manages a cleft-palate speech clinic in conjunction with a team of surgical, orthodontic, and other specialists. Another has a mobile speech clinic in a Western state financed by the Elks and travels continually with her trailer clinic over the hills and far away. Still another does her speech therapy in an orthopedic school for children with cerebral palsy. Another has shifted from speech therapy into audiology and heads that department in a university. Another has become a psychiatrist specializing in children's problems including those of speech. Another does private practice primarily

---

[1] The academic background, casework experiences, and other requirements for membership and certification, together with the Code of Ethics to which all members of American Speech and Hearing Association subscribe, may be found at the beginning of the current *Directory* of the Association. Further information is to be found in the various issues of the monthly periodical *ASHA*.

with actors who have voice problems. Many of them are directors of college speech clinics. But most (and we almost said "the best") of them are doing speech therapy in the public schools.

Speech Therapy in the Public Schools.   In the setting of the public schools, speech therapists find not only real interest and financial support but also an opportunity for service which is almost unique. A public school speech therapist is employed as a teacher, but she (remember again, please that many are men) is a very special sort of a teacher, a teacher-therapist. Her job is more like that of the school nurse than a classroom teacher. Children are referred to her for help, or she discovers them through screening testing. The case loads seem (and often are) very large. Many public-school therapists see one hundred children each week, and they therefore work with most of them in groups ranging from three to about seven children in a group. Fortunately, the majority of these children do not present very difficult problems. Most of them have mild articulatory defects and improve swiftly. A few of them need individual therapy and parental counseling. Usually one day each week is set aside for these purposes and for general coordination of the therapist's program with other school activities. One of the basic advantages of this setup is that it permits the child to have therapy in a natural rather than a clinical setting, and it makes possible a transfer of new skills from the therapy room into the child's daily life in the school. For the speech therapist, too, there are advantages. She is not frozen in the same room of the same school with the same children under the same principal day after day and month after month. She moves from school to school, often shifting midmorning from one to another. She prepares her own schedule, selects her own cases, designs her own therapy, and does not have to put on overshoes or collect the milk money. Somehow, her regime keeps her from having to wear the teacher's mask. She remains a pretty free agent. A good therapist can usually dismiss over a third of her cases each year, and most of the rest show improvement. Thus she has a sense of real achievement, which is augmented by the appreciation of parents, teachers, and the children themselves.

Speech Therapy in the Hospital Setting.   It is difficult to describe any typical program for this type of practice since programs vary widely. The hospital therapist generally sees the more severely impaired cases, especially those of organic origin. She works with patients such as those with aphasia, cleft palates, cerebral palsy, laryngectomees, stuttering, voice problems, and dysarthrias. A portion of her work is solely diagnosis; the rest is therapy, both individual and in small groups. The case load is small. Therapy is usually difficult, however, and often the prognosis may be poor. At times the amount of real improvement may be slight. Hospital therapy demands real competence on the part of the speech therapist. He (or she) must show that professional competence in the white glare of the hospital walls under the scrutiny of other specialists in rehabilitation. But hospital speech therapy is also very rewarding. One constantly learns more and more about the human being. There are ward rounds and staffings of cases of all types. There is close collaboration with the psychologists, the social worker, the occupational therapist, the physiotherapist, as well as with the medical profession.

Speech Therapy in Schools for Crippled Children.   In the ortho- pedic schools, we find a blend of the two types of therapy settings described above. The case loads are small and the problems are usually difficult. Much of the work is individual therapy, although small groups are also employed when socialization is needed. The therapist often must coordi- nate her own therapy with that of the other special teachers. For example, if the classroom teacher is having a social science project on the farmer's life, the speech therapist will use this theme in the communication used to work on smooth breathing in a child with cerebral palsy, or on the final sounds of the words *cows* and *chickens* as spoken by a postpolio child with a partially paralyzed tongue and a lateral lisp. Each child is studied very intensively from every angle by the staff members of such a school, and the speech therapist is a member of a teacher-therapist team.[2]

Speech Therapy in Community Speech and Hearing Centers.   Fairly recently we have seen the establishment of speech and hearing clinics sup- ported not by the schools, hospitals, or colleges but by the community health and welfare organizations. Preschool children are thereby provided with services, as are the aged adults, and these centers often provide a professional setting where the practice of speech pathology and audiology can be very rewarding. They also serve as diagnostic agencies to which workers in the public schools may refer their more difficult cases.

Private Practice.   Once a speech therapist has satisfied the clinical certification requirements of the American Speech and Hearing Association (not only certain strict academic requirements but also a professional examination and therapy experience under the supervision and sponsorship of a designated professional therapist) he may do private practice in this field. In this setting, the speech therapist often works with cases referred by physicians or other speech therapists and is paid for his work by the patient, insurance company or the government. He may have an office in a medical arts building or clinic, or may do the work in his own home. Many female speech therapists do some private practice in their homes once they are married and have small children of their own. There also

---

[2] An excellent account of some speech therapy casework in a school for crippled children is found in the article by George O. Egland, "An Analysis of an Exceptional Case of Retarded Speech," *Journal of Speech and Hearing Disorders*, XIX (1954), 233–43.

seems to be a growing trend for private summer speech clinics operated by public-school speech therapists in which intensive therapy is offered to the more severely handicapped children who could not be adequately served during the school year. The majority of the cases seen in private practice are those with delayed speech, stuttering, or the organic speech disorders. There are many problems that arise in private practice that should be seriously considered by individuals who plan such a career.[3] It is no bed of roses.

Audiology. We have already indicated that there are many other setting in which speech therapy is flourishing. However, most professional speech therapists begin their work either in the clinic or the public schools and then diverge later. So we will not describe these other types of work here. However, we must not forget to describe the way in which speech therapy serves as a beginning for other careers, especially those of audiology and special education. All speech therapists take some courses in hearing during their undergraduate preparation, and they take more when they continue in graduate school. Some of them find in audiology a smell of scientific certainty (illusory or not) which contrasts markedly with that of speech therapy where one must constantly deal with probabilities and the intangible. They find in audiometry and the research on hearing loss a definiteness which they crave. Audiology is a very fast-growing field, and the demand for workers is even greater than in speech therapy. All beginning students should give it serious consideration.

Special Education. In much the same way, beginning speech therapists usually take courses in special education as part of their undergraduate preparation, and those who later work in the public schools often come into close contact with other special teachers. As a result, some of them (the male therapists especially) find themselves active in such professional organizations as the Council for Exceptional Children, which serves all the fields of special education including the gifted child. Perhaps because of his experience in organizing and administering the speech therapy program and the public relations work which it often entails, the speech therapist becomes a marked man in the school system. He knows all the principles and the superintendent. He works with all the special teachers. Moreover, he already has an extensive academic background in not one but two fields of rehabilitation: speech and hearing. These experiences and qualifications often lead superintendents to encourage the speech therapist to do graduate work in special education in the areas in which his preparation was scanty so that he can be promoted to the directorship of all special education services. Those of us in speech therapy often regret

[3] See Paul D. Knight. "Advantages and Disadvantages of Private Practice," *Journal of Speech Disorders,* XII (1947), 199–201. See also *ibid* "Private Practice in Speech Pathology and Audiology," *ASHA,* III (November, 1961), 387–407.

our profession's loss when a competent therapist becomes an administrator, but when this occurs (and it has been happening more frequently each year), at least his newly hired replacement can find sympathetic understanding and support.

So we end this book with an invitation. We have helped you explore a portion of the forest of speech pathology. Strange at first, some parts of this forest are now familiar to you. Yet, there are many parts of this forest no man has entered. Perhaps you would like to join us in blazing a trail.

REFERENCES

Articles

1. American Speech and Hearing Association. *A Guide to Graduate Education in Speech Pathology and Audiology, 1967–1968.* Washington, D.C.: American Speech and Hearing Association, 1968.
    Outline the nature of this information provided in this booklet.
2. Black, M. E. "The Origins and Status of Speech Therapy in the Schools." *ASHA*, VIII (1966), 419–25.
    What are your impressions concerning the worldwide nature of the profession of speech pathology and audiology?
3. Brong, C. C. "Sigma Alpha Eta." *ASHA*, II (1960), 435–36.
    Describe this student organization and its purposes.
4. Johnson, W. "Communicology." *ASHA*, X (1968), 44–58.
    Why are professional titles of importance in defining the nature of our field?
5. Johnson, W., Brown, S. F., Curtis, J. F., Edney, C. W., and Keaster, J. *Speech Handicapped School Children.* 3d ed. New York: Harper & Row, Publishers, 1967.
    What is the clinical point of view in speech pathology? See pp. 95–110.
6. Klingbeil, G. M. "The Historical Background of the Modern Speech Clinic." *Journal of Speech Disorders*, IV (1939), 115–32.
    Give a brief summary of the history of our profession.
7. Lawrence, C. F. "Speech Pathology and Audiology in the United States." *British Journal of Disorders of Communication*, IV (1969), 89–95.
    How is our profession viewed from abroad?
8. McReynolds, L. "Contingencies and Consequencies in Speech Therapy." *Journal of Speech and Hearing Disorders*, XXXV (1970), 12–24.
    What motivating methods besides games can be used?
9. McWilliams, B. J. and Gluck, M. R. "Speech Clinic Joins Child Guidance Center: A Study in Interdisciplinary Collaboration." *Hospitals*, XXXVI (1962), 51–54.
    What sort of joint cooperation was achieved in this setting?
10. Moore, P. and Kester, D. G. "Historical Notes on Speech Correction in the Preassociation Era." *Journal of Speech and Hearing Disorders*, XVIII (1953), 48–53.
    What was speech therapy like during this early period?
11. Murphy, A. T. and Fitzsimons, R. M. *Stuttering and Personality Dynamics.* New York: The Ronald Press Company, 1960.
    Read Chapter 2 and tell what the characteristics of the good clinician should be.
12. Nelson, C. D. "The Therapist and Medical Specialists." *Western Speech*, (1961), 6–10.
    What suggestions does the author give for interacting with these specialists?
13. Newman, P. W. *Opportunities in Speech Pathology.* New York: Voca-

tional Guidance Manuals (235 East 45th St., New York City), 1968.
What are these opportunities?

14. Nichols, A. C. "Public School Speech and Hearing Therapy." In Rieber, R. W. and Brubaker, R. S., eds., *Speech Pathology* (Philadelphia: J. B. Lippincott Co., 1966).
Summarize the essential information provided in this chapter.

15. O'Toole, T. J. and Zaslow, E. L. "Public School Speech and Hearing Programs: Things Are Changing." ASHA, XI (1969), 499–501.
What changes are occurring in public-school speech therapy?

16. Panagos, J. M. and Hanna, S. J. "A Speech and Hearing Program in Appalachia." *Rehabilitation Literature,* XXIX (1968), 2–7.
Describe this mountain program.

17. Pendergast, K. "Speech Improvement and Speech Therapy in the Elementary School." ASHA, V (1963), 548–49.
Describe the differences between speech improvement and speech therapy.

18. Perkins, W. H. "Our Profession: What is It?" ASHA, IV (1962), 339–44.
How does the author answer this question?

19. Sandlin, R. E. "The Role of a Clinical Hearing and Speech Center." *National Hearing Aid Journal,* XXI (1968), 8–9, 21.
Describe how such a center works.

20. Walle, E. L. and Newman, P. W. "Rehabilitation Services for Speech, Hearing, and Language Disorders in an Extended Care Facility." ASHA, IX (1967), 216–19.
How are speech pathology and audiology services organized in such a setting?

21. Webb, C. C. and Parnell, J. "Unit Teaching in Speech and Hearing at the Elementary School Level." *Journal of Speech and Hearing Disorders,* XXV (1960), 302–4.
Describe this program.

22. Webster, E. J. "Parent Counseling by Speech Pathologists and Audiologists." *Journal of Speech and Hearing Disorders,* XXXI (1966), 331–34.
Why does the author feel that the speech therapist must also be able to counsel parents, and how should it be done?

23. ———. Perkins, W. H., Bloomer, H. H., and Pronovost, W. "Case Selection in the Schools." *Journal of Speech and Hearing Disorders,* XXXI (1966), 352–58.
What are some of the criteria suggested for picking out the children in the public schools who need speech therapy?

24. West, R. "An Historical Review of the American Literature in Speech Pathology." In Rieber, R. W. and Brubaker, R. S., eds., *Speech Pathology* (Philadelphia: J. B. Lippincott Co., 1966).
What were the essential contributions of each of the four decades in the development of our profession?

25. ———. "To Our New Members—Ave et Vale." ASHA, III (1961), 6–8.
What is the author saying to those who enter his profession?

Texts

26. Black, M. E. *Speech Correction in the Schools*. Englewood Cliffs, N.J.: Prentice-Hall, Inc., 1964.
    This book contains a clear account of the organization and administration of speech therapy in the public-school setting with many practical suggestions for the beginning speech clinician.
27. Eldridge, M. A *History of the Treatment of Speech Disorders*. London: Livingstone, 1968.
    Contains a fairly detailed account of the historical development of our profession in various parts of the world.
28. Rieber, R. W. and Brubaker, R. S., eds., *Speech Pathology*. Philadelphia: J. B. Lippincott Co., 1966.
    The final section of this book, "Part V: Current Trends in Other Countries," presents a review of the status and contributions of our profession in other lands, each one written by an authority from that country. The significant research is given.
29. Van Hattum, R. J., ed. *Clinical Speech in the Schools: Organization and Management*. Springfield, Ill.: Charles C Thomas, Publisher, 1969.
    Describes the organization of speech and hearing therapy in the schools.

GLOSSARY

Abracadabra: A magical set of words or sounds used as an incantation.

Acalculia: Loss of ability in using mathematical symbols due to brain injury.

Acoustic: Pertaining to the perception of sound.

Adenoids: Growths of lymphoid tissue on the back wall of the throat (nasopharynx).

Affricate: A consonantal sound beginning as a stop (plosive) but expelled as a fricative. The *ch* [tʃ] and the *j* [dʒ] sounds in the words *chain* and *jump* are affricates.

Agnosia: Loss of ability to interpret the meanings of sensory stimulation; due to brain injury; may be visual, auditory, or tactual.

Air wastage: The use of silent exhalation before or after phonation on a single breath.

Alexia: Difficulty in reading due to brain damage.

Allergy: Extreme sensitivity to certain proteins.

Alveolar: The ridges on the jaw bones beneath the gums. An alveolar sound is one in which the tongue makes contact with the upper-gum ridge.

Anomia: Inability to remember familiar words due to brain injury.

Anoxia: Oygen deficiency.

Antiexpectancy: A group of devices used by the stutterer to distract himself from the expectation of stuttering.

Aphasia: Impairment in the use of meaningful symbols due to brain injury.

Aphonia: Loss of voice.

Approach-avoidance: Refers to conflicts produced when the person is beset by two opposing drives to do or not to do something.

Approximation: Behavior which comes closer to a standard or goal.

Apraxia: Loss of ability to make voluntary movements or to use tools meaningfully; due to brain injury.

Articulation: The utterance of the individual speech sounds.

Aspirate: Breathy; the use of excessive initial airflow preceding phonation as in the *aspirate* attack.

Assimilation: A change in the characteristic of a speech sound due to the influence of adjacent sounds. In *assimilation nasality*, voiced sounds followed or preceded by a nasal consonant tend to be excessively nasalized.

Asymmetry: Unequal proportionate size of the right and left halves of a structure.

Atrophy: A withering; a shrinking in size and decline in function of some bodily structure or organ.

Athetosis: One of the forms of cerebral palsy characterized by writhing, shaking, involuntary movements of the head, limbs, or the body.

Ataxia: Loss of ability to perform gross motor coordinations.

Atresia: The blockage of an opening or canal.

Attack: The initiation of voicing.

Auditory memory span: The ability to recall a series of test sounds, syllables, or words.

Aural: Pertaining to hearing.

Auricle: The visible outer ear.

Autism: An emotional disturbance in children resulting in a detachment from their environmental surroundings; almost complete withdrawal from social interaction.

Avoidance: A device such as the use of a synonym or circumlocution to escape from having to speak a word upon which stuttering is anticipated; also a trick to escape from having to speak in a feared situation.

Babbling: A continuous, free experimenting with speech sounds.

Basal fluency level: A period of communication in which no stuttering appears. See *Desensitization therapy.*

Base-rate: The presumably stable rate of responding to a stimulus or stimuli.

Bicuspid: The fourth and fifth teeth, each of which has two cusps or points.

Bifid: Divided into two parts, as in a cleft or bifid uvula.

Binaural: Pertaining to both ears.

Bone conduction: The transmission of sound waves (speech) directly to the cochlea by means of the bones of the skull.

Bradylalia: Abnormally slow utterance.

C.A.T.: Children's Apperception Test, a projective test of personality.

Catharsis: The discharge of pent-up feelings.

Catastrophic response: A sudden change in behavior by the aphasic characterized by extreme irritability, flushing or fainting, withdrawal or random movements.

Cerebral palsy: A group of disorders due to brain injury in which the motor coordinations are especially affected. Most common forms are athetosis, spasticity, and ataxia.

Clavicular breathing: A form of shallow, gasping speech-breathing in which the shoulder blades move with the short inhalations.

Cleft lip or palate: See Chapter 8.

Cluttering: A disorder of time or rhythm characterized by unorganized, hasty spurts of speech often accompanied by slurred articulation.

Cochlea: The spiral-shaped structure of the inner ear containing the end organs of the auditory nerve.

Cognate: Referring to pairs of sounds which are produced motorically in much the same way, one being voiced (sonant) and the other unvoiced (surd). Some cognates are *t* and *d*, *s* and *z*.

Commentary: The verbalization of what is being perceived as in self-talk or parallel talk.

Conductive hearing loss: Hearing loss due to failure of the bone levers in the middle ear to transmit sound vibrations to the cochlea.

Configurations: (in articulation therapy) Patterning of sounds in proper sequence.

Contact ulcers: A breakdown in the tissues of the vocal cords, usually near their posterior attachments to the arytenoid cartilages.

Content words (Contentives): Words such as nouns and verbs that carry the major burden of meaningfulness.

Contingent: Following as a consequence of some preceding behavior.

Continuant: A speech sound which can be prolonged without distortion; e.g., *s* or *f* or *u*.

Covert: Hidden behavior; inner feelings, thoughts, reactions.

Creative dramatics: An improvised, unrehearsed playlet acted spontaneously by a group of children with the unobtrusive aid of an adult leader.

CV: A syllable containing the consonant-vowel sequence as in *see* or *toe* or *ka*.

CVC: A syllable containing the consonant-vowel-consonant sequence, as in the first syllable of the word *containing*.

Decibel: A unit of sound intensity.

Delayed auditory feedback: The return of one's own voice as an echo.

Dental: Pertaining to the teeth. A dentalized *l* sound is made with the tongue tip on the upper teeth.

Deep testing: The exploration of an articulation case's ability to articulate a large number of words, all of which include one specific sound, to discover those in which that sound is spoken correctly.

Desensitization: The toughening of a person to stress; increasing the person's ability to confront his problem with less anxiety, guilt, or hostility; a type of adaptation to stress therapy used for beginning stutterers. See Chapter 7.

Diadochokinesis: The maximum speed of a rhythmically repeated movement.

Differential diagnosis: The process of distinguishing one disorder from another.

Differentiation: The functional separation of a finer movement from a larger one with which it formerly coexisted.

Diphthong: Two adjacent vowels within the same syllable which blend together.

Distortion: The misarticulation of a standard sound in which the latter is replaced by a sound not normally used in the language. A lateral lisp is a distortion.

Dysarthria: Atriculation disorders produced by peripheral or central nerve damage.

Dyslalia: Functional (nonorganic) disorders of articulation.

Dysphasia: The general term for aphasic problems.

Dysphemia: A poorly timed control mechanism for coordinating sequential utterance. It is variously conceived as being due to a constitutional and hereditary difference or to psychopathology. It reflects itself in stuttering and cluttering.

Dysphonias: Disorders of voice.

Ear training: Therapy devoted to self-hearing of speech deviations and standard utterance.

Echolalia: The automatic involuntary repetition of heard phrases and sentences.

Echo speech: A technique in which the case is trained to repeat instantly what he is hearing, following almost simultaneously the utterance of another person. Also called "shadowing."

Egocentric: Self-centered; pertaining to the self and its display.

Ego strength: Morale or self-confidence.

Electroencephalogram (E.E.G.): The record of brain waves of electrical potential. Used in diagnosing epilepsy, tumors, or other pathologies.

Embolism: A clogging of a blood vessel as by a clot.

Empathy: The conscious or unconscious imitation or identification of one person with the behavior or feelings of another.

Encephalitis: A disease characterized by inflammation or lesions of the brain.

Epiglottis: The shield-like cartilage that hovers over the front part of the larynx.

Epilepsy: A neurological disease characterized by convulsions and seizures.

Esophageal speech: Speech of laryngectomized persons produced by air pulses ejected from the esophagus.

Esophagus: The tube leading from the throat to the stomach.

Etiology: Causation.

Eunuchoid voice: A very high-pitched voice similar to that of a castrated male adult.

Eustachian tube: The air canal connecting the throat cavity with the middle ear.

Expressive aphasia: The difficulty in sending meaningful messages, as in the speaking, writing, or gesturing difficulties of the aphasic. Executive aphasia.

Falsetto: Usually the upper and unnatural range of a male voice produced by a different type of laryngeal functioning.

Fauces: The rear side margins of the mouth cavity which separate the mouth from the pharynx.

Feedback: The backflow of information concerning the output of a motor system. Auditory feedback refers to self-hearing; kinesthetic feedback to the self-perception of one's movements.

Fixation: In stuttering, the prolongation of a speech posture.

Flaccid: Passively uncontracted, limp.

Frenum: The white membrane below the tongue tip.

Fluency: Unhesitant speech.

Fricative: A speech sound produced by forcing the airstream through a constricted opening. The *f* and *v* sounds are fricatives. Sibilants are also fricatives.

Function words (functors): Words which indicate action, arrangement, and relationship. Examples: prepositions, articles, adverbs, and conjunctions.

Glide: A class of speech sounds in which the characteristic feature is produced by shifting from one articulatory posture to another. Examples are the *y* [j] in *you*, and the *w* in *we*.

Glottal catch (or stop): A tiny cough-like sound produced by the sudden release of a pulse of voiced or unvoiced air from the vocal folds.

Glottal fry: A ticker-like continuous clicking sound produced by the vocal cords.

Glottis: The space between the vocal cords when they are not brought together.

Guttural voice: A low-pitched falsetto.

Hard contacts: Hypertensed fixed articulatory postures assumed by stutterers in attempting feared words.

Harelip: A cleft of the upper lip.

Hemiplegia: Paralysis or neurological involvement of one side of the body.

Hemorrhage: Bleeding.

Hyperactivity: Excessive and often random movements as often shown by a brain-injured child.

Hypernasality (Rhinolalia aperta): Excessively nasal voice quality.

Hyponasality: Lack of sufficient nasality, as in the denasal or adenoidal voice.

Identification: In articulation therapy, the techniques used to recognize the essential features of the correct sound or its error.

Idioglossia: Self-language with a vocabulary invented by the child.

Incidence: Frequency of occurrence.

Incisor: Any one of the four front teeth in the upper or lower jaws.

Infantile swallow: A form of swallowing in which the tongue is usually protruded between the teeth.

Inflection: A shift in pitch during the utterance of a syllable.

Interdental: Between the teeth. An interdental lisp would show itself in the substitution of the *th* for the *s* as in *thoup* for *soup*.

Interiorized stuttering: A form of stuttering behavior in which no visible contortions or audible abnormalities are shown, but a hidden struggle usually in the larynx or breathing musculatures is present. Also characterized by clever disguise reactions.

Isolation techniques: Activities used to locate the defective sound in utterance.

Jargon: Continuous but unintelligible speech.

Kernel sentences: The early primitive sentence forms from which other transformations later develop.

Kinesthesia: The perception of muscular contraction or movement.

Kinetic analysis: The analysis of error sounds in terms of their movement patterns.

Lalling: An articulatory disorder characterized by errors on sounds produced by lifting the tip of the tongue such as *l* and *r*.

Lambdacism: Defective *l* sound.

Lateral: A sound such as the *l* in which the airflow courses around the side of the uplifted tongue. One variety of lateral lisp is so produced.

Laryngeal: Pertaining to the larynx.

Laryngectomy: The surgical removal of the larynx.

Larnyx: The cartilaginous structure housing the vocal folds.

Laryngologist: A physician specializing in diseases and pathology of the larynx.

Lesion: A wound; broken tissue.

Lingual: Pertaining to the tongue. A lingual lisp is identical with an interdental lisp.

Lisp: An articulatory disorder characterized by defective sibilant sounds such as the *s* and *z*.

Malleus: The bone of the middle ear which rests against the eardrum.

Malocclusion: An abnormal bite.

Mandible: Lower jaw.

Maxilla: Upper jaw.

Medial: The occurrence of a sound within a word but not initiating or ending it.

Median: Midline, in the middle.

MMPI: Minnesota Multiphase Personality Inventory, a test of personality problems.

Monaural: Hear with one ear.

Monitoring: Checking and controlling the output of speech.

Monopitch: Speaking in a very narrow pitch range, usually of one to four semitones.

Motokinesthetic method: A method for teaching sounds and words in which the therapist directs the movements of the tongue, jaw, and lips by touch and manipulation.

Mucosa: The mouth and throat linings which secrete mucus.

Multiple sclerosis: A progressive and deteriorating muscular disability produced by overgrowth of the connective tissue surrounding the nerve tracts.

Muscular dystrophy: A disease of unknown origin characterized by progressive deterioration in muscle functioning and also by withering of the muscles.

Mutism: Without speech. Voluntary mutism: refusal to speak.

Myasthenia: Muscular weakness.

Nares: Nostrils.

Nasal emission: Airflow through the nose.

Nasal lisp: The substituting of a snorted unvoiced *n* for the sibilant sounds.

Nasopharynx: That part of the throat, pharynx, above the level of the base of the uvula.

Negative practice: Deliberate practice of the error or abnormal behavior.

Negative reinforcement: The cessation of unpleasantness when applied contingently.

Nerve deafness: Loss of hearing due to inadequate functioning of the cochlea, auditory nerve, or hearing centers in the brain.

Nonfluency: Pause, hesitation, repetition, or other behavior which interrupts the normal flow of utterance.

Nucleus: A central core. Nucleus situations are those in which the case tries especially hard to monitor his speech so as to improve it.

Obturator: An appliance used to close a cleft or gap.

Occluded lisp: The substitution of a *t* or a *ts* for the *s* or the *d* and *dz* for the *z*.

Omission: One of the four types of articulatory errors. The standard sound is replaced usually by a slight pause equal in duration to the sound omitted.

Operant conditioning: The differential reinforcement of desired responses.

Opposition breathing: Breathing in which the thorax (chest) and diaphragm work oppositely against each other in providing breath support for voice.

Optimal pitch level: The pitch range at which a given individual may phonate most efficiently.

Orthodontist: A dentist who specializes in repositioning of the teeth.

Oscillations: Rhythmic repetitive movements, repetitions of a sound, syllable, or posture.

Otologist: A physician who specializes in hearing disorders and diseases.

Overt: Clearly visible or audible behavior.

Palpation: Examining by tapping or touching.

Parallel talk: A technique in which the therapist provides a running commentary on what the case is doing, perceiving, or probably feeling.

Paraphasia: Aphasic behavior characterized by jumbled, inaccurate words.

Perseveration: The automatic and often involuntary continuation of behavior.

PFAGH: An acronym representing penalty, frustration, anxiety, guilt, and hostility.

Pharyngeal flap: A tissue bridge between the soft palate and the back wall of the throat.

Pharynx: The throat.

Phonation: Voice.

Phonemic: Refers to a group of very similar sounds represented by the same phonetic symbol.

Phonetic placement: A method for teaching a new sound by the use of diagrams, mirrors, or manipulation whereby the essential motor features of the sound are made clear.

Pitch breaks: Sudden abnormal shifts of pitch during speech.

Plosive: A speech sound characterized by the sudden release of a puff of air. Examples are *p, t, g.*

Polygraph: An instrument for recording breathing, heart beat, and other functions.

Preparatory set: An anticipatory readiness to perform an act.

Presbycusis: The hearing loss due to old age.

Primary reinforcer: A stimulus which satisfies a basic need and is not dependent upon learning. Examples: water, food, sex.

Proboscis: Nose.

Prognosis: Prediction of progress.

Propositionality: The meaningfulness of a message or utterance; its information content.

Proprioception: Sense information from muscles, joints, or tendons.

Prosthodontist: A dental specialist who makes prostheses.

Prosthesis: An appliance used to compensate for a missing or paralyzed structure.

Puberal: Pertaining to the period during which the secondary sexual characteristics begin to appear.

Pyknolepsy: A mild form of epilepsy characterized by stoppages in speech, among other things.

Receptive aphasia: Aphasia in which the major deficits are in comprehending.

Reciprocal inhibition: The mutual cancellation or inhibition produced by pairing incompatible response tendencies such as anxiety and anger.

Rhinolalia: Excessive nasality.

Rhotacism: Articulatory errors involving the production of the *r* sounds.

Rorschach: A test of personality involving the use of ink blots.

Schedules of reinforcement: The program for administering reinforcements. May be total (100%) in which reinforcement is given after each desired response, or partial (e.g., given for every five responses, etc.).

Secondary reinforcer: A stimulus which has been previously associated with a primary reinforcer.

Secondary stuttering: Refers to the advanced forms of stuttering in which awareness, fear, avoidance, and struggle are shown.

Self-talk: An audible commentary by the person describing what he is doing, perceiving, or feeling.

Semitone: A half-note, a half-step on the musical scale.

Septum: The partition between the right and left nasal cavities formed of bone and cartilage.

Shadowing: See *Echo talk.*

Sibling: Brother or sister.

Sigmatism: Lisping.

Sonant: A voiced sound.

Spastic: (*noun*) An individual who shows one of the varieties of cerebral palsy. (*adjective*) Characterized by highly tensed contractions of muscle groups.

Spastic dysphonia: A voice disorder in which phonation is produced only with great effort and strain.

Stabilization: The process of making a response permanent and unfluctuating.

Stapes: The innermost bone of the middle ear.

Stapedectomy: Surgical removal of the stapes.

Stigma: A mark or sign of defect or disgrace.

Stop consonant: A sound characterized by a momentary blocking of airflow. Examples are the *k, d,* and *p.*

Strident lisp: Sibilants characterized by piercing, whistling sounds.

Strident voice: Hash voice quality.

Surd: Unvoiced sound such as the *s* as opposed to its cognate *z* which is voiced or sonant.

Syntax: The grammatical structure of a language.

Tachylalia: Extremely rapid speech.

Tempo: Rate of utterance.

Thorax: Chest.

Time-outs: Intervals of silence administered contingently by the experimenter when an undesired speech response such as stuttering occurs.

Tinnitus: Ringing noises in the ears.

Tooth prop: A small wooden or plastic peg to be held between the teeth.

Trauma: Shock or injury.

Tremor: The swift, tremulous vibration of a muscle group.

Tympanic membrane: The eardrum.

Unilaterality: One-handedness; preference for one hand as contrasted with ambidexterity.

Uvula: The hanging portion of the soft palate. The velar tail.

Velum: Soft palate.

Velopharyngeal closure: The more or less complete shutting off of the nasopharynx.

Ventricular phonation: Voice produced by the vibration of the false vocal folds.

Vocal fry: See *Glottal fry.*

Vocal play: In the development of speech, the stage during which the child experiments with sounds and syllables.

Xanthippe: Why Socrates became a philosopher.

THE PHONETIC ALPHABET

Consonants

Phonetic Symbol	Key Words (English)	Phonetics	Phonetic Symbol	Key Words (English)	Phonetics
b	beg, tub	bɛg tʌb	p	paper, damper	pepɚ dæmpɚ
d	do, and	du ænd	r	run, far	rʌn fɑr
f	fan, scarf	fæn skɑrf	s	send, us	sɛnd ʌs
g	grow, bag	gro bæg	t	toe, ant	to ænt
dʒ	judge, enjoy	dʒʌdʒ ɪndʒɔɪ	ʃ	shed, ash	ʃɛd æʃ
h	hem, inhale	hɛm ɪnhel	tʃ	cheap, each	tʃip itʃ
k	kick, uncle	kɪk ʌŋkl	θ	thin, tooth	θɪn tuθ
l	let, pal	lɛt pæl	ð	then, breathe	ðɛn brið
l	apple, turtle	æpl tɝtl	v	vow, have	vau hæv
m	men, arm	mɛn ɑrm	w	wet, twin	wɛt twɪn
m	autumn, wisdom	ɔtm wɪzdm	hw	when, white	hwɛn hwart
n	nose, gain	noz gen	j	you, yet	ju jɛt
n̩	sudden, curtain	sʌdn̩ kɝtn̩	ʒ	pleasure, vision	plɛʒɚ vɪʒɛn
ŋ	wrong, anger	rɔŋ æŋgɚ	z	zoo, ooze	zu uz

443

* These sounds are only rarely used in General American speech, but are common in the East and South. General American speech uses [æ] for [a], [ɔ] for [ɒ], and [ɝ] for [ɜ].

This sheet is reproduced with the authors' permission from the text *An Introduction to General American Phonetics*, second eduction, by Charles G. Van Riper and Dorothy Edna Smith (New York: Harper & Row, Publishers, 1962), p. 8.

THE PHONETIC ALPHABET—Continued

Vowels

Phonetic Symbol	Key Words English	Phonetics	Phonetic Symbol	Key Words English	Phonetics
a *	ask, rather	ask raðɚ	ɒ *	log, toss	lɒg tɒs
ɑ	father, odd	faðɚ ɑd	ɝ	earn, fur	ɝn fɝ
e	make, eight	mek et	ɜ *	earn, fur	ɜn fɜ
æ	sat, act	sæt ækt	ɚ	never, percale	nevɚ pɚkel
i	fatigue, east	fətig ist	u	truth, blue	truθ blu
ɛ	red, end	rɛd ɛnd	ʊ	put, nook	pʊt nʊk
ɪ	it, since	ɪt sɪns	ʌ	under, love	ʌndɚ lʌv
o	hope, old	hop old	ə	about, second	əbaʊt sɛkənd
ɔ	sauce, off	ɔc scs			

Diphthongs

Phonetic Symbol	Key Words English	Phonetics	Phonetic Symbol	Key Words English	Phonetics
aɪ	sigh, aisle	saɪ aɪl	ɔɪ	coy, oil	kɔɪ ɔɪl
aʊ	now, owl	naʊ aʊl			

Index

Acalculia, in aphasia, 343
Acoustic deficiencies, in articulation defects, 184–99
Acoustic trauma, and noise, 408
Acute otitis media, 402
Adams, J., 102–3
Adenoidal voice, 46–47
Adults, role of. *See* Parental influence
Adverbs, in children's speech, 73
Aggression, in the speech defective, 11
Agnosia, visual and auditory, 343
Agraphia:
  in cerebral palsy, 343
  and delayed speech, 92
Air-conduction hearing, 395
Air-pressure controls, and cleft-palate speech, 370–72
Alaryngeal voice, 132, 136–38
Alexia:
  in cerebral palsy, 343
  and delayed speech, 92
American Speech and Hearing Association, 422–23, 425
Anal eroticism, and stuttering, 254
Anomia, and aphasia, 343
Anticipatory goal responses, in speech acquisition, 65

Antiexpectancy devices, in stuttering, 273
Anxiety, in the speech defective, 14–17
Anxiety reduction, in stuttering, 290–98, 317, 323, 327
Aphasia, 31, 47–48, 89, 91, 92–94, 112, 125, 342–56
Aphonia, 42, 45–46, 49, 131–41
Approach-avoidance conflicts, in stuttering, 265–66, 271–72
Apraxia, and agnosia, 343
Aronson, A. E., 142
Articulation, in children's speech, 74–77
Articulation, disorders of, 31–37, 171–243
  acoustic deficiencies, 184–99
  case histories, 175–78
  causes of, 174–84
  in cleft-palate speech, 376–79
  diagnostic examinations, 197–99
  dysarthria, 173–74
  dyslalia, 173–74
  isolated sound level therapy, 209–24
  organic abnormalities, 178–84

Articulation (*Cont.*):
  perceptual deficiencies, 184–99
  phonetic analysis, 185–92
  sentence level therapy, 232–43
  syllables, production of, 224–27
  tests for, 193–99
  treatment of, 199–243
  word level therapy, 227–32
Artificial larynx, 132–33, 135–36, 137–38
Assimilation nasality, 155
Ataxic cerebral palsy, 380
Athetoid cerebral palsy, 380, 381
Atresia, of external ear canal, 397, 400
Audiologists, in hearing rehabilitation, 413–14
Audiology, as a profession, 428
Auditory agnosia, 412–13
Auditory defects, and stuttering, 262
Auditory memory span, 93, 174–75, 184–85
Auditory stimulation, in articulation therapy, 218
Autism, 89, 126. *See also* Schizophrenia
  in delayed speech, 98–99
  and mutism, 102
  theory of, in speech acquisition, 60–61
Autohypnotic training, in stuttering, 281
Automatic speech, in aphasia, 345
Avoidance reactions, in stuttering, 251

Babbling:
  games, with cerebral palsy, 382
  and speech development, 57
  and stuttering, 256
Backus, O. L., 201
Bar, A., 97, 102
Baracz, J. C., 101
Bereiter, C., 100–101
Berlin, C. I., 136

Binaural auditory training units, 160, 164–65
Blake, J. N., 84–85
Blends, in articulation disorders, 36
Blowing exercises, in cleft-palate therapy, 374–76
Bluemel, C. S., 248
Bobath method, in cerebral palsy, 383
Body image integration, in aphasia, 355
Body postures, and pitch level, 152. *See also* Kinesthesia
Bone-conduction hearing, 395
Boone, D. R., 344
Brain damage, 94–101. *See also* Delayed speech; Cerebral palsy; Aphasia
Breathing abnormalities, in stuttering, 251–52
Breathy voice, 155–57
Brown, J. R., 142
Bruhn, M. E., 416
Brutten, E. J., 260–61
Buck, McKenzie, 317, 349
Bunger, A. M., 416

Catastrophic response, in brain-damaged children, 95–96
Central auditory impairments, 412–13
Central nervous system, deficits of, 91–101
Cerebral palsy, 31, 45, 49–50, 89, 91, 125, 379–86
  and dysarthria, 173
  and spastic dysphonia, 141–42
  speech therapy in, 382–86
Cerumenous glands, 393
Chicken pox, and hearing loss, 407–8
Childhood schizophrenia. *See* Autism; Schizophrenia
Children:
  articulation defects in, 175–78
  auditory memory span, 184–85

Children (*Cont.*):
  delayed speech in, 82–126
  early vocalization in, 54–60
  first words in, 60–67
  fluency, attainment of, 76–77
  hearing losses in, 184
  language learning in, 72–78
  minimal brain damage in, 94–101
  speech development in, 53–78
  and stuttering, 263–77, 286–313, 335
  vocabulary, acquisition of, 77–78
  vocal play, 58–59
Chomsky, Noam, 83
Chronic otitis media, 402–3
Cleft palates, 34–35, 49, 356–59
  articulation problems of, 376–79
  formation of, 56
  protheses for, 362–67
  speech therapy for, 366–79
  velopharyngeal competency in, 367–70
Cluttering, 41–42
  and delayed speech therapy, 125–26
  and stuttering, 262–63
Cochlea, of inner ear, 394
Comfort sounds, in infants, 54–57
Communicative stress, in stuttering, 293, 295–97, 317–18, 323, 326–27
Compensatory movements, in articulation defects, 180–81
Conductive hearing losses, 89–90, 395, 397–98
Conflict reinforcement, in stuttering, 258–61
Congenital aphasia, 48, 93
Consonants, in articulation disorders, 36
Constitutional theories, of stuttering, 261–62
Contact ulcers, and vocal folds, 158
Contingent reinforcement, 106–7

Corrective sets, in articulation therapy, 237–38
Covert penalties, for defective speech, 9–11
Creative dramatics, in stuttering therapy, 292
Crying sounds, in infants, 54–57
Curry, T., 59

Deafness, 49. *See also* Hearing disorders
  in children, 57, 89–91
  and mutism, 102
Deep tests, for articulation errors, 194–95, 208–9
Defective speech, handicaps of, 6–20
Delayed auditory feedback, 151–52, 262
Delayed speech, in children, 48–49, 82–126
  autism, 98–99
  causes of, 89–101
  childhood schizophrenia, 96–97
  emotional problems, 96
  experience deprivation, 100–101
  minimal brain damage, 94–101
  negativism, 99–100
  neurological dysfunctions, 91–101
Delayed speech, treatment of, 101–26
  aphasia, 92–94
  gesture language, use of, 115–16
  imitation, use of, 107–10
  jargon, elimination of, 110–11
  language, development of, 117–25
  motivation problems, 105–7
  parallel talk, use of, 111–13
  self-talk, use of, 111-13
  sounds and movements, use of, 121–22
  vocabulary acquisition, 116
  vocal phonics, 122–25
Denasality, 155

Dental abnormalities, and tongue-thrust habits, 57
Desensitization therapy, in stuttering, 299–302, 320–25
Developmental aphasia, 92, 93
Developmental dysarthria, 174 fn
Developmental dyspraxia, 174 fn
Deviant speech, cultural attitudes toward, 2–6
Diadochokinesis, in articulation defects, 182
Diehl, C. F., 148
Diplegia, in cerebral palsy, 381
Diphtheria, and hearing loss, 408
Diplophonia, 149
Displacement, in anxiety reactions, 16–17
Dwyer, J. H., 97, 102
Dysarthria, 91–92, 173–74
Dyslalia, 125, 173–74
Dysphasia, 47–49, 342–56
Dysphasia (Buck), 347
Dysphemia, and stuttering, 261–62
Dysphonia, 42–47, 141–42

Ear training:
    in articulation therapy, 212–16
    key-word method, 230–32
Echolalia:
    in aphasia, 93
    in infants, 67, 69–70, 113–15
Echo speech, 163, 234–36
Egland, George O., 299 fn
Ego strength, and stuttering, 285, 286–87, 297–98
Eisenson, J., 263, 345–46
Electrolarynges, 132, 133, 135, 137–38
Emotional conflicts:
    and articulation disorders, 176, 177
    in delayed speech, 96
    and mutism, 102
Engelmann, S., 100–101
English syntax, in children's speech, 71–78

Erickson, R., 196–97
Error, in articulation therapy:
    prediction of, 214–16
    voluntary practice of, 240–42
Escape devices, in stuttering, 273
Esophageal voice, vicarious, 132, 136–38
Eunuchoid voice, 150
Eustachian tube, 394
Examining for Aphasia (Eisenson), 345
Experience deprivation, in children, 89
External auditory canal, 392–93
External otitis, and hearing loss, 399–400
External vibrators, in esophageal speech, 132–33

Facial contortions, and stuttering, 266, 267
Falsetto voice, 44, 46–47, 144, 150–51, 152, 153–54, 159, 381
Fear, role of, in stuttering, 267–71
Figure-ground relationships, in brain-damaged children, 95
First words, in infancy, 60–67
Fitz-Simons, R. M., 276, 291
Fluency, attainment of, in children, 76–78
Fluency factor, in stuttering, 284, 286, 298–300
Fluent stuttering, technique of, 311–13, 333–35
Foreign accent, and articulation disorders, 49, 175
Freund, H., 276
Frontal lisp, 34
Frustration:
    in brain-damaged children, 95
    in the speech defective, 6, 12–14
    in stuttering, 287–90, 316–17, 322, 327
Frustration theory, and stuttering, 257–58

Gardner, M. H., 135
Gesell, A., 69
Gesture Language, and delayed speech therapy, 115–16
Gestures, and speech acquisition, 63–64
Global aphasia, 347
Glossopharyngeal press, in esophageal speech, 136–37
Goldman-Fristoe Test of Articulation, 194
Gray, B. B., 282
Greene, M. C. L., 136, 139–40
Gross sound discrimination, 414–15
Group counseling, in stuttering, 293, 306
Guilt:
  reduction of, in stuttering, 290–98, 317, 323, 327
  in the speech defective, 17–19
Guttural voice, 47

Habitual pitch level, 145–46
Harris, F. H., 104
Harris, H. E., 135
Hearing aids, 160, 417–19
Hearing disorders, 392–419
  acquired hearing loss, 398–400
  and articulation disorders, 184
  auditory training, 414–15
  central auditory impairments, 412–13
  in children, 89–91
  conductive hearing loss, 89–90
  drugs, effect of, 406–7
  hearing aids, 417–19
  hearing loss, classification of, 395–412
  mechanism of ear, 392–94
  middle ear abnormalities, 400–404
  noise-induced hearing loss, 408–9
  perceptive hearing loss, 89–90
  presbycusis, 409–12
  rehabilitation, 413–19
  speechreading, 415–17

Hemianopia, and aphasia, 347
Hemiplegia, 347, 381
Hesitant speech, and stuttering, 255–56, 293–95
Hess, E. H., 56
Hewett, F. M., 104–5
High-pitched voice, 44, 144, 145–47. *See also* Falsetto
Hostility, in the speech defective, 19–20
Hostility reduction, and stuttering, 290–98, 317, 323
Hyperactivity, in brain-damaged children, 95
Hypernasality, 46, 49, 154, 160–61
Hypnosis, in stuttering therapy, 304, 306
Hysterical aphonia, 138–41

Illinois Test of Psycholinguistic Abilities, 117
Imitation:
  and articulation disorders, 175
  in children's speech learning, 76
  and delayed speech therapy, 107–10
Imitation theory, of speech acquisition, 61–64
Imitative behavior, in infants, 60
Incus, in middle ear, 394
Infantile swallow, 56–57
Infants. *See* Children
Inflected vocal play, in infants, 59–60
Inhalation method, in esophageal speech, 136
Injection procedure, in esophageal speech, 136–37
Inner ear, mechanism of, 394
Instrumental response, in speech acquisition, 66
Intensity, disorders of, 45–46
Interdental lisp, 34
Interiorized stuttering, 251
International Association of Laryngectomees (IAL), 135

Interrupter devices, in stuttering, 273–74

"Introduction to Speech Problems: Physical Diagnosis" (Van Riper), 172

Irwin, John V., 162

Irwin, O. C., 59, 217

Isolated sound level, in articulation therapy, 209–24

Jargon:
    in aphasia, 94
    in infants, 67, 68–69, 110–11, 113–15, 124

Jargon aphasia, 347

Jaundice, and speech disorders, 47

Jetty, Albert, 392 fn

Johnston, M. K., 104

Jones, R. K., 261

Junkermann, E. R., 140–41

Kanomycin, and hearing loss, 405, 406

Karlin, I. W., 263

Key sentences, in articulation therapy, 234–37

Key word method, in articulation therapy, 220–22, 227–32

Kinesthesia, 152, 269

Kinetic analysis, in articulation defects, 189–91, 193–94

Kinzie, C. E., 416

Knutsen, Rigmor, 254

Lalling, 35, 186, 189
    in cerebral palsy, 383–85
    in cleft-palate speech, 377–78
    and infant feeding, 56

Lambdalalia, 27

Language, development of, in delayed speech therapy, 117–25

Language learning, in infants, 72–78

Language Master, use of, in aphasia, 349

Language Modalities Test for Aphasis (Wepman and Jones), 345–47

Laradon Articulation Scale, 194, 196

Laryngectomees, rehabilitation of, 132–38

Larynx, artificial, 132–33, 135–36, 137–38

Lateral lisp, 34, 186, 187

Learning theory, 64–66. *See also* Operant conditioning
    and articulation therapy, 202, 203
    in stuttering, 254–56, 258–61

Lee, L. L., 117

Lemert, E. M., 4

Lenneberg, E. H., 83

Lewis, M. M., 54

Liberman, A. M., 66

Linguistics, and articulation therapy, 202–3

Lipreading, 415–17

Lisping, 34–36
    reconfiguration techniques, 228–32
    sentence level therapy, 234–39
    and vocal phonics, 123

Long-echo talk, in articulation therapy, 235–36

Lost Cord Clubs, 134

Lovaas, O. L., 103–4

Low-pitched falsetto, 163

Low-pitched voice, 44, 145

McCurry, W. H., 217

McDonald Deep Test of Articulation, 194–95, 198

Malleus, in middle ear, 394

Marshall, R. C., 208

Martin, H., 133

Measles, and hearing loss, 407–8

Memory training, in aphasia, 351–52

Meningitis, and speech disorders, 47

Mental retardation. *See also* Delayed speech:

Mental retardation (*Cont.*):
and articulation defects, 176–77
and mutism, 102
Menyuk, P., 89
Michigan Picture Language Inventory, 117
Middle ear:
abnormalities, 400–404
mechanism of, 393–94
Milisen, R., 200
Minimal brain damage, in children, 94–101
Minnesota Test for Differential Diagnosis of Aphasia (Schuell), 345–46
Mixed type hearing loss, 395–97
Monoplegia, in cerebral palsy, 381
Monotone, as a voice disorder, 44–45, 144, 147–48
Morley, Muriel, 174
Motivation problems, and delayed speech, 105–7
Motokinesthetic method, 113–14, 200–201
Motor deficiencies, in articulation defects, 181–84
Motor Theory of Perception, 66–67
Mowrer, O. H., 60
Multiple speech disorders, 49–50
Mumps, and hearing loss, 407–8
Murphy, A. T., 276, 291
Muscle training, in cleft-palate therapy, 372–74
Musical tones, effect of, on infants, 90
Mutism:
in children, 86
in delayed speech, 96–100
treatment of, 101–26
voluntary, 16
Myasthenic cerebral palsy, 380, 381–82
Mykelbust, H., 97

Nasality, 42–43

Negative practice, in articulation therapy, 240–42
Negativism, in children, 89, 95, 99–100
Neurological dysfunctions:
in delayed speech, 89, 91–101
in spastic dysphonia, 141–42
Neuromuscular incoordinations, and articulation defects, 181–82
Neurosis, as a cause of stuttering, 253–54
New Voice Clubs, 134–35
Nitchie, E. B., 416
Noise-induced hearing loss, 408–9
Nonsense syllables, in articulation therapy, 225–26
Nonsense words, in articulation therapy, 226–27
Northwestern Syntax Screening Test (*NSST*), 117–18
Noun phrases, in children's speech, 73

Occluded lisp, 34
Open bite, in infants, 57
Open class words, in children's speech, 72
Operant conditioning:
in delayed speech, 103–5
and infant speech acquisition, 65–66
and stuttering, 260, 282
Operator words, in children's speech, 72
Oral eroticism, and stuttering, 254
Oral panendoscope, in cleft-palate therapy, 368
Organic speech disorders, 341–86. *See also* Speech disorders:
aphasia, 342–56
and articulation disorders, 178–84
cerebral palsy, 379–86
cleft-palate speech, 356–79
defined, 342–45

Orthodontia, with articulation defects, 179–84
Ossicular chain, in middle ear, 394
Otitis media, and hearing loss, 401–3
Otologists, and hearing rehabilitation, 413
Otosclerosis, 403–4
Oval window, in middle ear, 394
Overtones, in voice quality, 46

Pantomime technique, in vocal therapy, 165–66
Paradigmatic aphasia, 347
Paradoxical intention method, in stuttering, 281
Parallel talk:
    in aphasia, 350, 352, 353–54
    in delayed speech therapy, 111–13
    in stuttering, 254–59
Paralytic stroke, and voice disorders, 47
Paraphasia, 343
Parental influence:
    in articulation disorders, 175–78
    in speech learning, 75–78
    in stuttering, 256–57, 292–93, 296–98, 303
Partial reinforcement, in speech acquisition, 66
Pearson, J. S., 142
Penalties:
    for defective speech, 6–11
    in stuttering, 255, 267–68, 287, 314–16, 322, 327
Perceptive hearing loss, 89–90
Perceptual deficiencies, in articulation defects, 184–99
Perceptual handicaps, in children, 94–101
Perseveration:
    in aphasia, 343, 350–51
    in brain-damaged children, 95
Personality changes:
    in aphasia, 347–48
    in stuttering, 275–76

Phonasthenia, 142–44
Phonemic approximations, 186–87
Phonemic disorders, 33
Phonetic analysis, in articulation defects, 185–94
Phonetic discrimination, difficulties in, 185–86
Phonetic placement, in articulation therapy, 218–20
Photo-Articulation Test, 194
Physical therapy, with articulation defects, 179–84
Pitch, disorders of, 43–45, 144–45, 151–54
Pitch breaks, 144, 148–50
Pivot words, in children's speech, 72
Play therapy, and stuttering, 291–92
Possessives, teaching of, in delayed speech therapy, 120
Postponement devices, in stuttering, 272
Posture, in stuttering, 250
Predictive Screening Test of Articulation (PSTA), 196–97
Prepositional phrases, in children's speech, 73
Presbycusis, 409–12
Prespasm period, in stuttering, 329–32
Primary reinforcement, in speech acquisition, 66
Progressive approximation:
    in articulation therapy, 216–18
    in voice therapy, 164–65
Propositionality, and stuttering, 283, 285
Proprioceptive feedback, in articulation therapy, 239, 243
Prosody, disorders of, 37–42
Prostheses, for cleft palates, 362–67
Protest behavior, in the speech defective, 11
Protruding teeth, in infants, 57
Psychotherapy:
    for aphasics, 355–56
    with cerebral palsy, 386

Psychotherapy (*Cont.*):
  for cleft-palate patients, 369
  and hysterical aphonia, 139
  and phonasthenia, 142–43
  and stuttering, 275, 280–81, 283, 301, 304, 306
  and vocal pitch, 146, 150–51
Puberty, and voice pitch, 145, 147, 148–50
Pulse rate abnormalities, in stuttering, 251–52
Putney, F. J., 135

Raph, J. B., 101
Reading, elimination of, in therapy, 106–7
Reconfiguration techniques, in articulation therapy, 228–29
Referential spread, in infant speech, 67–71
Reinforcement theory, of speech acquisition, 64–66. *See also* Operant conditioning
Relaxation technique, in stuttering, 280, 281–82, 306–7
Resistance, in correcting vocal disorders, 162–63
Resistance therapy, in stuttering, 333–35
Rheingold, H. L., 65
Rhinolalia aperta, 46
Rhinolalia clausa, 46
Rhotacism, 27
Riddle of Stuttering, The (Bluemel), 248
Rimland, B., 98
Role-playing, in articulation therapy, 238–39
Rubella, and hearing loss, 405–6
Rubin, H., 97, 102
Rutherford, D., 379

Scarlet fever, and hearing loss, 408

Schizophrenia:
  in childhood, 89, 96–97
  and vocal pitch level, 148
Schlanger, B. B., 83
Schuell, H., 345–46
Scrapbooks, use of, with children, 78
Screening tests, for articulation errors, 195–96
Secondary reinforcement, in speech acquisition, 66
Self-correction, in articulation therapy, 204–5, 212–16
Self-hearing, in articulation therapy, 213–16
Self-language, in children, 85–86
Self-perception, of pitch level, 152–53
Self-talk:
  in aphasia, 350, 353–54
  and delayed speech therapy, 106, 109, 111–13, 115–16
  in stuttering, 254
Semantic aphasia, 347
Semantic theory, of stuttering, 256–57
Semicircular canals, of inner ear, 394
Sensori-neural hearing loss, 395, 404–6, 418
Sensory deprivation, in delayed speech, 89–91
Sentence level therapy, in articulation disorders, 232–43
Sentences, in children's speech, 73
Serous otitis media, 401–2
Sex ratio, in stuttering, 262
Sexual characteristics, secondary, and voice pitch, 145, 147, 148–50
Shadowing techniques:
  in articulation therapy, 234–35
  in stuttering, 281
Sheehan, J. G., 259–60, 270
Shoemaker, D. J., 260–61
Signaling techniques, in articulation therapy, 229–30
Sign language. *See* Gesture language
Simple speech, use of, with children, 76–78
Sloane, H. M., 104

Slow-motion speech, in articulation therapy, 234
Smith, Svend, 58
Socialized vocalization, in infants, 38
Socioeconomic factors, in learning speech, 74
Sokolowsky, R. R., 140–41
Sound discrimination, in articulation therapy, 210–13
Sound prolongations, in stuttering, 250
Sound stabilizing, in articulation therapy, 222–24
Sounds, use of, in delayed speech therapy, 121–22
Spasmophemia, 27
Spastic dysphonia, 141–42
Spastic paralysis. *See* Cerebral palsy
Specific language disability (SLD), 125
Speech, development of, in children, 53–78. *See also* Delayed speech
Speech assignments:
    in articulation therapy, 239
    in stuttering, 313–16
Speech deviancy, cultural attitudes toward, 2–6
Speech disorders, 27–50
    of articulation, 31–37
    classification of, 31–50
    defined, 29–31
    handicaps of, 6–20
    historical treatment of, 20–23
    multiple speech disorders, 49–50
    organic disorders, 341–86
    present attitude toward, 23–24
    symbolization, disorders of, 47–49
    time and prosody, disorders of, 37–42. *See also* Stuttering
    voice disorders, 42–47
Speech pathology, as a profession, 422–29
Speech perception, deficiencies in, 82–126
Speechreading, 415–17

Stabilization:
    of new voice, 165–66
    of response, in stuttering, 332–33
Stapedectomy, and otosclerosis, 403–4
Stapes, in middle ear, 394
Starting devices, in stuttering, 272
Stereotyped inflections, 45, 145, 147, 151
Streptomycin, and hearing loss, 405, 406
Strident voice, 45, 157–58, 159
Struggle reactions, in stuttering, 251
Stuttering, 3–4, 7, 31, 37–41, 71, 76, 248–335
    approach-avoidance conflicts, 265–66, 271–72
    in children, 39–41, 286–313
    and cluttering, 41–42, 262–63
    conflict reinforcement, 258–60
    defined, 248–50
    and delayed speech therapy, 126
    desensitization therapy, 299–302, 320–25
    development of, 263–77
    fear, role of, 267–71
    fluent stuttering, technique of, 333–35
    forms of, 41–42
    frequency of, 283–86
    frustration theory of, 257–58
    and learning theory, 254–56, 258–61
    neurological basis of, 261–63
    as a neurosis, 253–54
    operant conditioning theories, 202, 260
    origins of, 252–63
    parental influences in, 256–57, 292–93, 296–98, 303
    personality changes in, 275–76
    physiological reactions of, 251–52
    semantic theory of, 256–57
    severity of, 283–86
    and situation fears, 265, 270–71, 318, 323–24, 326

Stuttering *(Cont.)*:
social penalties of, 267–68, 314–16, 322
therapist, role of, 308–13, 321–22
treatment of, 278–335
two-factor learning theories of, 260–61
and unison speech, 281, 328–29
and word fears, 265, 269–70, 318–19, 324, 325–26
Subject-predicate sentences, in delayed speech, 87–88
Surgery:
in articulation defects, 179–84
for cleft palates, 360–62
Syllable repetition, 58, 250
Syllables, in articulation therapy, 224–27
Symbolization, disorders of, 47–49
Symptom reinforcement, in stuttering, 266–67
Syntactic aphasia, 347
Syntax, in children's speech, 71–78

Talking-and-writing techniques, in articulation therapy, 223–24, 225–26, 229
Telegrammic speech, 87, 94
Templin-Darley Tests of Articulation, 194, 198
Time, disorders of, 37–42, 248–335
Time-beat methods, in stuttering, 281
Todd, G. A., 65
Tongue, behavior of, in infants, 55–57
Tongue depressors, in articulation therapy, 219
Tongue exercises:
for articulation defects, 183–84
in cleft-palate speech, 377–78
Tooth props, in articulation therapy, 219
Transformations, in children's grammar, 74
Travis, L. E., 199

Treacher-Collins Syndrome, and hearing loss, 397–98
Tremor syndrome, and spastic dysphonia, 141–42
Tremulous voice, 145, 151
Trojan, F., 281
Two-factor learning theories, in stuttering, 260–61
Tympanic membrane, 392, 393–94, 400–401

Unintelligibility, in children, 86
Unison speech:
in articulation therapy, 236–37
in stuttering, 281, 328–29
Uranoscolalia, 27

Van Riper, Charles, 162, 196–97
Ventricular phonation, 158–59
Verb phrases, in children's speech, 73
Verb tenses, teaching of, in delayed speech therapy, 120
Vestibule, in inner ear, 394
Vibrators, external, in esophageal speech, 132–33
Vicarious esophageal voice, 132, 136–38
Vocabulary:
acquisition of, in children, 77–78
and delayed speech therapy, 116
Vocal fry technique, 141
Vocal intensity, disorders of, 131–44
Vocal nodules, and husky voice, 156, 159
Vocal phonics, and delayed speech therapy, 122–25
Vocal play, in infants, 58–59, 67, 69–70
Vocal stuttering (dysphonia), 141–42
Voice disorders, 42–47, 130–66
hysterical aphonia, 139–41
of intensity, 45–46, 131–44
phonasthenia, 142–44

Voice disorders (*Cont.*):
  of pitch, 43–45, 144–45, 148–50,
    151–54
  spastic dysphonia, 141–42
  vicarious voice, methods for pro-
    ducing, 132–36
  of voice quality, 46–47, 154–66
Voluntary mutism, 16, 255
Vowels, formation of, in infants, 59–
  60

Weber, J. L., 202–3
Weisberg, P., 65
Weiss, A., 262–63

Westlake, H., 379
White, William, 134
Whooping cough, and hearing loss,
  408
Williams, D., 273
Wingate, M. E., 255–56
Winitz, H., 65–66, 174
Wood, N. E., 86–87
Word level therapy, in articulation
  disorders, 227–32
Wright, Gilbert, 132 fn
Wyatt, G., 256

Young, Edna Hill, 113, 200–201